OBSTETRICS ILLUSTRATED

OBSTETRICS ILLUSTRATED

Alistair W.F. Miller FRCOG, FRCS (Glas)
Consultant Obstetrician and Gynaecologist, The Queen Mother's Hospital
and Royal Samaritan Hospital for Women, Glasgow; Royal Samaritan Lec-
turer in Gynaecology, University of Glasgow

Robin Callander FFPh, FMAA, AIMBI
Formerly Director of Medical Illustration, Glasgow University

FOURTH EDITION

CHURCHILL LIVINGSTONE
EDINBURGH LONDON MELBOURNE AND NEW YORK 1989

CHURCHILL LIVINGSTONE
Medical Division of Longman Group UK Limited

Distributed in the United States of America by
Churchill Livingstone Inc., 650 Avenue of the
Americas, New York, N.Y. 10011, and by associated
companies, branches and representatives throughout
the world.

First Edition 1969
Second Edition 1974
Third Edition 1980
Fourth Edition 1989
  Reprinted 1992
  Reprinted 1993

ISBN 0 443 04016 8

British Library Cataloguing in Publication Data
A catalogue record for this book is available from the British Library

Library of Congress Cataloging in Publication Data
Miller, Alistair W. F.
    Obstetrics illustrated.

    Rev. ed. of: Obstetrics illustrated/Matthew M.
Garrey ... [et al.]. 3rd ed. 1980.
    Includes index.
    1. Obstetrics—Outlines, syllabi, etc.
I. Callander, Robin. II. Obstetrics illustrated.
III. Title. [DNLM: 1 Obstetrics—atlases. WQ 17
M647o]
RG533.M55 1989 618.2   88-25811

The
publisher's
policy is to use
**paper manufactured
from sustainable forests**

Produced by Longman Singapore Publishers Pte Ltd
Printed in Singapore

It is both an honour and a great responsibility for a new author to be invited to join the team preparing another edition of a successful textbook. In this instance the three original authors have all retired from practice and the revision of the text has been almost entirely in the hands of the new author. He has been greatly helped by the experience and continuity provided by the original illustrator.

It is a tribute to the thoroughness of Drs Garrey, Govan and Hodge that few completely new topics have been introduced. The text, however, has been updated and, in some sections, completely re-written to bring it into line with today's practice. Some excisions have also been made, reducing the overall length of the book. The contents have been considerably rearranged to produce a more logical progression through the book and new headings and typeface have been employed which, we hope, will make the book easier to use and improve its clarity and appearance. The original emphasis on a clinical, and necessarily didactic, approach has been retained.

The author is particularly grateful to his colleagues Dr Margaret McNay, Dr Tom Turner and Dr Martin Whittle for advice on their specialties—ultrasound, neonatal paediatrics and fetal medicine—and to his secretary Mrs Mary Gray for her unfailing speed and accuracy in preparing his efforts. We hope this edition is worthy of its predecessors and will continue to meet the needs of medical students, midwives and others learning the art and science of obstetrics.

Alistair W.F. Miller
Robin Callander

1989

PREFACE

CONTENTS

CONTENTS

CONTENTS

CHAPTER 1

PHYSIOLOGY OF REPRODUCTION

OVULATION AND MENSTRUATION

CYCLICAL OVARIAN CHANGES

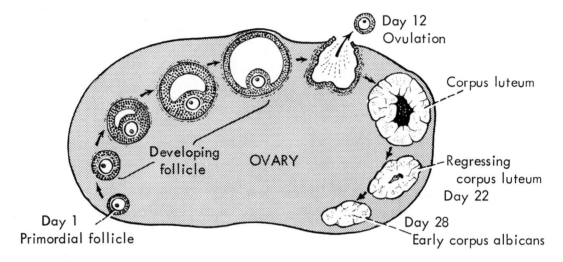

During the normal 28 day cycle a sequence of changes occurs in the ovary aimed at the production of a mature ovum, capable of being fertilized. This sequence also controls the quantity and quality of steroids necessary for the preparation of the uterus for reception of the ovum.

PITUITARY CONTROL OF OVARY

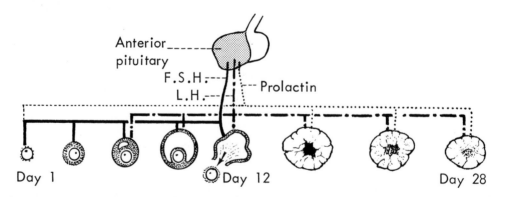

The ovarian changes are controlled mainly by the anterior pituitary which produces 3 hormones — follicle stimulating hormone (F.S.H.) which initiates follicle growth; luteinising hormone (L.H.) which stimulates ovulation and causes luteinisation of granulosa cells after escape of the ovum; and prolactin, the effect of which is uncertain.

OVULATION AND MENSTRUATION

ENDOMETRIAL CHANGES

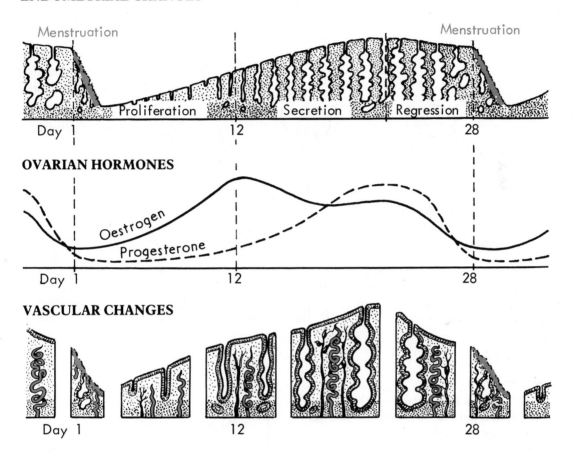

OVARIAN HORMONES

VASCULAR CHANGES

PROLIFERATIVE PHASE — Stimulated by oestrogen, the endometrium is reconstructed. Glands are straight and do not secrete.

SECRETORY PHASE — Stimulated mainly by progesterone, and endometrium is highly vascularized. Glands enlarge and become tortuous and secrete or store glycogen, mucin and other substances which can nourish a fertilized ovum. Blood vessels become more coiled.

PREMENSTRUAL (REGRESSIVE) PHASE — Endometrial growth ceases 5 – 6 days before menstruation. Before menstruation it shrinks due to decreased blood flow and discharge of secretion. This increases the tortuosity of glands and blood vessels.

OVULATION AND MENSTRUATION

The secretion of pituitary gonadotrophins is under the dual control of the ovary and a centre in the hypothalamus.

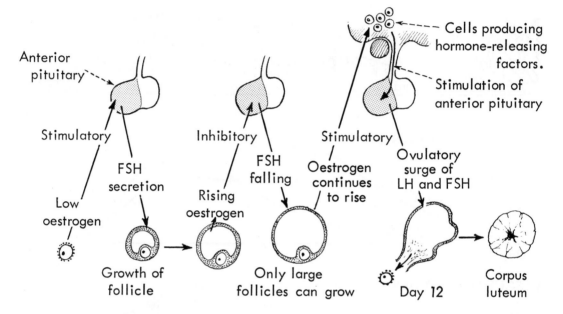

At the end of a menstrual cycle the plasma oestrogen is low, causing secretion of FSH which stimulates follicular growth.

Growing follicles secrete oestrogen which partially inhibits FSH secretion (negative feedback). Only large follicles possessing large numbers of FSH receptors continue to grow.

Blood oestrogen continues to rise and ultimately stimulates the hypothalamus to secrete LH releasing factors (positive feedback), causing a surge of FSH and LH, thus inducing ovulation.

The changes in the blood levels of the essential hormones are shown in the accompanying diagram.

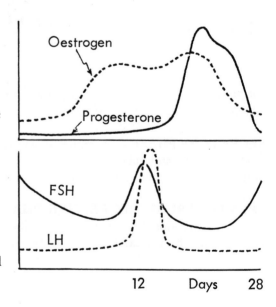

FERTILIZATION AND NIDATION

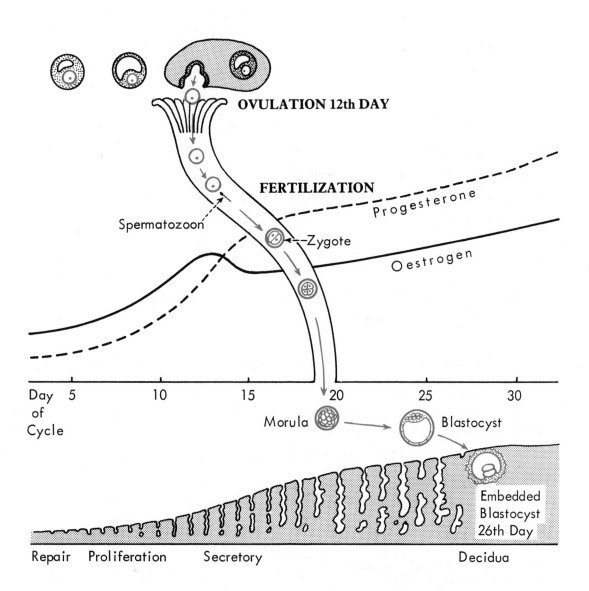

After fertilization in the fallopian tube the zygote (fertilized ovum) divides repeatedly to form a solid sphere of cells — the morula. It reaches the uterine cavity by the 7th day after ovulation and is fully embedded by the 14th day after ovulation.

HORMONAL RELATIONSHIPS IN EARLY PREGNANCY

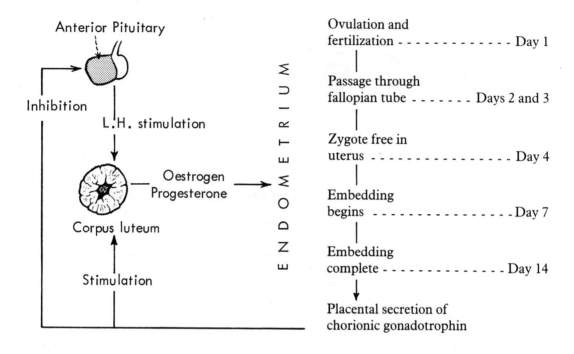

During the first 14 days of pregnancy the growth of the uterus and decidua (the endometrium of pregnancy) is maintained by the corpus luteum under the influence of hypophysial luteinizing hormone. After 14 days the primitive chorion secretes a luteinizing hormone (chorionic gonadotrophin) which assumes control of the corpus luteum and inhibits pituitary gonadotrophic activity.

QUANTITATIVE RELATIONSHIPS

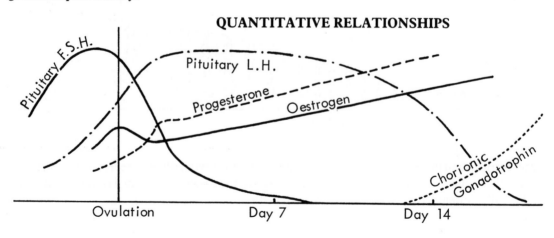

HORMONAL RELATIONSHIPS IN EARLY PREGNANCY

Under the influence of placental luteinizing hormone the corpus luteum continues to grow and secrete steroids for the maintenance of uterine decidual growth. Chorionic gonadotrophin output reaches a peak around 10 – 12 weeks and then declines to an almost constant level until term. With this decline the corpus luteum activity fails but placental steroid production commences to replace it so that the output of oestrogens and progesterone rises steadily.

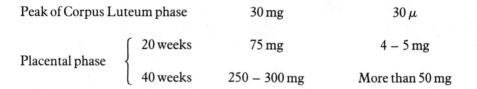

OVARIAN and PLACENTAL STEROID OUTPUT

	Progesterone/24 hr	Urinary Oestrogens/24hr
Peak of Corpus Luteum phase	30 mg	30 μ
Placental phase { 20 weeks	75 mg	4 – 5 mg
40 weeks	250 – 300 mg	More than 50 mg

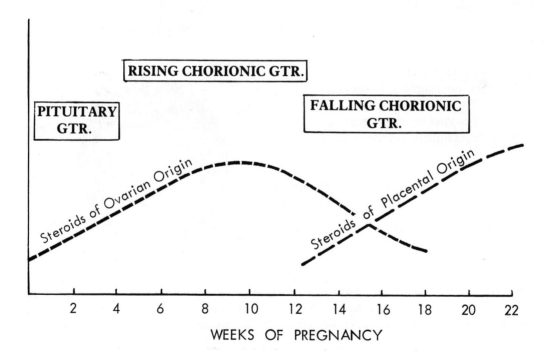

RISING CHORIONIC GTR.

PITUITARY GTR.

FALLING CHORIONIC GTR.

Steroids of Ovarian Origin

Steroids of Placental Origin

2   4   6   8   10   12   14   16   18   20   22

WEEKS OF PREGNANCY

DEVELOPMENT OF THE EMBRYO

While still in the fallopian tube the fertilized ovum divides repeatedly to form a round mass of cells — the morula.

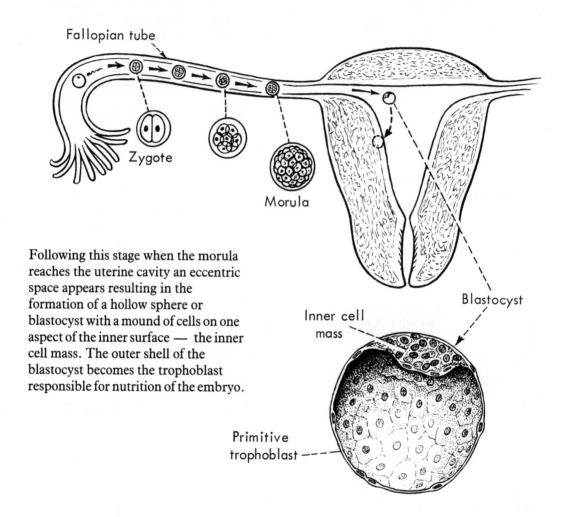

Following this stage when the morula reaches the uterine cavity an eccentric space appears resulting in the formation of a hollow sphere or blastocyst with a mound of cells on one aspect of the inner surface — the inner cell mass. The outer shell of the blastocyst becomes the trophoblast responsible for nutrition of the embryo.

Up to this point the secretions within the tube and uterus have been sufficient for the initial growth of the zygote. Further development demands an increased supply of food and oxygen, and the zygote must gain access to the maternal blood supply by embedding in the decidua.

DEVELOPMENT OF THE EMBRYO

The inner cell mass differentiates and forms two distinct masses, the outer or ectodermal layer and the inner or entodermal. A further differentiation produces a third layer, the mesoderm, between these two. This grows outwards and eventually lines the blastocyst. The combination of trophoblast and primitive mesoderm is termed the chorion.

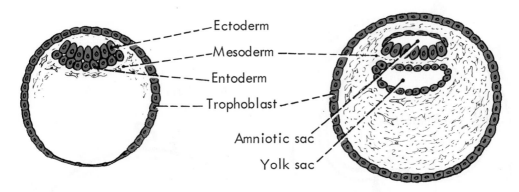

Ectoderm
Mesoderm
Entoderm
Trophoblast
Amniotic sac
Yolk sac

Two small cavities appear, one in the ectoderm forming the amniotic sac, the other in the entoderm — the yolk sac.

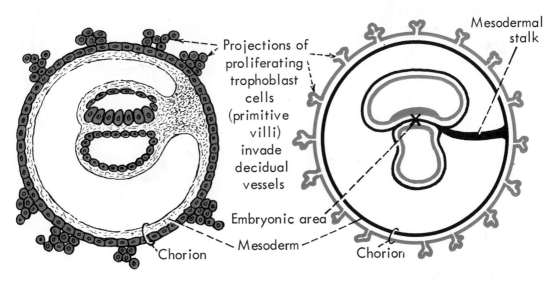

Projections of proliferating trophoblast cells (primitive villi) invade decidual vessels

Mesodermal stalk

Embryonic area

Mesoderm

Chorion

Chorion

The two small spheres, covered by mesoderm, move into the middle of the blastocyst cavity, the mesoderm forming the connecting stalk. The two opposing layers of ectoderm and entoderm together with the interposed mesoderm are destined to form the actual embryo. Expansion of the amniotic sac takes place.

9

DEVELOPMENT OF THE EMBRYO

Expansion of the amniotic cavity continues until the amnion reaches the wall of the blastocyst. At the same time it enfolds the yolk sac. Part of the yolk sac becomes enclosed within the embryo while the remainder forms a vestigial tube applied to the original mesodermal stalk.

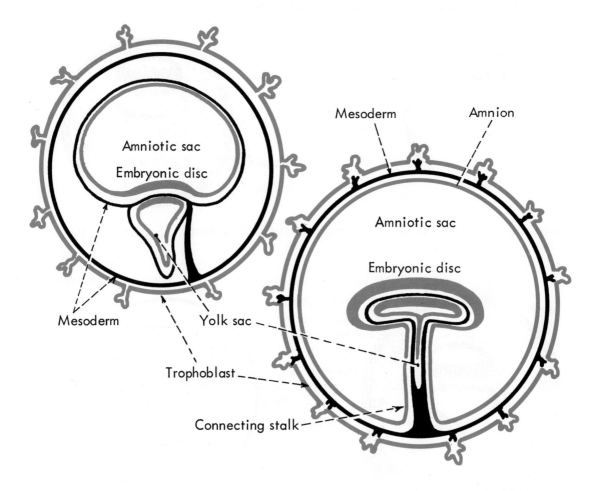

Blood vessels develop in the embryonic mesoderm and in the mesoderm of the trophoblast. Extension of these vessels along the connecting stalk results in the formation of the umbilical arteries and vein.

DEVELOPMENT OF THE EMBRYO

Within the embryo the vessels at the cephalic end differentiate to form the heart. Fetal blood formation occurs within the primitive blood vessels of the trophoblast and fetus. Interchange between mother and fetus is facilitated by the formation of this feto-trophoblastic circulation. The formation and differentiation of the haemopoietic vascular system occurs between the third and fourth weeks of pregnancy. From then on full development of the fetus can take place.

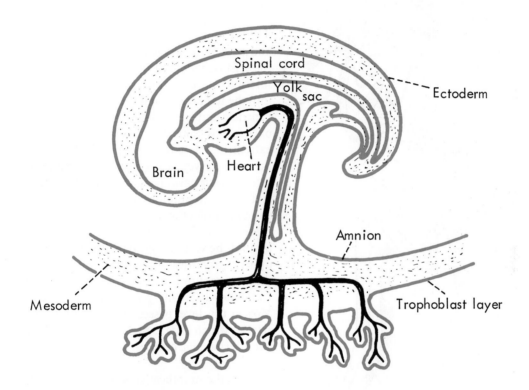

STRUCTURES DERIVED FROM PRIMARY LAYERS

ECTODERM — Skin and appendages, nervous system including medulla of adrenal, glands such as anterior pituitary and salivary.

ENTODERM — Gastro-intestinal tract, liver, gall bladder, biliary tract, pancreas, respiratory tract, germ cells of gonads.

MESODERM — Bone, muscle, cartilage, connective tissue, serous linings, cardio-vascular system, kidneys and most of genital tract.

11

DEVELOPMENT OF THE FETUS — CIRCULATION

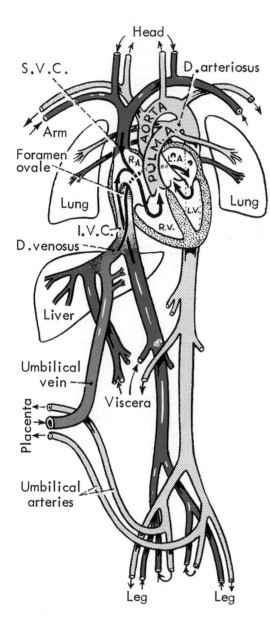

Oxygenated blood from the placenta returns to the fetus via the umbilical vein. This vessel penetrates the liver and gives off small branches to that organ. Most of the blood is directed via the ductus venosus into the inferior vena cava which is carrying the returning non-oxygenated blood from the lower limbs, kidneys, liver etc.

There is only partial mixing of the two streams and most of the oxygenated blood is directed to the crista dividens at the upper end of the inferior vena cava through the foramen ovale into the left atrium and thence to the left ventricle and aorta. This relatively well oxygenated blood supplies the head and upper extremities. The remainder of the blood from the superior vena cava mixes with that of the inferior vena cava, passes to the right ventricle and thence to pulmonary artery. A very small amount of blood goes to the lungs. Most of it passes on via the ductus arteriosus into the aorta beyond the vessels supplying the head and upper extremities. Thereafter it passes down the aorta to supply the viscera and lower limbs. Little blood actually goes to the lower limbs. Most at this level passes into the umbilical arteries which arise as branches of the right and left internal iliac arteries.

At birth the umbilical vessels contract. Breathing helps to create a negative thoracic pressure thus sucking more blood from the pulmonary artery into the lungs and diverting it from the ductus arteriosus which gradually closes. The foramen ovale is a valvular opening, the valve functioning from right to left. The left atrial pressure rises and closes this valve.

DEVELOPMENT OF THE ORGANS — TIMETABLE

ORGAN	DIFFERENTIATION	COMPLETE FORMATION
Spinal Cord	3 – 4 weeks	20 weeks
Brain	3	28
Eyes	3	20 – 24
Olfactory apparatus	4 – 5	8
Auditory apparatus	3 – 4	24 – 28
Respiratory system	5	24 – 28
Heart	3	6
Gastro-intestinal system	3	24
Liver	3 – 4	12
Renal system	4 – 5	12
Genital system	5	7
Face	3 – 4	8
Limbs	4 – 5	8

OSSIFICATION CENTRES

HEAD	Weeks	UPPER LIMB	Weeks
Mandible	7	Humerus	8
Occipital bone	8 – 10	Radius	8
Maxilla	8	Ulna	8
Temporal bone	9	Phalanges	9 – 16
Sphenoid bone	9 – 14	Metacarpals	9 – 12
Nasal bone	10		
Frontal bone	9 – 10	LOWER LIMB	
Bony labyrinth	17 – 20	Femur	9
Teeth	17 – 28	Tibia	9
Hyoid bone	28 – 32	Fibula	9
		Epiphysis around	
BODY		knee joint	35 – 40
Clavicle	7	Calcaneum	21 – 29
Scapula	8 – 9	Talus	24 – 32
Ribs 5,6,7.	8 – 9	Cuboid	40
2,3,4; 8,9,10,11.	9	Metatarsals	9 – 12
1 and 12.	10		
Sternum	21 – 24	VERTEBRAE	9 – 12

13

PLACENTA — DEVELOPMENT

The primitive trophoblast of the chorion frondosum erodes the decidua, destroying glands and stroma but leaving the maternal arterioles and venules. These dilate to form sinusoids. The chorionic villi, now lying in a pool of maternal blood, divide repeatedly to form complex tree-like structures in which branches of the umbilical vessels form vascular cascades closely related to the surface trophoblast ephithelium.

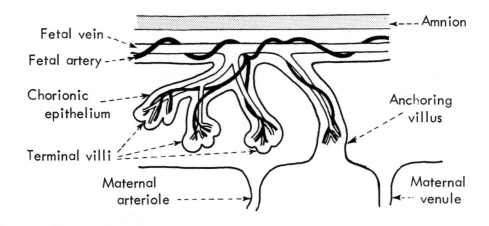

The branches of the original villi, now themselves termed villi, are of two types. The majority float freely in the maternal blood and are known as terminal villi. A number are attached to the maternal tissue — anchoring villi.

The trophoblastic epithelium lines the whole cavity containing the maternal blood in which the terminal villi are suspended.

The syncytiotrophoblast possesses, among other properties, some of the characteristics of vascular endothelium thus preventing the possibility of thrombosis.

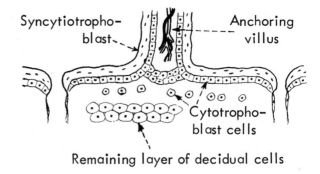

PLACENTA — DEVELOPMENT

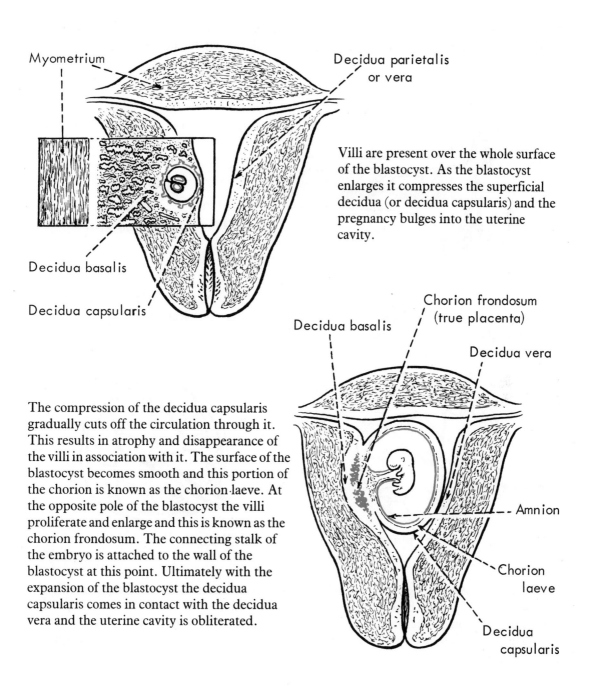

Myometrium

Decidua parietalis
or vera

Decidua basalis

Decidua capsularis

Villi are present over the whole surface of the blastocyst. As the blastocyst enlarges it compresses the superficial decidua (or decidua capsularis) and the pregnancy bulges into the uterine cavity.

Decidua basalis

Chorion frondosum
(true placenta)

Decidua vera

Amnion

Chorion
laeve

Decidua
capsularis

The compression of the decidua capsularis gradually cuts off the circulation through it. This results in atrophy and disappearance of the villi in association with it. The surface of the blastocyst becomes smooth and this portion of the chorion is known as the chorion laeve. At the opposite pole of the blastocyst the villi proliferate and enlarge and this is known as the chorion frondosum. The connecting stalk of the embryo is attached to the wall of the blastocyst at this point. Ultimately with the expansion of the blastocyst the decidua capsularis comes in contact with the decidua vera and the uterine cavity is obliterated.

15

PLACENTA — DEVELOPMENT OF THE CORD

The fully formed placenta is a disc, approximately one inch in thickness, tapering towards the edges. It weighs roughly 500g and is dark red, the colour being due mainly to the maternal blood in the intervillous spaces.

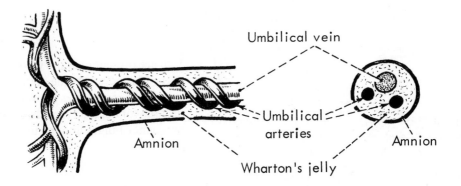

The umbilical cord has two arteries and one vein, embedded in Wharton's jelly which is a loose myxomatous tissue of mesodermal origin. This jelly acts as a physical buffer and prevents kinking of the cord and interference with circulation.

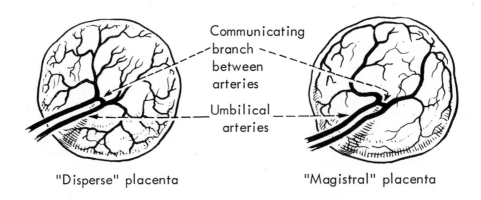

The umbilical vessels are generally attached to the placenta near its centre. They immediately divide repeatedly to form branches all over the surface. This is known as the 'disperse' type of placenta. Occasionally the main vessels may extend almost to the margins of the placenta before dividing (although they give off small branches in their course). This is the 'magistral' type of placenta.

There is a short communicating branch between the two umbilical arteries just as they reach the placental surface. This serves to equalise the pressure and flow to each half of the placenta.

PLACENTA — FUNCTIONS

The functions of the placenta depend on the structure and health of the placental villi. These villi are bathed in maternal blood but there is no direct connection between fetal and maternal blood. The structures between the two circulations make up the so-called placental barrier.

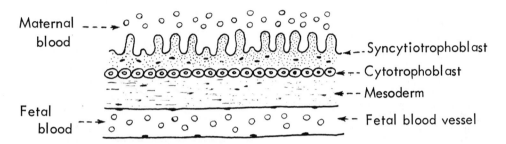

The barrier effect is reduced in two ways. Tiny polypoid extensions of the syncytial cytoplasm — microvilli – increase the surface for absorption, secretion and interchange between the two circulations. Secondly, as the pregnancy increases in size, especially after the 16th week, the syncytiotrophoblast is reduced in thickness without alteration of its microvillous structure. The fetal mesoderm is reduced in amount and the vessels of the villi dilate.

Thickness of placental barrier: At 12 weeks...0.025mm; at term...0.002mm.

The functions of the placenta are:

A. RESPIRATORY

The fall in pressure as the maternal blood enters the placenta and the resulting slow flow aid the feto-maternal interchange. Maternal blood has a relatively high O_2 and a low CO_2 content. The passage of O_2 to the fetus and of CO_2 to the mother thus occurs by a process of simple diffusion. In addition fetal haemoglobin has a greater ability to take up O_2 than adult haemoglobin.

B. EXCRETORY

Little is known of the excretory mechanism across the placenta. Urea is present in the same concentration in both fetal and maternal bloods.

C. NUTRITIONAL

Carbohydrates, simple lipids and proteins (as amino acids) are all transferred across the placenta. This occurs either by a diffusion process, as with glucose, or by special transport mechanisms, as with amino acids.

PLACENTA — FUNCTIONS

D. ENDOCRINE

The placenta produces:

1. Oestrogens
2. Progesterone
3. Chorionic gonadotrophin (HCG)
4. Placental lactogen (HPL)
5. Corticosteroids

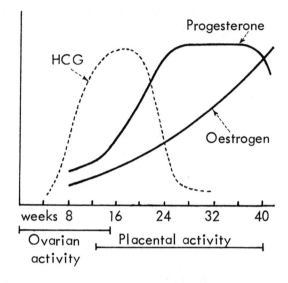

Oestrogens and progesterone are produced by the ovary in the first 12 weeks of pregnancy. Chorionic gonadotrophin is secreted in large quantities to maintain the corpus luteum. Thereafter oestrogens and progesterone are produced by the placenta, the corpus luteum regresses and the secretion of chorionic gonadotrophin is greatly reduced.

Oestrogens and progesterone maintain the growth of the uterus and control its activity during pregnancy. They are also responsible for changes in the mother such as growth of the breasts.

Levels of placental lactogen rise steadily throughout pregnancy although the exact function of this hormone remains uncertain.

Measurements of the levels of oestrogens, progesterone and placental lactogen are used as tests of placental function. Their physiological effects are discussed in more detail in Chapter 2.

OTHER PREGNANCY-ASSOCIATED SUBSTANCES

A number of proteins and enzymes such as heat-stable alkaline phosphatase and cystine amino-peptidase are produced by the placenta. Some of the proteins are identified simply by names such as Pregnancy associated Plasma Proteins A and B. Their functions and importance remain unclear.

DEVELOPMENT OF MEMBRANES

The membranes are derived from that part of the trophoblast which atrophies as the blastocyst expands — the chorion laeve — plus the amnion.

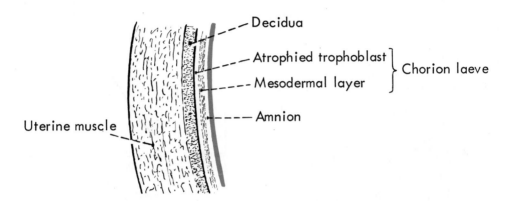

The amnion is easily stripped from the chorion and this helps to distinguish dizygotic (binovular) from monozygotic (monovular) twins.

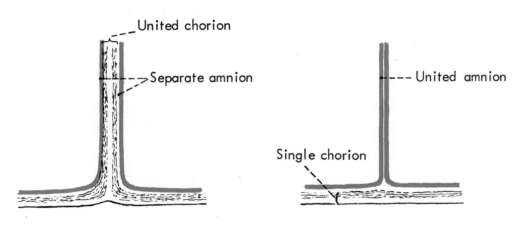

**BINOVULAR
(OR MONOVULAR DICHORIONIC)**

If the membranes are in three distinct layers over the surface in apposition, the twins may be either monovular or binovular.

MONOVULAR

When the membranes in apposition consist only of two layers — the two amnions — the twins are definitely monovular.

AMNIOTIC FLUID

VOLUME

This increases up to the 38th week, falls slightly up to term and then more rapidly thereafter.

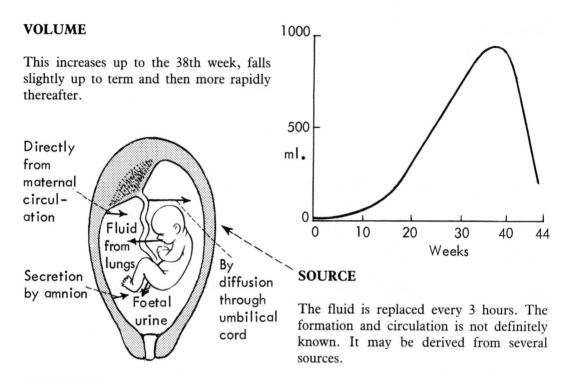

SOURCE

The fluid is replaced every 3 hours. The formation and circulation is not definitely known. It may be derived from several sources.

COMPOSITION

It is not a simple transudate. The concentrations of substances are seldom the same as those found in maternal plasma, although some may rise or fall in concert with the maternal blood.

	Concentration per 100 ml	Ratio $\frac{\text{Amniotic Fluid}}{\text{Maternal Plasma}}$
Protein	0.375g	1/20
Creatinine	2–4mg	2/1
Urea	40–60mg	2/1
Uric acid	6.0mg	2/1
Glucose	10–60mg	1/8–3/5
Total lipids	49–59mg	1/20
Cholesterol	2–10mg	1/30
Phospholipids	3–5mg	1/40
Electrolytes	as in mother	1/1

As pregnancy progresses the fetal urine is a relatively greater component of the liquor. The content of the liquor, therefore, may reflect fetal renal function. Creatinine levels in the liquor, which rise sharply at about 38 weeks, have been used as a test of fetal maturity.

AMNIOTIC FLUID

HORMONES

Chorionic gonadotrophin, placental lactogen, oestrogens, progesterone and hydroxycorticosteroids are found in considerable quantities.

Prostaglandins of two types are found. Type E is found in early pregnancy, whereas at term it is type F which is present.

ENZYMES

A wide variety of enzymes has been demonstrated in amniotic fluid and its cells. These may be measured in tests for certain metabolic disorders.

CYTOLOGY

Three cell types are found in early pregnancy, large eosinophilic, large basophilic and small basophilic. These are derived from fetal skin, mouth, vagina and bladder.

After the 36th week anucleate polygonal eosinophilic cells are found which stain orange with Nile blue sulphate and which are squames from fetal skin. This may be used as a test to confirm rupture of the membranes.

A more detailed account of tests to examine the liquor is given in Chapter 6.

CHAPTER 2

MATERNAL PHYSIOLOGY

WEIGHT INCREASE

WEIGHT

There is an increase in weight during pregnancy equivalent to 25 per cent of non-pregnant weight: approximately 12.5 kg in the average patient.

There is marked variation in normal women but the main increase occurs in the second half of pregnancy and is usually around 0.5kg per week. Towards term the rate of gain diminishes and weight may fall after 40 weeks.

The increase is due to growth of the conceptus, enlargement of maternal organs, maternal storage of fat and protein and increase in the maternal blood volume and interstitial fluid.

DISTRIBUTION OF WEIGHT INCREASE

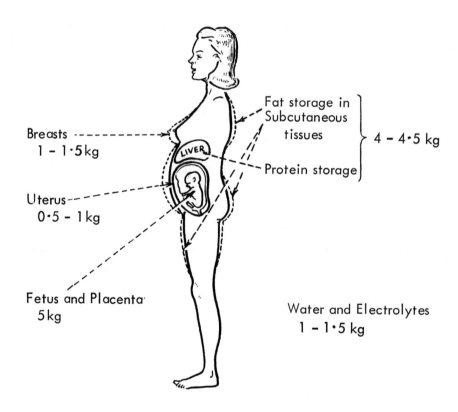

Breasts
1 – 1·5kg

Fat storage in Subcutaneous tissues

Protein storage

4 – 4·5 kg

Uterus
0·5 – 1kg

Fetus and Placenta
5kg

Water and Electrolytes
1 – 1·5 kg

METABOLISM

The demands for energy derive from:-

A. BASIC PHYSIOLOGICAL PROCESSES. Respiration, circulation, digestion, secretion, maintenance of body temperature, growth and repair. These account for 66 per cent of total energy requirements in the non-pregnant female .... 1,440 kcal/day

B. EVERYDAY ACTIVITIES. Walking, maintaining posture, speech, other movements — e.g. eating. Equivalent to 17 per cent of total in non-pregnant state. .... 360 kcal/day

C. WORK. This varies greatly. Probably 7 – 10 per cent of total ..150 – 200 kcal/day

D. SPECIFIC DYNAMIC ACTION OF FOOD. Metabolism appears to be stimulated by the taking of food. In the region of 7 per cent of total .... 144 kcal/day

TOTAL ENERGY REQUIRED IN NON-PREGNANT STATE .... 2,100 kcal/day

IN PREGNANCY

There is a marked increase in 'A' due to the demands of fetus, placenta, uterus, breasts etc.

A slight reduction in 'B' may occur as pregnancy advances, and it is assumed that 'C' will play only a minor role, at least in the third trimester.

There ought to be an increased intake of food and therefore an increase in 'D'.

The total energy required by the patient in advanced pregnancy will be around 2,500 kcal/day.

During lactation a further increase is required for milk production and the total requirements will be in the region of 3,000 kcal/day.

METABOLISM

The total metabolism is increased in pregnancy due largely to the fetus.

Oxygen consumption is raised by 20 percent and thus the basal metabolic rate, expressed as kilocalories per square metre per hour, is increased in proportion.

To maintain the increased total metabolism there is an increased activity in control mechanisms.

The anterior pituitary probably secretes more thyroid stimulating hormone.

The thyroid gland hypertrophies and is palpably enlarged in 70 per cent of patients.

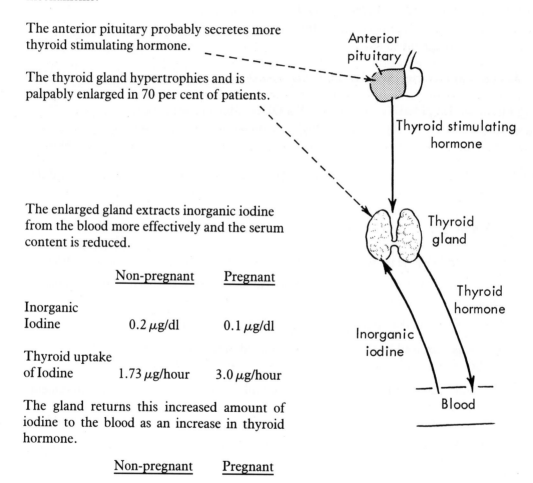

The enlarged gland extracts inorganic iodine from the blood more effectively and the serum content is reduced.

	Non-pregnant	Pregnant
Inorganic Iodine	0.2 µg/dl	0.1 µg/dl
Thyroid uptake of Iodine	1.73 µg/hour	3.0 µg/hour

The gland returns this increased amount of iodine to the blood as an increase in thyroid hormone.

	Non-pregnant	Pregnant
Protein bound Iodine	400 nmol/litre	620–800 nmol/litre

CARBOHYDRATE METABOLISM

In the non-pregnant state ingested glucose is dealt with in four ways. Under the influence of insulin it may be deposited in the liver as glycogen. Some escapes into the general circulation and a proportion of this is metabolised directly by the tissues: some is converted to depot fat and a further portion is stored as muscle glycogen again with the aid of insulin.

The blood sugar is maintained between 4.5 and 5.5 mmol/litre (80–100 mg/dl). Sugar which passes out in the renal glomerular filtrate is never in excess of the amount which can be reabsorbed by the tubules, and none appears in the urine.

A marked alteration in carbohydrate metabolism occurs in pregnancy. There is a demand on the part of the fetus for an easily convertible source of energy. At the same time there is a need to store energy for future demands such as lactation and the steadily increasing growth of the pregnancy and also to provide a more steady source of energy in the form of a high energy fuel. This the maternal body achieves by storage of fat. The major portion of the diet is carbohydrates and this requires to be redirected to satisfy the above requirements. The first noticeable change occurs in the blood sugar and this can be demonstrated by an oral glucose tolerance test. It can be seen from this that the blood sugar, after a meal, remains high thus facilitating placental transfer.

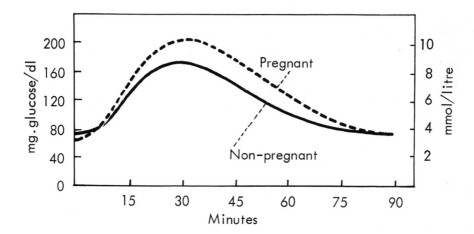

The mechanism governing the changes is not clearly understood but may be as in the following diagram on page 28.

CARBOHYDRATE METABOLISM

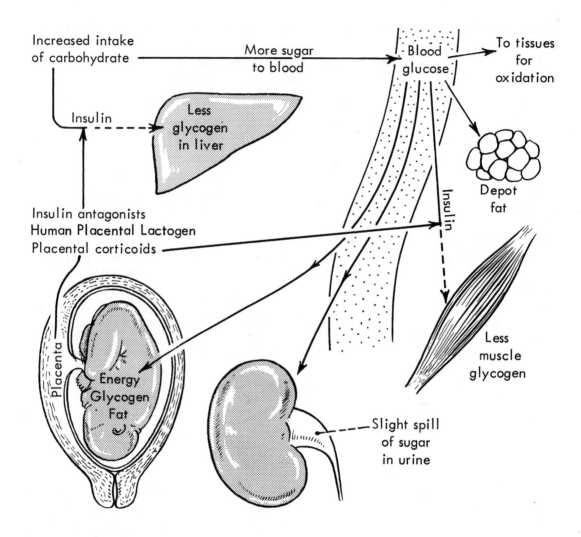

In pregnancy there is an increase in antagonists to insulin. These are the raised levels of steroids, corticoids and human placental lactogen (HPL) produced by the placenta. Less glycogen is deposited in the maternal liver and muscles. More sugar circulates for a longer time in the maternal blood. The placenta is able to pass more to the fetus. At the same time rather more passes the glomerulus than can be reabsorbed by the renal tubule and a small amount appears in the urine of many pregnant women.

PROTEIN METABOLISM

The overall picture is one of positive nitrogen balance. This reaches its peak at the 28th week.

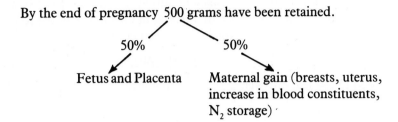

By the end of pregnancy 500 grams have been retained.

50%

50%

Fetus and Placenta

Maternal gain (breasts, uterus, increase in blood constituents, N_2 storage)

This is achieved by a complicated series of interlocking mechanisms, not all of them understood.

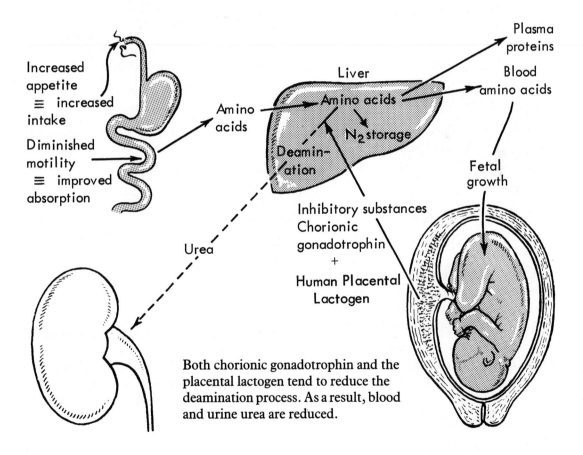

Increased appetite ≡ increased intake

Diminished motility ≡ improved absorption

Amino acids

Liver

Amino acids

Plasma proteins

Blood amino acids

N_2 storage

Deamin-ation

Fetal growth

Urea

Inhibitory substances Chorionic gonadotrophin + Human Placental Lactogen

Both chorionic gonadotrophin and the placental lactogen tend to reduce the deamination process. As a result, blood and urine urea are reduced.

PROTEIN METABOLISM

PLASMA PROTEINS

The concentration values are altered by haemodilution thus masking the fact that the total amounts are increased in most instances. In the case of urea however the reduction in concentration is greater than can be explained by haemodilution.

	Non-pregnant	Pregnant
Blood amino acid nitrogen	3.5 nmol/litre (5.0 mg/dl)	2 – 3.5 nmol/litre (3.4 – 5.0 mg/dl
Plasma proteins	81 g/litre	75 g/litre
Albumin/globulin ratio	1.32/l	0.84/l
Blood urea	2.5 – 7.0mmol/litre (20 – 40 mg/dl)	1.5 – 4.2mmol/litre (10 – 25 mg/dl)
Urates	0.16 mmol/litre (3.0 mg/dl)	0.16 mmol/litre (3.0 mg/dl)
Creatinine	88 – 176 μmol/litre (1 – 2 mg/dl)	88 – 176 μmol/litre (1 – 2 mg/dl)

Changes occur in the concentration of several plasma proteins, notably a fall in albumin and a rise in β-globulin and fibrinogen.

	Non-pregnant	Pregnant
Albumin	4.25 g/litre	3.25 g/litre
β-globulin	10.0 g/litre	13.0 g/litre
Fibrinogen	2.6 g/litre	4.0 g/litre

As a result the albumin/globulin ratio falls. Globulins act as transport mechanisms for many substances in the blood such as hormones and iron. Cortisol, oestrogens, progesterone, aldosterone and other steroids are greatly increased in pregnancy, so also is the transport of iron. This may account for some of the protein changes.

URINARY NITROGEN

	Non-pregnant (grams)	Pregnant (grams)
Total nitrogen/24 hours	12 – 16	8 – 12
Urea as percentage of total N_2	80 – 90	70 – 85
Ammonia N_2 as percentage of total	2.5 – 4.5	3 – 5

FAT METABOLISM

Fat would appear to be the main form of maternal stored energy during pregnancy. By 30 weeks some 4 kg are stored. Little is stored thereafter. Most of this is in the form of depot fat, in the abdominal wall, back and thighs, and perhaps retroperitoneally. Despite the enlargement only some 12 – 20 g are deposited in the breasts.

Blood fat increases from 3rd month

	Total lipoid	Cholesterol
Non-pregnant	700 mg/dl	3.1 mmol/litre (120mg/dl)
Pregnant at term	1,050 mg/dl	7.2 mmol/litre (280mg/dl)

The high blood levels and increased deposition are due partly to increased intake and partly to increased conversion of glucose to fat.

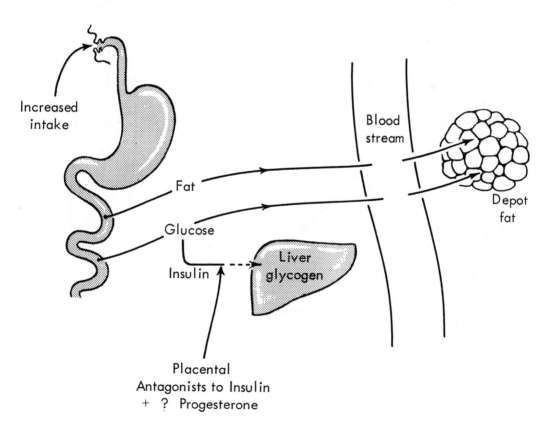

FAT METABOLISM

Three facts have to be related:

1. The total metabolism and demand for energy are increased in pregnancy.
2. Glycogen stores are diminished and therefore energy obtained directly from carbohydrate will be reduced.
3. Although blood fat is greatly increased only a moderate amount is laid down in fat stores.

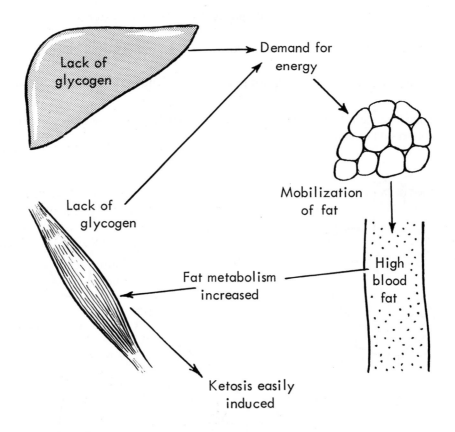

It is well recognised that the pregnant patient easily becomes ketotic whenever any strain, such as labour, is imposed. This is probably directly related to the poor glycogen stores.

RESPIRATORY CHANGES

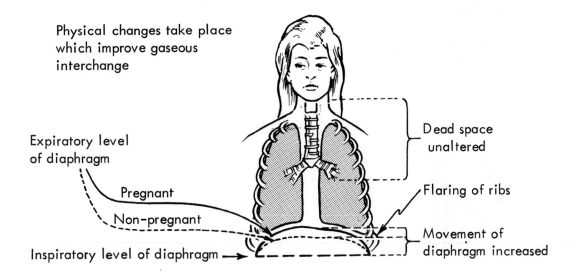

Physical changes take place which improve gaseous interchange

Dead space unaltered

Expiratory level of diaphragm

Pregnant

Non-pregnant

Inspiratory level of diaphragm →

Flaring of ribs

Movement of diaphragm increased

The increased movement of the diaphragm and the flaring of ribs increase the tidal movement of air. Expiration is more complete so that an increased volume of fresh air can be taken in. This increase is approximately 2 dl . The dead space is unaltered and this increase in moving air is accommodated in the alveoli. The minute ventilation rises from 7.25 litres to 10.5 litres.

The increase in inspiration and expiration results in several changes:-

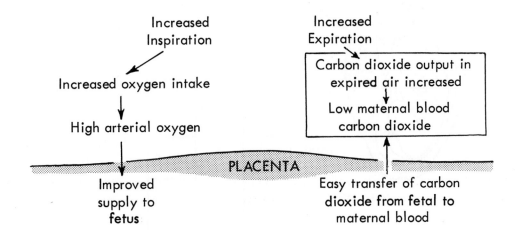

Increased Inspiration

Increased Expiration

Increased oxygen intake

High arterial oxygen

Carbon dioxide output in expired air increased

Low maternal blood carbon dioxide

PLACENTA

Improved supply to fetus

Easy transfer of carbon dioxide from fetal to maternal blood

The diaphragmatic excursion is reduced in late pregnancy and the increased respiratory exchange is maintained by thoracic movement.

33

RESPIRATORY CHANGES

Fetal plasma carbon dioxide tension exceeds that of maternal plasma by 4 – 8 mm mercury. Therefore it passes easily into the maternal blood. Despite this, due to the pulmonary hyperventilation, the concentration of carbon dioxide in maternal plasma is 6 – 10% less than that of the non-pregnant female.

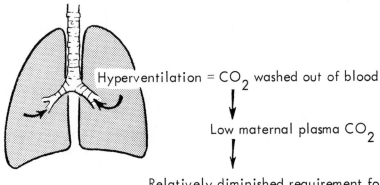

Hyperventilation = CO_2 washed out of blood

Low maternal plasma CO_2

Relatively diminished requirement for circulating cations

Flow of cations (sodium, potassium, and calcium) to fetus for growth.

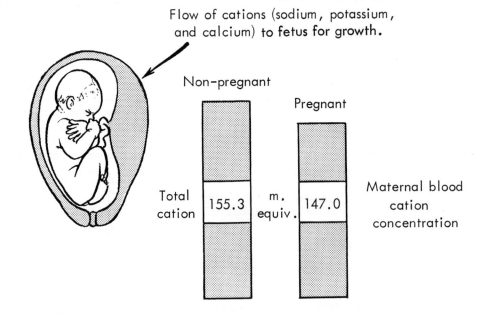

Non-pregnant

Pregnant

Total cation | 155.3 | m. equiv. | 147.0 | Maternal blood cation concentration

CATION CHANGES

The diminution in maternal circulating cation is only relative, that is, in concentration. The total circulating cation is raised.

SODIUM

850 m-equivalents are retained during pregnancy. This is divided in almost equal proportions between mother and conceptus.

Mother	850 m-equiv	Conceptus

m-equiv		m-equiv
Maternal blood _ _ _ _ 145		Fetus _ _ _ _ _ _ _ _ _ 280
Interstitial fluid_ _ _ _ 155	413 m-equiv 437 m-equiv	Liquor amnii _ _ _ _ _ 100
Uterus _ _ _ _ _ _ _ _ _ 78		Placenta _ _ _ _ _ _ _ 57
Breasts _ _ _ _ _ _ _ _ _ 35		

POTASSIUM

316 m-equivalents are stored during pregnancy. The conceptus receives almost twice as much as the mother.

Mother	316 m-equiv	Conceptus

m-equiv		m-equiv
Maternal blood _ _ _ _ 28		Fetus _ _ _ _ _ _ _ _ _ 154
Interstitial fluid _ _ _ _ 5	117 m-equiv 199 m-equiv	Liquor amnii _ _ _ _ _ 42
Uterus _ _ _ _ _ _ _ _ 49		Placenta _ _ _ _ _ _ _ 3
Breasts _ _ _ _ _ _ _ _ _ 35		

CALCIUM

29.5 m-equivalents are stored late in pregnancy. Almost all of this goes to the fetus (or conceptus).

CARDIOVASCULAR SYSTEM

Marked demands are made on this system, mainly as a result of the growth of the conceptus and the increase in metabolism.

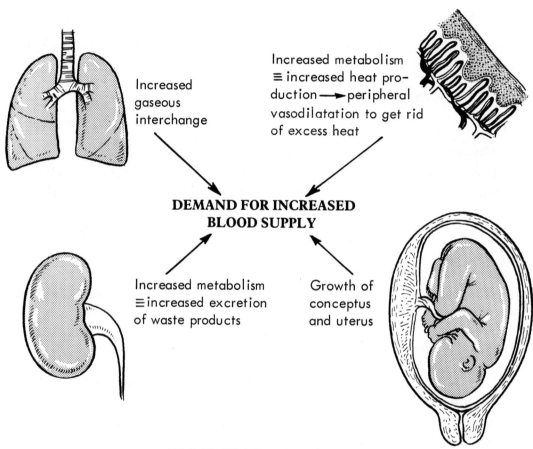

Increased gaseous interchange

Increased metabolism ≡ increased heat pro-duction ⟶ peripheral vasodilatation to get rid of excess heat

DEMAND FOR INCREASED BLOOD SUPPLY

Increased metabolism ≡ increased excretion of waste products

Growth of conceptus and uterus

BLOOD FLOW PER MINUTE

	Non-pregnant	Pregnant	
Pulmonary	5,800 ml	8,330 ml	
Peripheral (hand)	2 ml	7 ml	(per dl of hand volume)
Renal	880 ml	1,200 ml	
Uterine	51.7 ml	185 ml	

CARDIOVASCULAR SYSTEM

The demand for an increased blood supply to many parts of the body is met by an increase in blood volume. The mechanism whereby this is achieved is not understood but may be as follows:

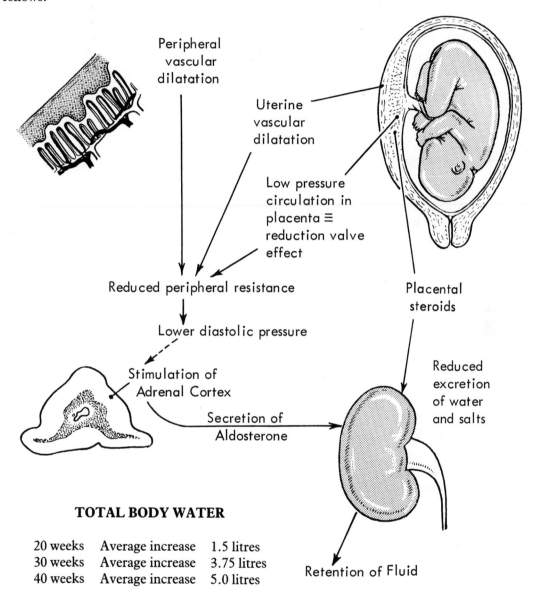

Peripheral vascular dilatation

Uterine vascular dilatation

Low pressure circulation in placenta $\equiv$ reduction valve effect

Reduced peripheral resistance

Lower diastolic pressure

Stimulation of Adrenal Cortex

Secretion of Aldosterone

Placental steroids

Reduced excretion of water and salts

Retention of Fluid

TOTAL BODY WATER

20 weeks	Average increase	1.5 litres
30 weeks	Average increase	3.75 litres
40 weeks	Average increase	5.0 litres

BLOOD VOLUME CHANGES

In the non-pregnant state, water $\equiv$ 72% body weight. Of this 5% is intravascular, intracellular fluid makes up 70% and interstitial fluid accounts for the remaining 25%.

In pregnancy, intracellular water appears to be unchanged but both blood and interstitial fluid are increased.

The plasma volume starts to increase early in pregnancy and reaches a peak around the 32nd week. Thereafter it is maintained until towards term when a slight fall occurs. The increase varies from individual to individual but is most marked in multigravid patients.

Average non-pregnant volume = 2,600 ml

Peak volume in primigravida   = 3,850 ml = 41% increase

Peak volume in multigravida   = 4,100 ml = 57% increase

This increase in plasma volume results in a reduction in blood viscosity as the red cell mass and protein content rise less relatively.

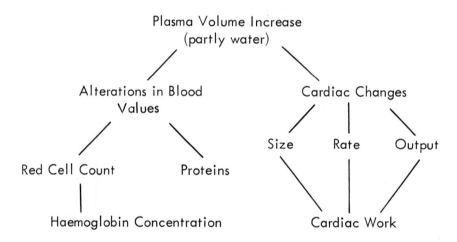

CARDIAC CHANGES

The work-load of the heart is increased by the demands made upon it.

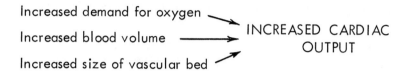

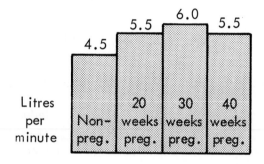

This increase in output is brought about <u>partly</u> by a rise in heart rate

	Heart Rate
Non-pregnant	70/min
20 weeks pregnant	78/min
Late pregnancy	85/min

and <u>partly</u> by an increased stroke volume.

Non-pregnant	64 ml.
20 weeks pregnant	70 ml.
30 weeks pregnant	70 ml.
40 weeks pregnant	64 ml.

The heart itself is enlarged, partly due to dilatation and partly to hypertrophy. Its volume increases from an average of 670ml to 750ml.

The increase in work-load is modified by changes in the composition of the blood and peripheral dilatation.

39

CARDIAC CHANGES

The work-load balance may be summarised as follows:

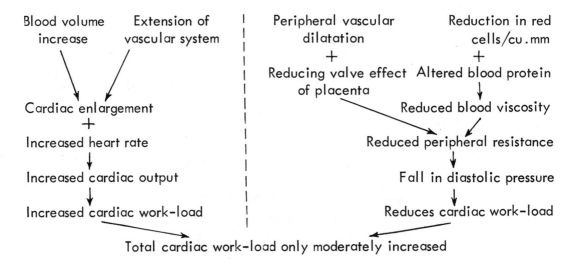

Blood volume increase   Extension of vascular system

Cardiac enlargement
+
Increased heart rate
↓
Increased cardiac output
↓
Increased cardiac work-load

Peripheral vascular dilatation
+
Reducing valve effect of placenta

Reduction in red cells/cu.mm
+
Altered blood protein
↓
Reduced blood viscosity

Reduced peripheral resistance
↓
Fall in diastolic pressure
↓
Reduces cardiac work-load

Total cardiac work-load only moderately increased

LOCAL VASCULAR CHANGES

Local changes are most apparent in the lower limbs and are due to the pressure exerted by the enlarging uterus on the pelvic veins. Since one-third of the total circulating blood is distributed to the lower limbs the increased venous pressure may produce varicosities and oedema of the vulva and legs. These changes are most marked during daytime due to the upright posture. They tend to be reversed at night when the patient retires to bed: oedema fluid is reabsorbed, venous return increased and renal output rises, resulting in nocturnal frequency.

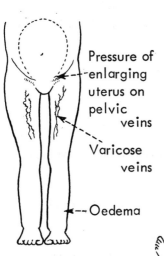

Pressure of enlarging uterus on pelvic veins

Varicose veins

Oedema

If the patient adopts the supine position however, the uterine pressure on the veins increases and this may lead to reduced venous return to the heart. This in turn leads to a reduction in cardiac output. An extreme example of this is the **SUPINE HYPOTENSIVE SYNDROME.**

This term describes the situation when the mother feels faint or even becomes unconscious due to a fall in cardiac output secondary to caval compression.

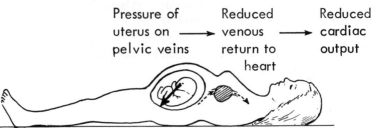

Pressure of uterus on pelvic veins ⟶ Reduced venous return to heart ⟶ Reduced cardiac output

BLOOD VALUES

The change in blood values such as haemoglobin content is the result of demands of the growing pregnancy modified by the increase in plasma volume.

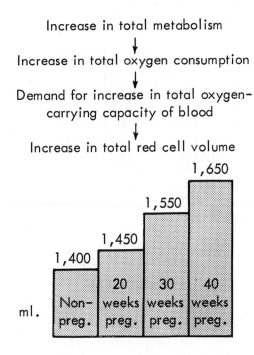

This represents a maximum increase of 18 per cent. The plasma volume increases by 40 – 45 per cent. Thus there is a reduction in the red cell count per cubic millimetre from 4.5 million to around 3.8 million. Towards term as the plasma volume diminishes the red cell count rises slightly.

Similarly the haematocrit falls during pregnancy with a slight rise at term.

	Packed cell volume (per cent)
Non-pregnant	40 – 42
20 weeks pregnant	39
30 weeks pregnant	38
40 weeks pregnant	40

41

BLOOD VALUES

Changes in haemoglobin run parallel with those in red cells. The mean cell haemoglobin concentration in the non-pregnant = 34 per cent, that is each dl. of red cells contain 34 g haemoglobin. This does not alter in pregnancy, therefore, as with the total red cell volume, the total haemoglobin rises throughout pregnancy.

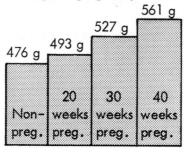

This is a total increase of 85 g, equivalent to 18 per cent.

The increasing plasma volume, however, produces an apparent reduction in haemoglobin. The haemoglobin concentration falls throughout pregnancy until the last four weeks when there may be a slight rise. The fall is apparent by the 12th week and the minimum value is reached at 32 weeks.

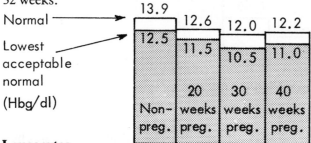

It will be seen from this that no single value can be taken as normal throughout pregnancy. This is important in diagnosing anaemia. At 30 weeks a haemoglobin reading of 10.5 is normal but the same reading at 20 weeks indicates anaemia.

Leucocytes

There is a marked increase in these cells during pregnancy from 7 x 10⁹/litre in the non-pregnant to 10.5 x 10⁹/litre in late pregnancy. The increase is due almost entirely to neutrophil polymorphonuclears.

Blood platelets

Increase continuously during pregnancy and in the puerperium.
>(Counts/litre) Non-preg. 187 x 10⁹; 20 weeks preg. 250 x 10⁹;
>30 weeks preg. 275 x 10⁹; 40 weeks preg. 316 x 10⁹; Puerperium 600 x 10⁹.

This may be related to the need to prevent haemorrhage but the mechanism is obscure.

COAGULATION SYSTEM

Changes in the coagulation system occur to make pregnancy a hypercoagulable state, presumably to meet the dangers of bleeding at placental separation.

Fibrinogen shows a steady rise in concentration throughout pregnancy, from a non-pregnant level of 2.6g per litre to 4g per litre. This is equivalent to more than 100 per cent increase in total circulating fibrinogen.

Levels of most of the other clotting factors also rise and platelet levels increase as already noted.

GASTRO-INTESTINAL TRACT

Changes in the gastro-intestinal tract appear to be of minor degree but may have a marked cumulative effect in some cases. The main change is one of decreased motility which may be due to the effect of increased circulating progesterone.

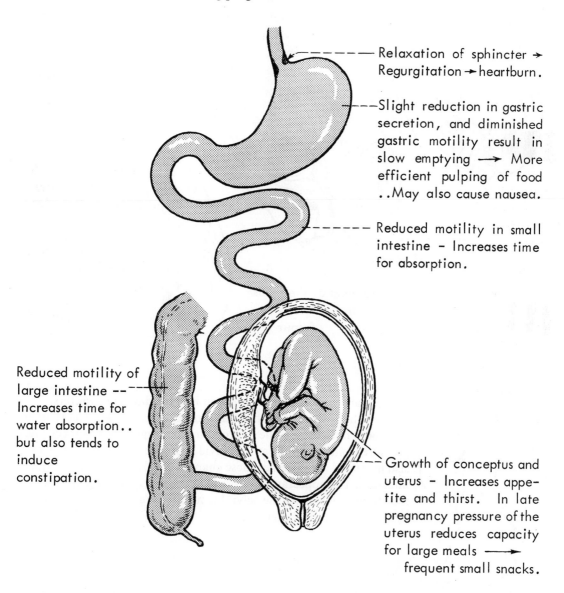

Relaxation of sphincter → Regurgitation → heartburn.

Slight reduction in gastric secretion, and diminished gastric motility result in slow emptying ⟶ More efficient pulping of food ..May also cause nausea.

Reduced motility in small intestine – Increases time for absorption.

Reduced motility of large intestine -- Increases time for water absorption.. but also tends to induce constipation.

Growth of conceptus and uterus – Increases appetite and thirst. In late pregnancy pressure of the uterus reduces capacity for large meals ⟶ frequent small snacks.

43

RENAL SYSTEM

Frequency of micturition is a common symptom in early pregnancy and again at term. This is due to changes in pelvic anatomy and is a 'normal' feature of pregnancy.

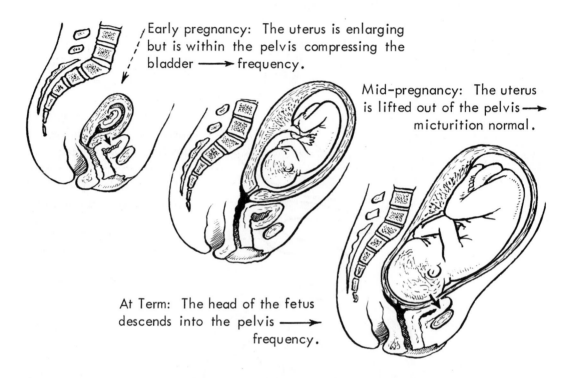

Early pregnancy: The uterus is enlarging but is within the pelvis compressing the bladder ⟶ frequency.

Mid-pregnancy: The uterus is lifted out of the pelvis ⟶ micturition normal.

At Term: The head of the fetus descends into the pelvis ⟶ frequency.

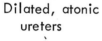

Dilated, atonic ureters

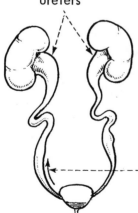

Vesico-ureteric reflux

Striking anatomical changes are seen in the kidneys and ureters. A degree of hydronephrosis and hydro-ureter exist. These result from loss of smooth muscle tone due to progesterone, aggravated by mechanical pressure from the uterus at the pelvic brim. Vesico-ureteric reflux is also increased and together these changes predispose to urinary tract infection. The appearances improve in the latter part of pregnancy as the uterus grows above the pelvic brim and rising oestrogen levels cause hypertrophy of the ureteric muscle.

RENAL SYSTEM

Urinary output on a normal fluid intake tends to be slightly diminished. This seems paradoxical in view of the increased flow of blood to the kidneys.

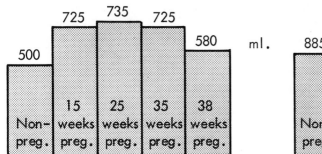

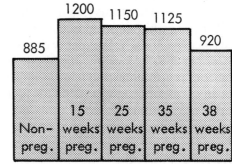

ml.

Renal plasma flow per minute is greatly increased.

Total renal blood flow runs almost parallel with plasma flow but with increasing haemodilution the red cell volume/dl decreases and this alters the figures.

As a result the amount of fluid filtered off the plasma through the renal glomeruli is similarly increased and 100 extra litres of fluid pass into the renal tubules each day. Despite this the urinary output is diminished. Obviously there must be an increased tubular reabsorption. It is estimated that extracellular water is increased by 6 to 7 litres during pregnancy. Along with this water sodium and other electrolytes are reabsorbed by the tubules to maintain body osmolarity. Under test the pregnant patient only excretes 80 per cent of the total found in the urine of non-pregnant subjects.

The mechanism whereby this is achieved is not yet known, but it is thought that the increased amounts of aldosterone, progesterone and oestrogen are responsible.

Glycosuria of mild degree occurs in 35–50 per cent of all pregnant women. Increased glomerular filtration leads to more sugar reaching the tubules than can be reabsorbed. Glycosuria occurs therefore with lower blood sugar levels than in the non-pregnant, the so-called lowered renal threshold.

REPRODUCTIVE SYSTEM

BREASTS

Each breast is made up of 15–20 glandular lobules separated by fat. The glands lead into tubules and then into ducts which open on to the nipple. The breasts increase in size in pregnancy due to proliferation of the glands and ducts under the influence of progesterone and oestrogen. The secretion of colostrum may begin in the first trimester and continues to term.

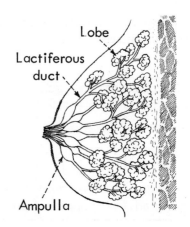

BODY OF UTERUS

The uterus grows enormously under the influence of oestrogen by hyperplasia and hypertrophy of its muscle fibres. Its weight increases from the non-pregnant level of 50g up to 1000g. The lower segment is formed from the isthmus, the area between the uterine cavity and the endocervical epithelium.

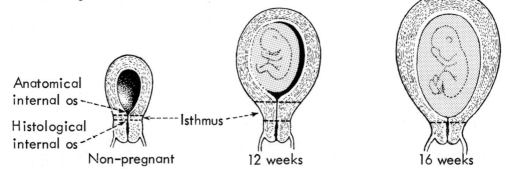

CERVIX

The cervix softens due to increased vascularity and changes in its connective tissue, due mainly it seems to oestrogen. There is increased secretion from its glands and the mucus becomes thick and forms a protective plug in the os, the operculum.

VAGINA AND PELVIC FLOOR

The changes of increased vascularity, muscular hypertrophy and softening of connective tissue are seen. The vaginal capacity is increased by hyperplasia and hypertrophy to allow distension of the vagina at birth.

PELVIC LIGAMENTS

There is softening of the ligaments of the pelvic joints, presumably due to oestrogen. The effect is to make the pelvis more mobile and increase its capacity.

ENDOCRINE CHANGES IN PREGNANCY

The following is a summary of the changes in maternal and placental hormones in pregnancy and their supposed effects.

PROGESTERONE is produced by the corpus luteum in the first few weeks of pregnancy. Thereafter it is derived from the placenta. Levels rise steadily during pregnancy with, it has been suggested, a fall towards term. Output reaches a maximum of at least 250mg per day.

Possible actions:-

1. Reduces smooth muscle tone. Stomach motility diminishes — may induce nausea. Colonic activity reduced — delayed emptying — increased water reabsorption — constipation. Reduced uterine tone — diminished uterine activity. Reduced bladder and ureteric tone — stasis of urine.
2. Reduces vascular tone — diastolic pressure reduced. Venous dilatation.
3. Raises temperature
4. Increases fat storage.
5. Induces over-breathing — alveolar and arterial carbon dioxide tension reduced.
6. Induces development of breasts.

OESTROGENS. In early pregnancy the source is the ovary. Later oestrone and oestradiol are probably produced by the placenta and are increased a hundredfold. Oestriol, however, is a product resulting from the interaction of the placenta and the fetal adrenals and is increased one thousandfold. The output of oestrogens reaches a maximum of at least 30 – 40 mg per day. Oestriol accounts for 85 per cent of this total. Levels increase up to term.

Possible actions:-

1. Induce growth of uterus and control its function.
2. Responsible, together with progesterone, for the development of the breasts.
3. Alter the chemical constitution of connective tissue, making it more pliable — stretching of cervix possible, joint capsules relax, pelvic joints mobile.
4. Cause water retention.
5. May reduce sodium excretion.

CORTISOL. The maternal adrenals are the sole source in early pregnancy but later considerable quantities are thought to be produced by the placenta. Some 25 mg are produced each day. Much of this is protein bound and therefore may not be generally active.

Possible actions:-

1. Increases blood sugar.
2. Modifies antibody activity.

ALDOSTERONE is almost certainly wholly derived from the maternal adrenals. The amounts produced during pregnancy are much increased. It promotes the retention of sodium and water.

ENDOCRINE CHANGES IN PREGNANCY

HUMAN CHORIONIC GONADOTROPHIN (HCG) is produced by the trophoblast and peak levels are reached before 16 weeks of gestation. From 18 weeks onwards, levels remain relatively constant. Apart from the early maintenance of the corpus luteum, the physiological role of HCG remains unclear. It appears to have a thyrotrophic action and to initiate testosterone secretion from the Leydig cells.

HUMAN PLACENTAL LACTOGEN (HPL). Levels of HPL (or chorionic somato-mammotrophin) rise steadily with the growth of the placenta throughout pregnancy. It is lactogenic and antagonistic to insulin.

RELAXIN is a hormone produced by the corpus luteum. It can be detected throughout pregnancy but highest levels are in the first trimester. Its physiological role is uncertain but it has been used clinically in cervical ripening.

PITUITARY HORMONES. Maternal FSH and LH levels are suppressed during pregnancy but prolactin levels rise throughout. Lactation does not start, however, until after delivery when high prolactin levels persist in association with falling oestrogen levels.

CHAPTER 3

OBSTETRICAL ANATOMY

PELVIC ORGANS

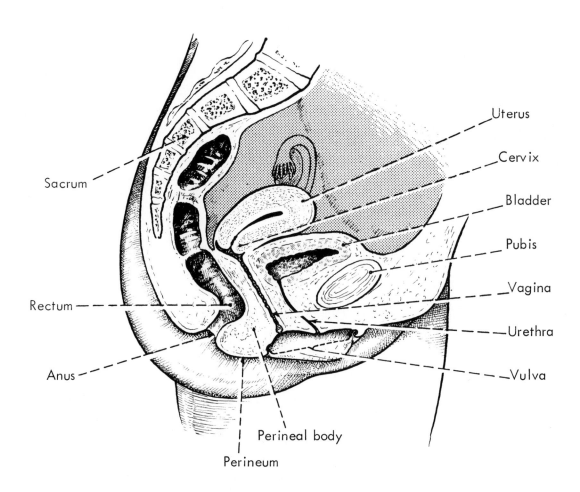

Uterus

Cervix

Bladder

Pubis

Vagina

Urethra

Vulva

Sacrum

Rectum

Anus

Perineal body

Perineum

VULVA

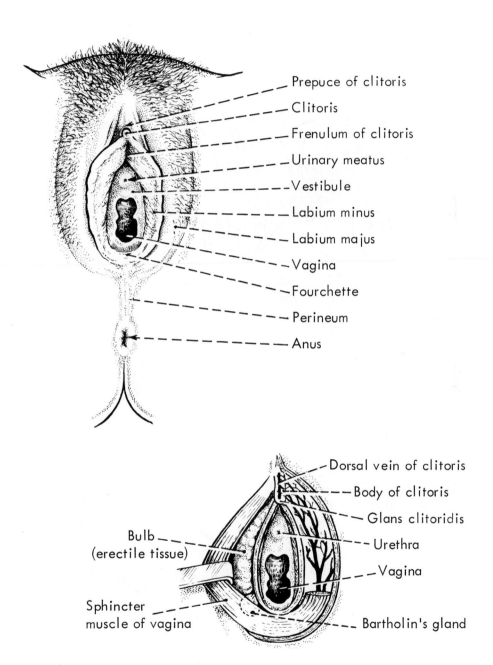

Prepuce of clitoris

Clitoris

Frenulum of clitoris

Urinary meatus

Vestibule

Labium minus

Labium majus

Vagina

Fourchette

Perineum

Anus

Dorsal vein of clitoris

Body of clitoris

Glans clitoridis

Urethra

Vagina

Bartholin's gland

Bulb
(erectile tissue)

Sphincter
muscle of vagina

PELVIC FLOOR

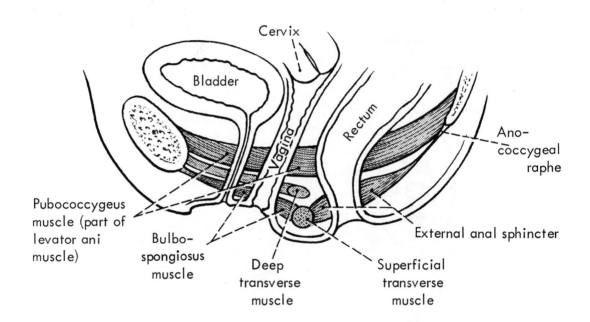

Cervix

Bladder

Vagina

Rectum

Ano-coccygeal raphe

Pubococcygeus muscle (part of levator ani muscle)

Bulbo-spongiosus muscle

Deep transverse muscle

Superficial transverse muscle

External anal sphincter

SOFT TISSUES OF THE OBSTETRIC PELVIS (Schematic)

A muscular basin with an opening below at the front. The muscular tissues are supported by and enclosed in the pelvic bones.

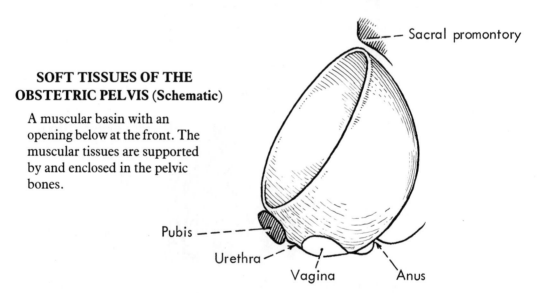

Sacral promontory

Pubis

Urethra

Vagina

Anus

PELVIC FLOOR

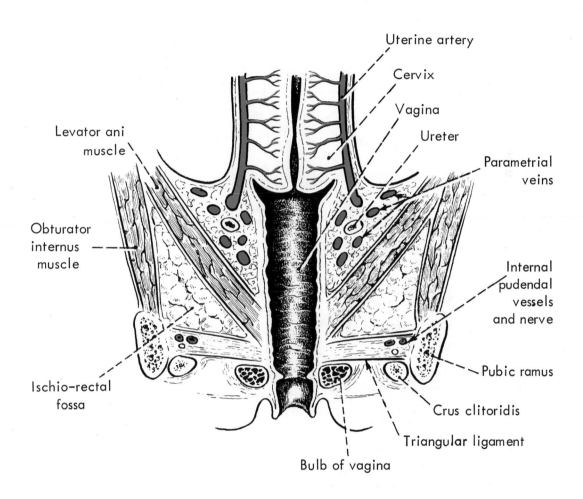

Uterine artery

Cervix

Vagina

Ureter

Parametrial veins

Levator ani muscle

Obturator internus muscle

Internal pudendal vessels and nerve

Ischio-rectal fossa

Pubic ramus

Crus clitoridis

Triangular ligament

Bulb of vagina

ISCHIORECTAL FOSSA

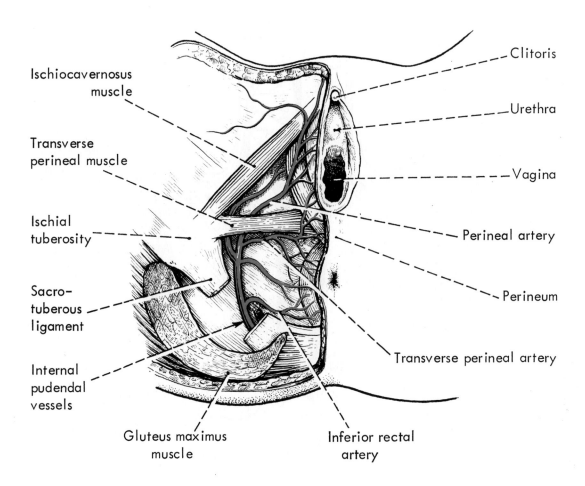

Ischiocavernosus muscle

Transverse perineal muscle

Ischial tuberosity

Sacro-tuberous ligament

Internal pudendal vessels

Clitoris

Urethra

Vagina

Perineal artery

Perineum

Transverse perineal artery

Gluteus maximus muscle

Inferior rectal artery

ISCHIORECTAL FOSSA

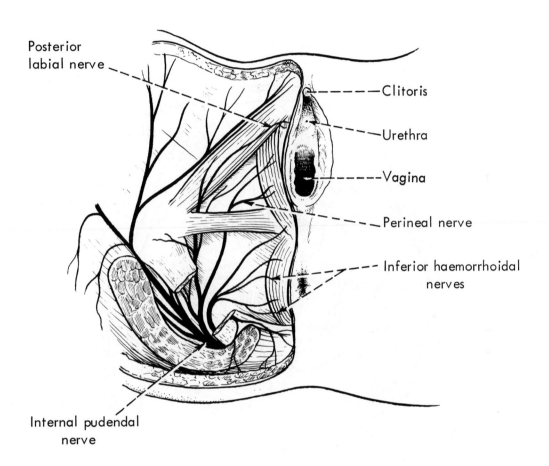

Posterior labial nerve

Clitoris

Urethra

Vagina

Perineal nerve

Inferior haemorrhoidal nerves

Internal pudendal nerve

PERINEUM

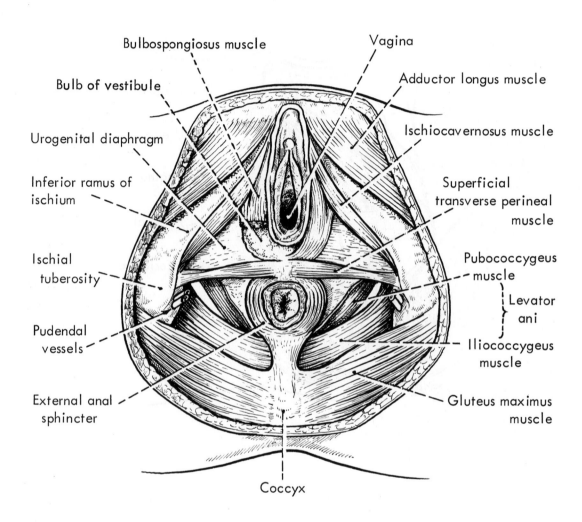

Bulbospongiosus muscle

Vagina

Bulb of vestibule

Adductor longus muscle

Urogenital diaphragm

Ischiocavernosus muscle

Inferior ramus of ischium

Superficial transverse perineal muscle

Ischial tuberosity

Pubococcygeus muscle

Levator ani

Pudendal vessels

Iliococcygeus muscle

External anal sphincter

Gluteus maximus muscle

Coccyx

PELVIC BLOOD SUPPLY

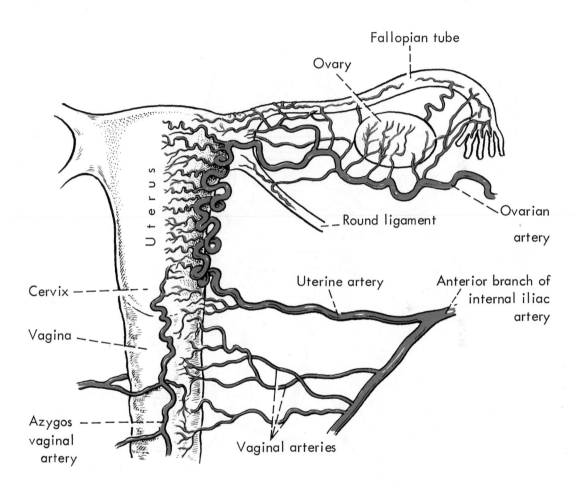

Note coiling of vessels to allow stretching as uterus grows in pregnancy.

PELVIC SYMPATHETIC NERVES

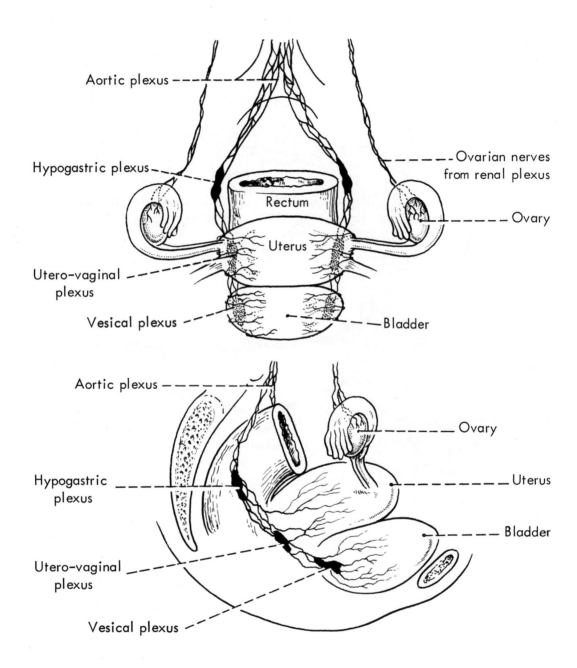

SUPPORTS OF UTERUS

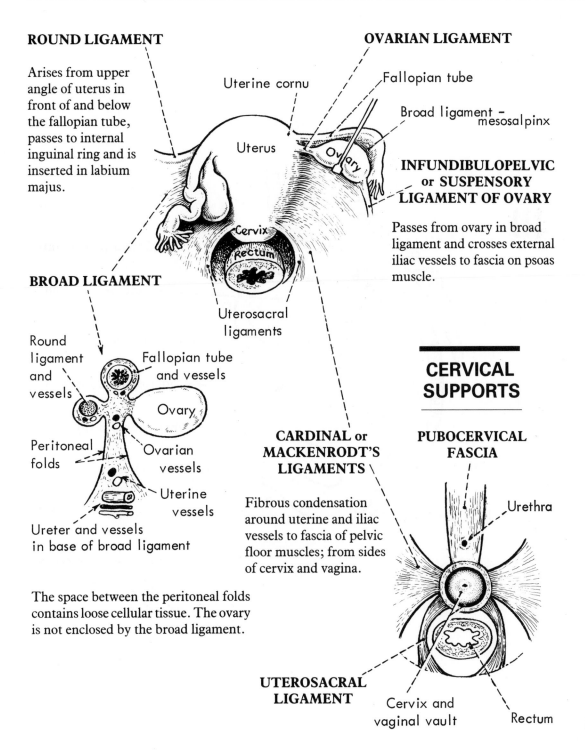

ROUND LIGAMENT

Arises from upper angle of uterus in front of and below the fallopian tube, passes to internal inguinal ring and is inserted in labium majus.

Uterine cornu

Uterus

Cervix

Rectum

OVARIAN LIGAMENT

Fallopian tube

Broad ligament – mesosalpinx

Ovary

INFUNDIBULOPELVIC or SUSPENSORY LIGAMENT OF OVARY

Passes from ovary in broad ligament and crosses external iliac vessels to fascia on psoas muscle.

BROAD LIGAMENT

Round ligament and vessels

Fallopian tube and vessels

Ovary

Peritoneal folds

Ovarian vessels

Uterine vessels

Ureter and vessels in base of broad ligament

Uterosacral ligaments

The space between the peritoneal folds contains loose cellular tissue. The ovary is not enclosed by the broad ligament.

CARDINAL or MACKENRODT'S LIGAMENTS

Fibrous condensation around uterine and iliac vessels to fascia of pelvic floor muscles; from sides of cervix and vagina.

CERVICAL SUPPORTS

PUBOCERVICAL FASCIA

Urethra

UTEROSACRAL LIGAMENT

Cervix and vaginal vault

Rectum

59

BONY PELVIS — SAGITTAL VIEW

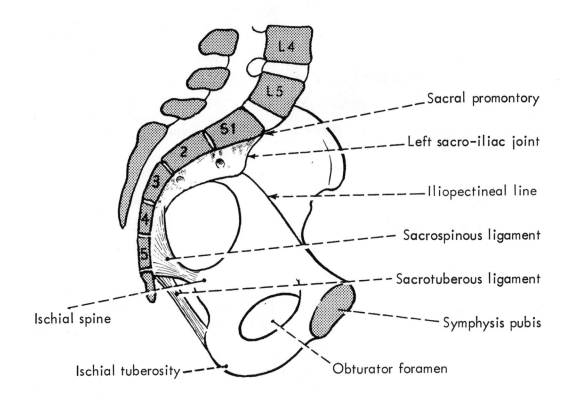

Sacral promontory

Left sacro-iliac joint

Iliopectineal line

Sacrospinous ligament

Sacrotuberous ligament

Symphysis pubis

Ischial spine

Ischial tuberosity

Obturator foramen

BONY PELVIS — BRIM

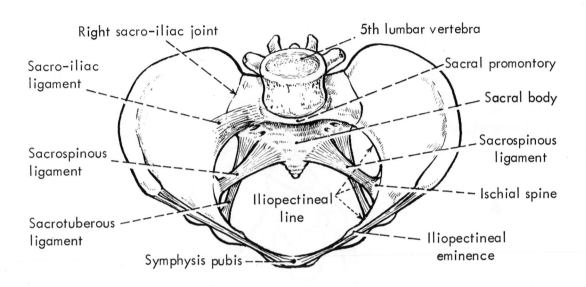

Right sacro-iliac joint

5th lumbar vertebra

Sacro-iliac ligament

Sacral promontory

Sacral body

Sacrospinous ligament

Sacrospinous ligament

Ischial spine

Sacrotuberous ligament

Iliopectineal line

Iliopectineal eminence

Symphysis pubis

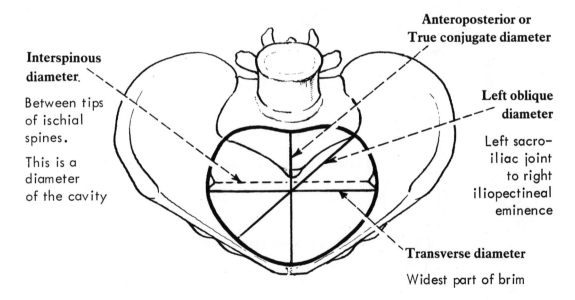

Interspinous diameter.

Between tips of ischial spines.

This is a diameter of the cavity

Anteroposterior or True conjugate diameter

Left oblique diameter

Left sacro-iliac joint to right iliopectineal eminence

Transverse diameter

Widest part of brim

The Plane of the Brim is bounded

Anteriorly by the Pubis,
Laterally by the Iliopectineal lines,
Posteriorly by the Alae and
Promontory of the Sacrum.

61

BONY PELVIS — CAVITY

The Pelvic Cavity is bounded
  Above by the Plane of the Brim,
  Below by the Plane of the Outlet,
  Posteriorly by the Sacrum,
  Laterally by Sacrosciatic ligaments and
    Ischial bones and
  Anteriorly by Obturator Foramina,
    Ascending Rami of Ischia and Pubis

Plane of mid cavity or plane of greatest pelvic diameters

Mid pubis to junction of second and third sacral vetebrae.

Plane of least pelvic diameters

Symphysis pubis through ischial spines to end of sacrum.

Note that pelvic outlet plane is in two parts angled to each other.

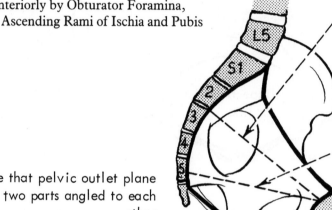

True conjugate of brim

From sacral promontory to upper and inner border of symphysis pubis.

Diagonal conjugate diameter of brim

From sacral promontory to under border of symphysis pubis.

Antero-posterior diameter of outlet

Under body of symphysis pubis to end of sacrum or coccyx if fused.

Inclination of pelvic brim 50° – 60° (Usually 55°)

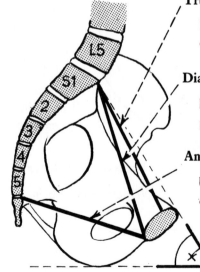

BONY PELVIS — OUTLET

The Plane of the Outlet is bounded
  Anteriorly by Pubic Arch
  Laterally by Great Sacrosciatic Ligaments
    and Ischial Tuberosities
  Posteriorly by Tip of Coccyx if fused or
    to End of Sacrum

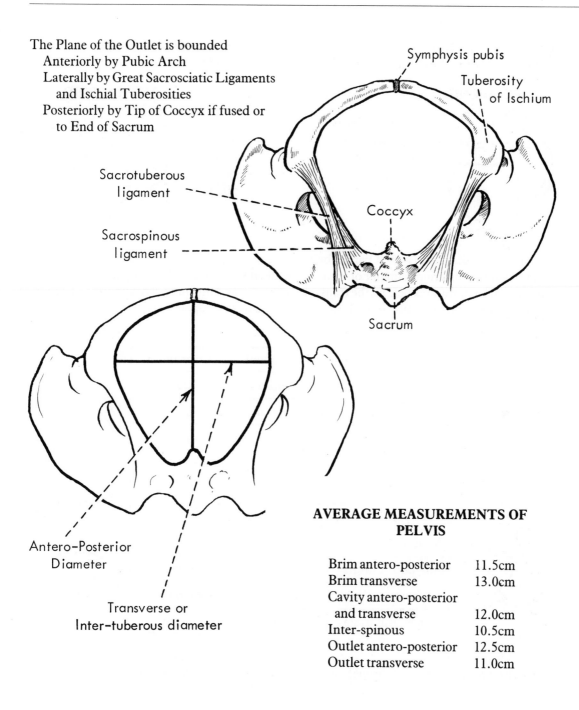

AVERAGE MEASUREMENTS OF PELVIS

Brim antero-posterior	11.5cm
Brim transverse	13.0cm
Cavity antero-posterior and transverse	12.0cm
Inter-spinous	10.5cm
Outlet antero-posterior	12.5cm
Outlet transverse	11.0cm

63

PELVIC TYPES

Four types of pelvis are described — Gynaecoid (50%), Anthropoid (25%), Android (20%), Platypelloid or Flat (5%). In many cases the pelvis is of mixed type.

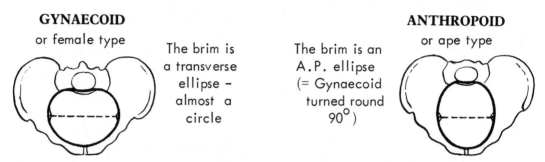

GYNAECOID
or female type

The brim is a transverse ellipse – almost a circle

The brim is an A.P. ellipse (= Gynaecoid turned round 90°)

ANTHROPOID
or ape type

The transverse diameter (widest part of brim) and the available transverse diameter (at mid-point of antero-posterior diameter of brim) coincide in the gynaecoid and anthropoid pelves. The hind pelvis is the area behind the transverse diameter and the fore pelvis the area in front. These areas are roughly equal in both the gynaecoid and anthropoid pelves.

Gynaecoid

Anthropoid

	Gynaecoid	Anthropoid
Sacral angle	Approximately 100°	
Sacral line	Parallel to pubis	
Sacrosciatic notch	Shallow, wide	Shallow, wider
Ischial spines	Not prominent	
Sacrum	Broad, shallow, concave	
Cavity side walls	Parallel	
Pubis	Light, shallow	
Sub-pubic angle	At least 85°	More than 80°
Bituberous diam.	Wide	Narrower
Outlet A.P. diam.	Long	Longer

The delivery of the fetal head through these types of pelvis has equal mechanical problems at all levels, i.e. if it is easy at brim it should be easy in cavity and outlet.

PELVIC TYPES

ANDROID

or male type

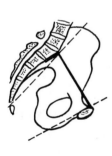

Brim is roughly triangular. Trans.diameter near sacrum. 'Available trans.' diameter is shortened.

Brim is kidney shaped. Transverse and 'available transverse' diameters coincide.

PLATYPELLOID

type

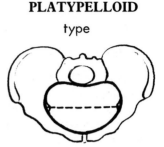

The area of the hind pelvis is reduced and shallow. Area of the fore pelvis is reduced and narrowed at front.

The hind pelvis is shallow and the area reduced. Fore pelvis is shallow and the area reduced.

	Android	**Platypelloid**
Sacral angle	90° or less	more than 90°
Sacral line	convergent	divergent
Sacrosciatic notch	narrowed	wide, shallow
Ischial spines	prominent, heavy	not prominent
Sacrum	flattened, narrow, long	broad, short, concave
Cavity side walls	converge	diverge
Pubis	heavy, deep	shallow
Sub-pubic angle	narrowed	more than 85°
Bituberous diam.	reduced	increased
Outlet A.P.diam.	narrow	longer

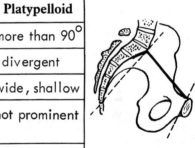

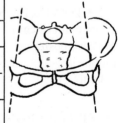

The delivery of a fetal head through this pelvis gives increasing problems the further it descends.

The delivery of a fetal head through this pelvis meets problems at the brim but thereafter the difficulties decrease with descent.

65

FETAL SKULL

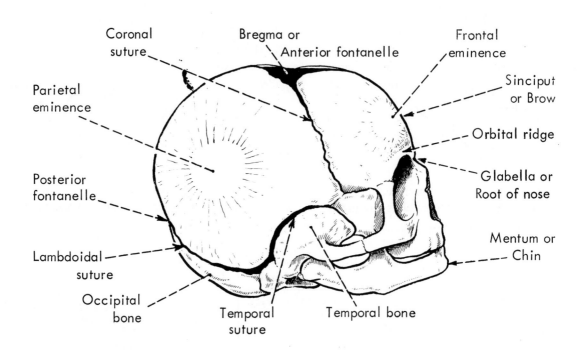

Coronal suture
Bregma or Anterior fontanelle
Frontal eminence
Parietal eminence
Sinciput or Brow
Orbital ridge
Posterior fontanelle
Glabella or Root of nose
Lambdoidal suture
Mentum or Chin
Occipital bone
Temporal suture
Temporal bone

(Diameters)

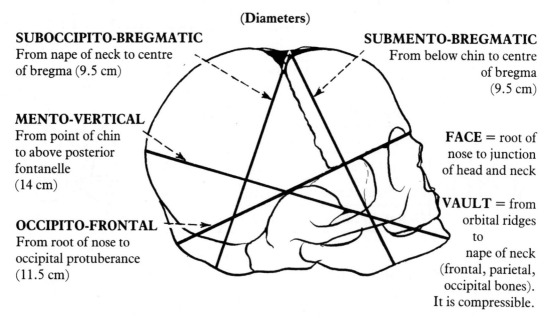

SUBOCCIPITO-BREGMATIC
From nape of neck to centre of bregma (9.5 cm)

MENTO-VERTICAL
From point of chin to above posterior fontanelle (14 cm)

OCCIPITO-FRONTAL
From root of nose to occipital protuberance (11.5 cm)

SUBMENTO-BREGMATIC
From below chin to centre of bregma (9.5 cm)

FACE = root of nose to junction of head and neck

VAULT = from orbital ridges to nape of neck (frontal, parietal, occipital bones). It is compressible.

(Measurements shown in brackets)

66

FETAL SKULL

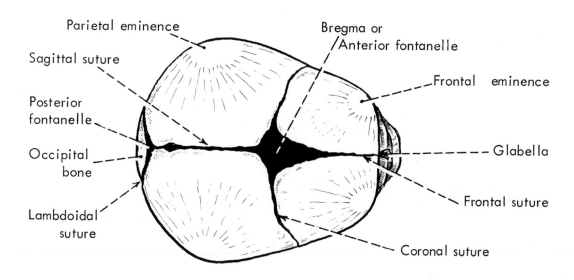

The **VERTEX** is the area bounded by the anterior and posterior fontanelles and the parietal eminences.

(Diameters)

BIPARIETAL (9.5 cm)
Between two parietal eminences

BITEMPORAL (8.5 cm)
Greatest distance between two halves of coronal suture

(Circumferences)

SUBOCCIPITO-BREGMATIC x BIPARIETAL (28 cm)
These are engaging diameters of well flexed vertex presentation.

OCCIPITO-FRONTAL x BIPARIETAL (33 cm)
These are engaging diameters of deflexed vertex presentation and found in Occipito-posterior positions.

MENTO-VERTICAL x BIPARIETAL (35.5 cm)
This is the largest circumference of the head and is found in Brow presentation.

CHAPTER 4

DIAGNOSIS OF PREGNANCY

SYMPTOMS, SIGNS AND TESTS OF PREGNANCY

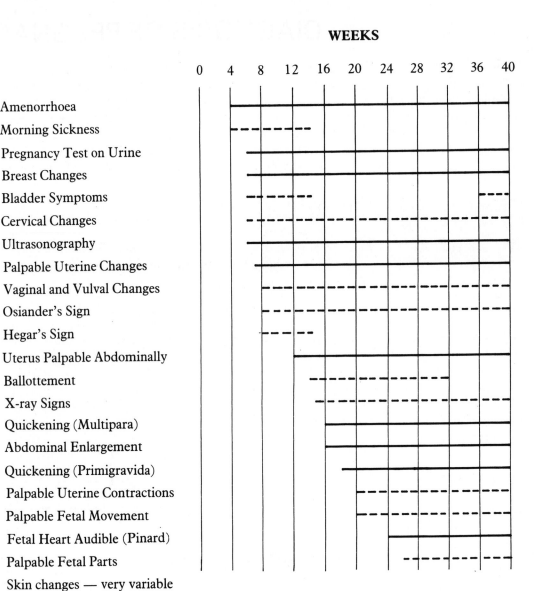

WEEKS

	0	4	8	12	16	20	24	28	32	36	40

Amenorrhoea

Morning Sickness

Pregnancy Test on Urine

Breast Changes

Bladder Symptoms

Cervical Changes

Ultrasonography

Palpable Uterine Changes

Vaginal and Vulval Changes

Osiander's Sign

Hegar's Sign

Uterus Palpable Abdominally

Ballottement

X-ray Signs

Quickening (Multipara)

Abdominal Enlargement

Quickening (Primigravida)

Palpable Uterine Contractions

Palpable Fetal Movement

Fetal Heart Audible (Pinard)

Palpable Fetal Parts

Skin changes — very variable

(The more useful symptoms, signs and tests are shown in full line.)

TESTS FOR PREGNANCY

IMMUNOLOGICAL TESTS

These tests depend on the fact that, 14 days after fertilisation, the chorion of the blastocyst secretes Human Chorionic Gonadotrophin (HCG). A peak is reached in 10 to 12 weeks, and the hormone is excreted in the mother's urine. An antiserum to HCG will detect the presence of the hormone in the urine but it is necessary to make the reaction visible, commonly using red cells coated with HCG. The antiserum and urine are added to the red cells. If the urine contains HCG the antiserum is neutralised and the red cells are deposited (positive test); if there is no HCG in the urine a diffuse sedimentation is seen due to the reaction between the antiserum and the coated cells (negative test)

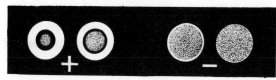

A positive result can be obtained from 8–9 days after a missed period.

BETA-HCG ASSAY - - - - - - - - - - - ->

Radio-immunoassay for Beta-HCG can be carried out on plasma or urine. It provides a very sensitive, early test of pregnancy. This may be particularly helpful in suspected ectopic pregnancy.

ULTRASOUND

A gestation sac may be detected at 5–6 weeks' amenorrhoea and fetal heart movements from 7 weeks.

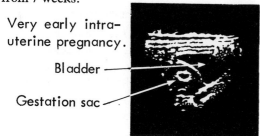

Very early intra-uterine pregnancy.

Bladder

Gestation sac

No fetal pole is seen

URINARY B-HCG

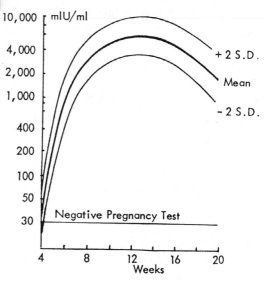

X-RAYS

X-rays are not normally used nowadays in the diagnosis of pregnancy. They may still however be employed occasionally in late pregnancy especially where multiple pregnancy is suspected.

SYMPTOMS AND SIGNS

4 WEEKS AMENORRHOEA

Causes such as ovarian-pituitary imbalance, the use of the contraceptive pill and emotional upset must be considered. Ovulation may have occurred earlier or later in the cycle than normal. Women do not always recall the date of their last menstrual period with precision.

4 WEEKS MORNING SICKNESS

Many women suffer some gastric upset in the early months, from nausea and anorexia to repeated vomiting, especially in the morning. The cause is unknown and raised levels of both oestrogen and HCG in the circulation have been blamed. Gastric motility is reduced, and in early pregnancy the lower oesophageal sphincter is relaxed.

6 WEEKS BLADDER SYMPTOMS

Increased frequency of micturition in the second and third months is due to a combination of increased vascularity and pressure from the enlarging uterus. Near term, frequency may again appear, due mainly to pressure of the fetal head on the bladder.

- -

CLINICAL SIGNS

(These are of less importance since the development of quick, sensitive laboratory tests for pregnancy.)

Cervical softening	6 weeks
Increased pulsation in lateral fornices (Osiander's sign)	8 weeks
Darkening of vaginal skin (Jacquemier's sign)	8 weeks

SYMPTOMS AND SIGNS

7 WEEKS

PALPABLE UTERINE ENLARGEMENT

At 7 weeks the uterus is the size of a large hen's egg

At 10 weeks it is the size of an orange

At 12 weeks it is the size of a grapefruit

8 WEEKS

HEGAR'S SIGN

This is the sensation experienced by the fingers, in bimanual examination, of almost meeting. It is due to the extreme softening of the lower segment.

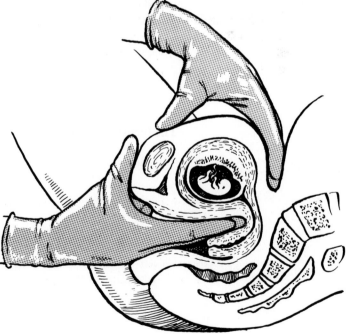

73

SYMPTOMS AND SIGNS

6–8 WEEKS

The earliest symptoms and signs — increased
vascularity and sensation of heaviness, almost
of pain — appear at 6 weeks. By 8 weeks the
nipple and surrounding area — the **Primary
areola** — have become more pigmented.

Montgomery's tubercles — sebaceous glands
which become prominent as raised pink-red
nodules on the areola.

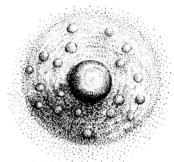

The breast at 8 weeks

16 WEEKS

By 16 weeks a clear fluid (colostrum) is secreted
and may be expressed. By 20 weeks the
secondary areola — a mottled effect due to
further pigmentation — has become
prominent.

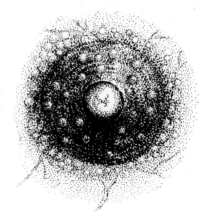

The breast at 16 weeks.

SYMPTOMS AND SIGNS

14 WEEKS   INTERNAL BALLOTTEMENT

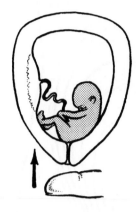 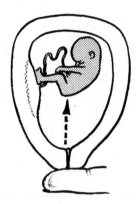 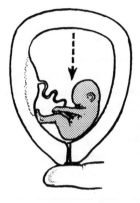

Tap gently upwards and
hold finger against cervix

The fetus is displaced
upwards

The fetus sinks and
a gentle tap is felt on
the finger.

24 WEEKS   EXTERNAL BALLOTTEMENT

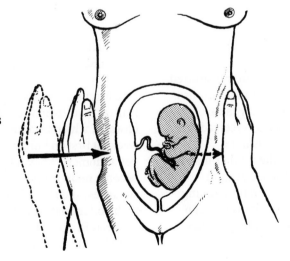

One hand taps the
abdomen and sends
the fetus across
the uterine
cavity.

The other hand lying
on the uterus per-
ceives the impulse.

These tests have almost disappeared from clinical practice with the widespread use of
ultrasound.

SYMPTOMS AND SIGNS

15 WEEKS

ABDOMINAL ENLARGEMENT

The uterus becomes abdominal by 12 weeks and increase in abdominal size is apparent by 15 weeks.

The reduction in fundal height which occurs between 38 and 40 weeks is called 'lightening', and is due to the descent of the fetus as the lower segment and cervix prepare for labour. It may not occur in women who have had a previous pregnancy; and the fundal height is an uncertain guide to maturity.

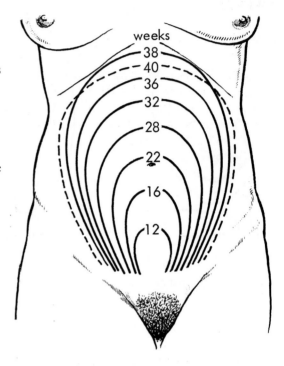

16–18 WEEKS

QUICKENING ('FEELING LIFE')

The sensation of fetal movement transmitted as far as the parietal peritoneum which has somatic innervation. It is a very faint sensation to begin with and is perceived more readily by the multipara. It is not a completely reliable sign; the mother may be unwilling to admit its absence even to herself; and hysterical women undergoing imaginary pregnancy ('pseudocyesis') can easily convince themselves of its presence.

20 WEEKS

PALPABLE UTERINE CONTRACTIONS (Braxton Hicks' sign)

The uterus undergoes irregular painless contractions from the 9th to 10th week onward, which become palpable by the 20th week, at first on bimanual examination, later per abdomen. They have no rhythm, but become more frequent as pregnancy advances, and in the last weeks may interfere with abdominal palpation. The distinction between Braxton Hicks' contractions and early labour is not always clear.

SYMPTOMS AND SIGNS

24 WEEKS

AUSCULTATION OF THE FETAL HEART

The fetal heart is heard with a fetal stethoscope (Pinard) pressed on the abdomen over the back of the fetus. Sounds are most clearly heard over the left fetal scapula so the point of maximum intensity will vary with the position of the fetus.

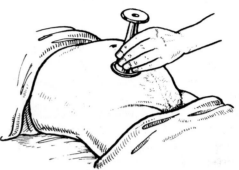

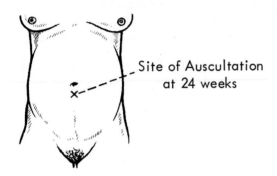

Site of Auscultation at 24 weeks

The rate varies between 120 and 140/minute and the rhythm should be regular.

Sounds to be distinguished from fetal heart:-
1. The maternal pulse, transmitted by aorta.
2. The uterine souffle, a blowing sound caused by the pulsation of blood through enlarged uterine arteries.

The Doppler flowmeter allows prolonged auscultation of the fetal heart from an early stage in pregnancy. (See Chapter 6)

20 WEEKS

PALPABLE FETAL MOVEMENTS

This sensation is felt at first as a faint flutter. Movements are stronger in the later months, and may be perceived as a definite impulse on the examiner's ear when the fetal stethoscope is being used.

26 WEEKS

PALPABLE FETAL PARTS

The outlines of the fetus, the head and limbs, begin to be palpable at this time. A fibromyoma is the only tumour that may falsely suggest fetal parts: but diagnosis of pregnancy cannot be made on this sign alone.

SKIN CHANGES

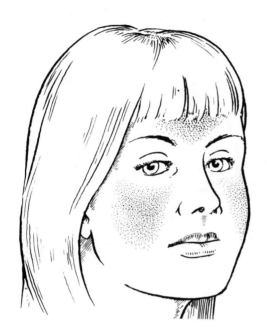

Areas already pigmented become more so (nipples, external genitalia and anal region). Some fresh pigmentation appears on the face (chloasma) and on the abdomen (linea nigra). These changes are thought to be due to deposition of melanin. Melanocyte stimulating hormone is elevated from early pregnancy.

('Chloasma' is from a Greek word meaning the greenish tint of a growing shoot or bud.)

Striae gravidarum are depressed streaks on the skin of the fat areas (abdomen, breasts and thighs). After delivery they regress and persist as striae albicantes. They are due to stretching, but may also be associated with increased secretion of ACTH affecting connective tissue.

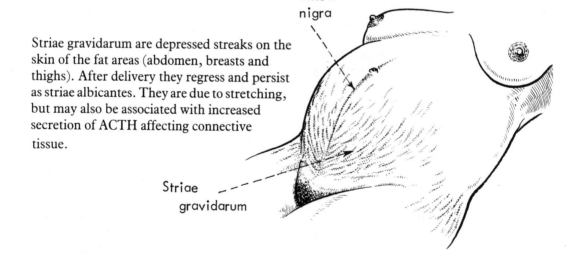

Linea nigra

Striae gravidarum

CHAPTER 5

ANTENATAL CARE

PRE-PREGNANCY COUNSELLING

Good antenatal care may begin before pregnancy. Even for an apparently normal, healthy couple planning a pregnancy, there may be advantages in discussing this with a professional adviser — specialist, general practitioner (GP), family-planning doctor, community midwife or health visitor. Such pre-pregnancy counselling would cover:

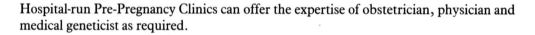

Medical and Family History.
General Health.
Diet.
Smoking.
Alcohol Intake.
Discontinuation of Hormonal Contraception.
Baseline Observations of Weight and Blood Pressure.
Rubella Immunity.

In some cases, specialist advice may be indicated:
Obstetric history — may indicate special management.
Familial or hereditary disorder — recurrence risks.
Known medical disorders e.g. diabetes, epilepsy —
    effect of pregnancy on disease and vice versa.
Regular medication e.g. anticonvulsants, steroids — risk of fetal damage.

Hospital-run Pre-Pregnancy Clinics can offer the expertise of obstetrician, physician and medical geneticist as required.

Planning for pregnancy should be emphasised in school health and health education programmes.

CARE IN PREGNANCY

PURPOSE

1. To maintain mother and baby in the best possible state of health by identifying problems, actual and potential, at an early stage and instituting appropriate management.
2. To educate the mother and her husband/partner about pregnancy and labour and dispel fears and ignorance.

RESPONSIBILITY

This usually begins with the patient's doctor and involves the specialist obstetrician, midwife, health visitor and physiotherapist. In this country supervision is usually shared between the specialist and the GP, together with their midwife colleagues. Arrangements vary according to local circumstances but good communication by means of a co-operation card is essential.

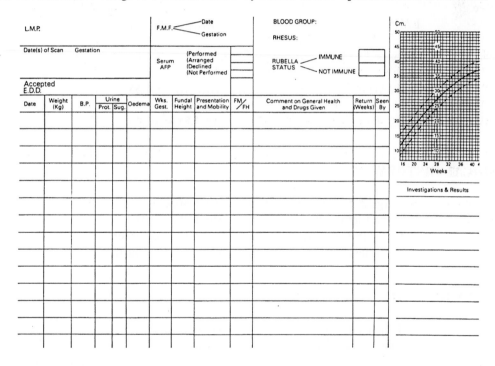

Domiciliary midwifery is at present a rarity in the UK. The choice will normally lie between a specialist unit and a GP unit associated, preferably directly, with a specialist unit. Women suitable for delivery under GP supervision are those without abnormality, having their second, third or fourth babies. Among specialist units the facilities will vary, especially in respect of paediatric care, and this must be taken into account in choosing the appropriate delivery place for high-risk patients.

THE FIRST VISIT

Ideally all pregnant women should be assessed early in pregnancy by a specialist and a plan made for their antenatal care and delivery.

The clinic atmosphere should be relaxed and welcoming. Facilities for accompanying husbands and children should be available.

A detailed history is required:

MENSTRUAL HISTORY

Date and certainty of last menstrual period (LMP).

Regularity of cycle.

Recent hormonal contraception.

Calculate expected date of delivery (EDD) as follows (280 days from first day of LMP): e.g.

LMP 9.7.87

Go back 3 months 9.4.87

Add a year 9.4.88

Add 7 days .... 16.4.88 = EDD

MEDICAL HISTORY

Surgical procedures.	Medication.
Anaesthetic difficulties.	Medical disorder.
Blood transfusion.	Psychiatric disorder.
Allergies.	Thrombo-embolism.

FAMILY HISTORY

Hypertension.	'Genetic' disorder.
Diabetes in 1° relative.	Twins.

SOCIAL HISTORY

Marital status.	Smoking.
Home and family situation.	Alcohol.

THE FIRST VISIT

OBSTETRIC HISTORY

Detailed enquiry is needed to identify any point which may influence management in the present pregnancy.

PREVIOUS OBSTETRIC HISTORY

Preg. No.	Date	Place	Gest.	Onset sp/ind	Dur. Hrs.	Mode of Delivery	Sex	Weight	LB/SB 1st week Death	Name and Unit No.
1	23/1/87	Maternity	40	S	10½	SVD	M	3·3k	LB	JOHN
	Complications: HBP at 38 weeks						Feeding: BREAST			
2	20/4/88	Maternity	8							
	Spontaneous abortion - D+C									
3										

The patient shown is described as para 1+1 (i.e. 1 delivery and 1 abortion). She might also be described as gravida 3 (i.e. pregnant for the 3rd time). Note, however, that this convention does not take account of the outcome of the delivery, e.g. a woman who has had a single pregnancy ending in a live birth or a still-birth or the delivery of twins is still a para 1+0.

CONTRACEPTIVE HISTORY

Details of contraceptive method used.
Was the pregnancy planned?
Length of time trying to conceive.

RISK FACTORS

Any factor from the above lists liable to increase maternal or fetal morbidity should be highlighted in the case sheet.

83

THE FIRST EXAMINATION

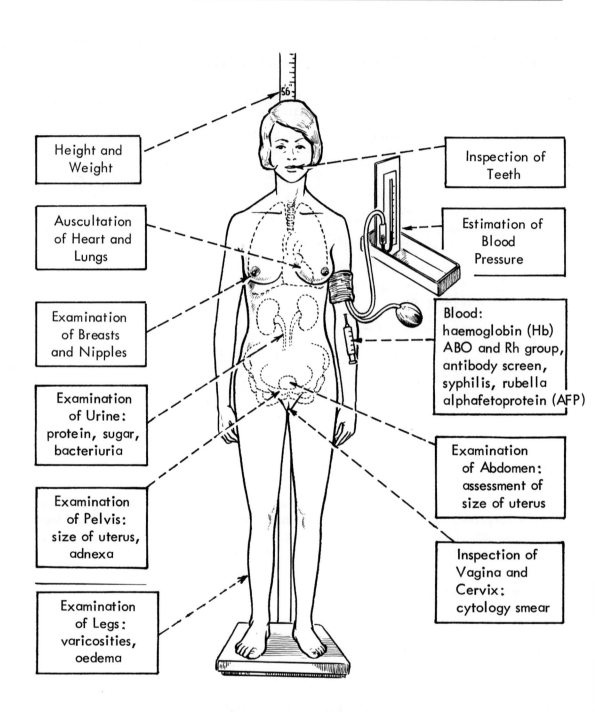

Height and
Weight

Auscultation
of Heart and
Lungs

Examination
of Breasts
and Nipples

Examination
of Urine:
protein, sugar,
bacteriuria

Examination
of Pelvis:
size of uterus,
adnexa

Examination
of Legs:
varicosities,
oedema

Inspection of
Teeth

Estimation of
Blood
Pressure

Blood:
haemoglobin (Hb)
ABO and Rh group,
antibody screen,
syphilis, rubella
alphafetoprotein (AFP)

Examination
of Abdomen:
assessment of
size of uterus

Inspection of
Vagina and
Cervix:
cytology smear

THE FIRST EXAMINATION

Wherever possible an ultrasound scan should be carried out in the first trimester. This may be at the first visit or subsequently, often at 16 weeks.

The advantages of a routine first trimester scan are:

Confirmation of continuing pregnancy.
Exclusion of twins.
Precise estimation of maturity (on which many obstetric assessments and decisions are based).
Recognition of major anomalies.

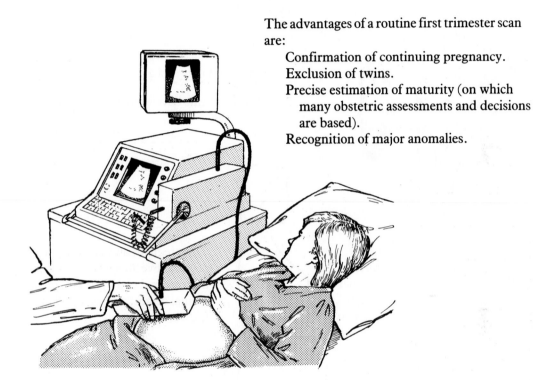

Real-time scanning

GENERAL HEALTH IN PREGNANCY

Some or all of the following topics will be discussed at the first visit or subsequently.

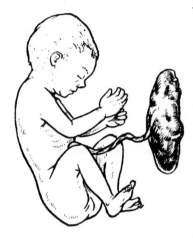

DIET

The body of a 3.4 kg (7½lb) baby at birth contains:-

400 g	Protein	25 g	Ca		The Placenta
220 g	Fat	16 g	P		contains
80 g	CHO	0.4 g	Fe		55 g Protein

Two-thirds of this development takes place in the last 3 months.

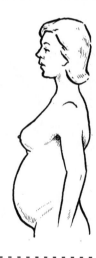

The mother also lays down new protein in the uterus and breasts (perhaps up to 500g) and at term her basal metabolism has increased by 20% or about 350 kcal/day. If she is breast-feeding, the baby will at one month require 7.0g Protein, 0.2g Ca and 300kcal daily.

The pregnant and lactating woman needs above all else a substantial increase in dietary protein, mostly of animal origin, and especially in the third trimester.

Estimated **Daily** requirements for Diet in Pregnancy:-

Protein	100 g	410 kcal
Fat	100 g	920 kcal
CHO	300 g	1230 kcal
		———
		2560 kcal

P 1.9 g
Ca 1.5 g
Fe 15 mg
Vit.A 6,000 I.U.
B complex 25 mg
Vit.C 100 mg
Vit.D 600 I.U.

Phosphorous requirements are always met when a good protein diet is taken.

The object should be to provide a good mixed diet palatable to the mother. Additional fat soluble vitamins (A, D), ascorbic acid, iron and folic acid may be indicated.

Cow's milk is the only naturally balanced food containing nearly 20g of first-class protein per pint, minerals, all the vitamins and fat.

GENERAL HEALTH IN PREGNANCY

EXERCISE

Mothers should be encouraged to see pregnancy as a healthy state and, within reason, normal activities, both domestic and recreational, should be encouraged.

CLEANLINESS

Good general hygiene should be encouraged. There is inevitably an increase in sweating and vaginal discharge during pregnancy.

COITUS

Coitus during pregnancy is normal in the human species and its frequency should depend on the mother's inclination. A previous history of abortion might be an indication for avoiding coitus during the first 3 months.

SMOKING

Women who are heavy smokers should be advised to cut down the number of cigarettes they smoke each day, or stop altogether if possible. Impairment of fetal growth, an increased risk of pre-term delivery and adverse effects on intellectual development have been described.

ALCOHOL

A fetal alcohol syndrome has been described (see Chapter 16), attributable to excess drinking. What constitutes a safe intake is uncertain at present and it seems sensible to advise mothers to be cautious, restricting themselves to occasional social drinking.

DRUGS

The mother should be advised to avoid any form of medication unless authorised by her doctor. See Chapter 7.

CLOTHING

Clothing should be loose and comfortable and attractive maternity wear is widely available today. Constricting garments and garters should be avoided.

BOWELS

Constipation is common in pregnancy and should not be a cause for concern. A diet high in fibre and fruit helps and mild laxatives may be taken if required.

TEETH

Teeth require the same care as in the non-pregnant state. A full dental check early in pregnancy should be recommended and the treatment in the United Kingdom is free to pregnant women. There is no objection to the use of local anaesthesia for dental treatment.

WORK

Most women may continue outside employment until the end of the second trimester. There should be ample opportunity for rest in the third trimester.

SUBSEQUENT ANTENATAL EXAMINATION

The traditional pattern, a monthly examination until 28 weeks, then fortnightly until 36 weeks and weekly thereafter, has much to commend it. These visits are shared between hospital and family doctor. Antenatal care remains a screening process for impaired fetal growth, malpresentation, anaemia, pre-eclampsia and other disorders. Special investigations are employed only when indicated by the routine examinations.

BLOOD PRESSURE

This should be measured at each visit and should be 120/80 or less and not above 145/90.

URINE

The urine should be tested at each visit for protein and sugar. When protein is detected, contamination and infection should be excluded before the observation is significant. Glycosuria is common but if persistent or recurrent a glucose tolerance test is indicated.

HAEMOGLOBIN

Dietary anaemia is now less common and prophylaxis with iron (100mg daily) and folic acid (300 micrograms daily) is commonly given. Haemoglobin levels should be estimated early in pregnancy and at about 30 and 36 weeks. Levels below 11g are indicative of anaemia.

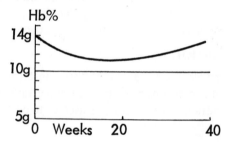

This is the normal Hb curve which reflects haemodilution. However, the amount of fluid retained during pregnancy is very variable.

RHESUS TESTING

Rhesus negative women are identified at the booking visit. A screening test for antibodies is also carried out. This should be repeated regularly throughout the pregnancy (see Chapter 8).

ABDOMINAL EXAMINATION

Regular abdominal palpation remains an important part of antenatal care.
1. It is the easiest and cheapest method of fetal monitoring.
2. Repeated examinations by the same obstetrician may give a first indication of retarded fetal growth or excessive increase in uterine size due to polyhydramnios or multiple pregnancy.
3. This requires the personal involvement of the obstetrician and continuity is clearly important. In this respect the organisation of many hospital clinics leaves much to be desired.

ABDOMINAL PALPATION

DEFINITIONS

The **Presentation** is that part of the fetus in the lower pole of the uterus overlying the pelvic brim, e.g. cephalic, vertex, breech etc.

The **Attitude** is the posture of the fetus.

Flexion   Deflexion   Extension

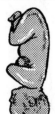
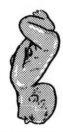

The **Lie** of the baby is the relation of the long axis of the fetus to the mother. Only a longitudinal lie is normal.

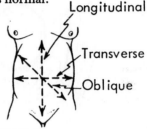

Longitudinal

Transverse

Oblique

The **Position** of the baby is the relationship of the presenting part to the mother's pelvis. It is conveniently expressed by referring to the position of one area of the presenting part known as the denominator.

The **Pelvis** is divided into eight parts for the purpose of description:

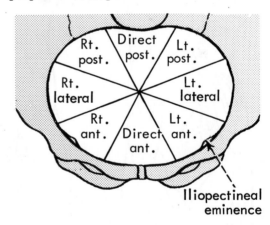

Iliopectineal eminence

The **Denominator** is an arbitrary part of the presentation;
   occiput in vertex presentation,
   sacrum in breech presentation,
   mentum in face presentation
and is used to denote the position of the presenting part with reference to the pelvis.

The denominator is in one of these segments and takes its position from it. Thus in a vertex presentation if the denominator, which is the occiput, is close to the left iliopectineal eminence, the position is described as Left Occipito-Anterior or LOA.

89

ABDOMINAL PALPATION

This examination must be made systematically.

Remember that the following tissue layers may interpose between your fingers and the fetal head.

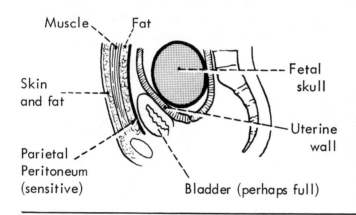

Muscle, Fat

Skin and fat

Parietal Peritoneum (sensitive)

Fetal skull

Uterine wall

Bladder (perhaps full)

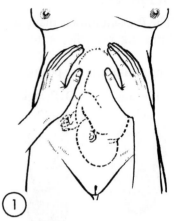

①

The fundus is palpated and its contents (here the breech) identified.

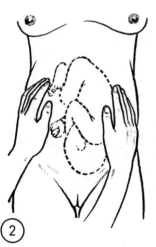

②

The hands palpate the contours of the uterus, identifying the back and the limbs.

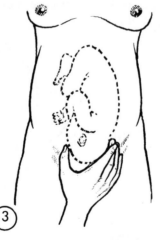

③

The head should be palpated, and it should be noted whether it is mobile or fixed in the pelvic brim.

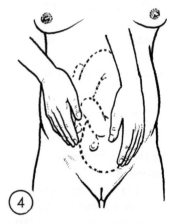

④

The examiner faces the patient's feet and gently pushes two fingers towards the pelvis. This is the best method of palpating the fetal head and determining whether it is fixed or mobile

ABDOMINAL PALPATION

The examiner must ask himself, and answer, **SIX** questions.

(1) Is the **FUNDAL HEIGHT** consistent with the estimation of maturity?

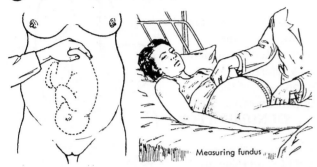

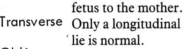

Measuring fundus

The height of the fundus in centimetres should equal approximately the weeks of gestation.

(2) Is the **LIE** Longitudinal? The Lie is the relation of the long axis of the fetus to the mother. Only a longitudinal lie is normal.

Transverse

Oblique

(3) Is the **CEPHALIC PRESENTATION** a **VERTEX**? This depends on the **ATTITUDE** of the fetus i.e. the relationship of its different parts to each other. The normal attitude is **FULL FLEXION**.

In full flexion, every fetal joint is flexed.

Sometimes the head may be extended.

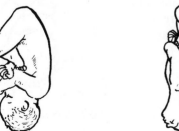

This gives a **VERTEX** presentation, the only normal presentation.

This gives a **FACE** presentation, which is highly abnormal.

(4) Is the **PRESENTATION** Breech?

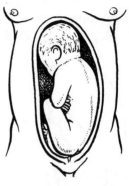

or Cephalic?

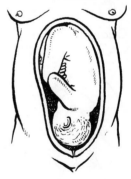

The presenting part is that part of the fetus which occupies the lower pole of the uterus. Only a cephalic presentation is normal after 32 weeks. At 30 weeks, however, up to 25% of babies present by the breech.

91

ABDOMINAL PALPATION

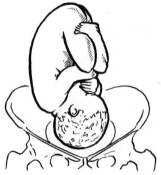

R. Occipito-Lateral
(R.O.L.)   25%

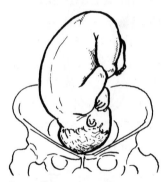

R. Occipito-Anterior
(R.O.A.)   10%

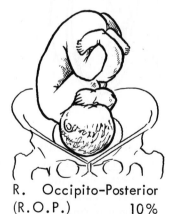

R. Occipito-Posterior
(R.O.P.)   10%

⑤ What is the **POSITION** of **VERTEX**?

The position is the relationship of the presenting part to the mother's pelvis. It is conveniently expressed by referring to the position of one area of the presenting part known as the **DENOMINATOR**.

The denominator of the vertex is the **OCCIPUT**; and there are eight recognised positions. (Direct anterior or posterior positions, not shown here, rarely occur).

The percentages given here refer to the position at the pelvic brim, and transverse and anterior are regarded as normal.

Position is important in obstetrics because if the fetus takes up a posterior position in the pelvis (i.e. if the occiput rotates towards the sacrum and the fetus faces forwards) the labour is likely to be long and difficult. There may be some analogy with the experience of trying to put a right foot into a left shoe.

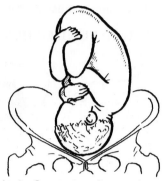

Left Occipito-Lateral
40%   (L.O.L.)

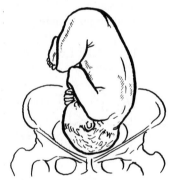

Left Occipito-Anterior
12%   (L.O.A.)

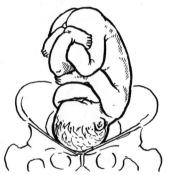

Left Occipito-Posterior
3%   (L.O.P.)

ABDOMINAL PALPATION

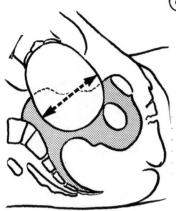

(6) Is the **VERTEX ENGAGED?**

Engagement means the descent of the biparietal diameter through pelvic brim. If the vertex is at the level of the ischial spines, the head must be engaged unless there is caput formation. Engagement can only be diagnosed with certainty by vaginal examination.

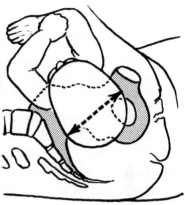

The head is 'fixed'
(3/5 palpable)

The head is 'engaged'
(2/5 palpable)

A convenient way to describe the amount of head above the brim is to identify the number of 'fifths' palpable. When the head is engaged not more than 2/5 will be felt abdominally.

Although it is discussed as a pre-labour phenomenon, engagement seldom occurs until after labour is established, and the term as now used really means that the presenting part is 'fixed' — entering the pelvis — as opposed to 'mobile' or still above the brim.

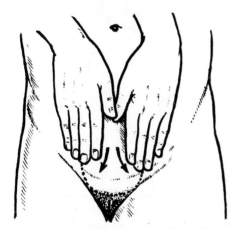

This presenting part is 'fixed'

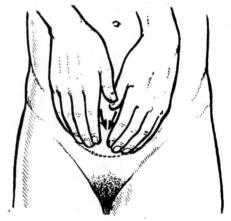

This presenting part is 'mobile'

93

VAGINAL EXAMINATION IN PREGNANCY

Bimanual examination is no longer a routine part of antenatal examination but is still sometimes required:

1. To assess maturity in early pregnancy.

2. To exclude suspected abnormalities such as incarcerated retroversion of the uterus or ovarian tumour.

3. To identify a presenting part which cannot be confidently identified abdominally.

4. To exclude or confirm gross degrees of contraction (in very small patients).

5. To assess the ripeness of the cervix near term.

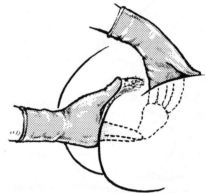

A bimanual examination in early pregnancy. Two fingers are shown in the vagina, but often one finger will give as much inform-ation as the patient will be more relaxed.

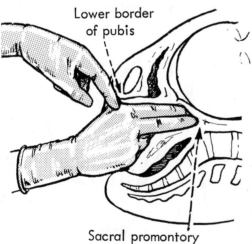

Lower border of pubis

Sacral promontory

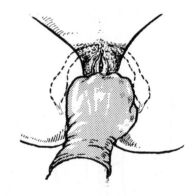

6. To assess pelvic capacity. The dia-gonal conjugate may be measured if the sacral promontory can be reached, in which case the pelvis is smaller than normal. The intertuberous diameter should be as wide as the normal fist. Prominence of the ischial spines and the width of the subpubic arch can be assessed. There is no doubt that some idea of pelvic shape and size can be obtained after much practice by this palpation, but there is a wide margin of error.

COMMON COMPLAINTS

SUBJECTIVE COMPLAINTS

Fatigue, somnolence, headache, 'blackouts', are often noticed in the early months and their cause is uncertain. Hypotension, secondary to peripheral vasodilatation, may be responsible for feelings of faintness

MORNING SICKNESS

Nausea and vomiting are due probably to the effect of large amounts of circulating steroids, especially oestrogens, and they seldom last beyond the sixteenth week. They can occur at any time of the day and are aggravated by cooking and fatigue. Mild cases are treated by light carbohydrate diet (biscuits and milk) in the morning and sometimes by anti-emetics. If the condition worsens it becomes hyperemesis gravidarum and is best treated in hospital (see Chapter 8).

CONSTIPATION

This is due in part to the effect of progesterone on smooth muscle, and in part due to obstruction by the large gravid uterus. A bowel motion every second or third day is perfectly consistent with good health, but sometimes laxatives are required. Any of the commonly used drugs may be taken with safety.

HEARTBURN

The enlarging uterus encourages some degree of hiatus hernia as pregnancy advances, and the symptom is due to oesophageal reflux of gastric acid. Sleeping in a semi-recumbent position is helpful, and antacids or compound preparations with alginates can be safely prescribed.

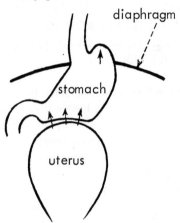

PRESSURE IN THE PELVIS

This gradually obstructs venous return and may lead to haemorrhoids, and varicose veins of the legs, vulva and abdominal wall. The legs can be clothed in special elastic stockings, and haemorrhoids are helped by suppositories.   Only in rare cases is haemorrhoidectomy required. Nothing can be done for varicosities of the vulva, beyond advising the patient to rest.

PELVIC JOINT PAINS

PELVIC ARTHROPATHY

The ligaments of the pelvic joints are softened and relaxed during pregnancy by the steroid induced oedema and the increased vascularity which occur in all the soft tissues. The pelvis becomes less rigid which may be of some advantage in labour; but movements can now take place in joints which are normally immovable; and various symptoms may arise.

BACKACHE, SACROILIAC STRAIN, LEG CRAMPS, SCIATIC OR FEMORAL NERVE PAIN

As well as the slackening of the ligaments, these complaints probably have a connection with postural changes — the 'Pride of Pregnancy' whereby the alteration in centre of gravity — — — — — — → 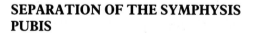 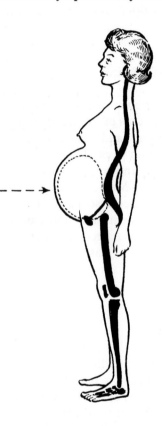 causes a characteristic lordosis. Muscle spasm develops along with pressure on nerve roots (leading to cramping pains and neuralgia) but there is no clearcut neurological condition. Treatment is directed towards resting the muscles and preventing undue flexion of the spinal joints, by getting the patient to sleep with boards under her mattress.

SEPARATION OF THE SYMPHYSIS PUBIS

Separation of up to 1cm is accepted as normal, but if there is symphyseal pain and the separation is beyond 1cm, a diagnosis of subluxation of the symphysis is made. There is usually sacro-iliac pain as well, and this condition can be crippling. The only treatment is complete rest in bed, and if the tenderness is not relieved as term approaches, epidural anaesthesia is required for the labour.

COCCYDYNIA

This condition is more likely to be met with in the puerperium as a result of pressure or even fracture during delivery. It rarely develops in the antenatal period, and the best treatment is rest, often with a rubber ring to avoid painful pressure points. If the pain persists, a peri-articular injection of a corticosteroid will give some relief.

NEUROPATHY IN PREGNANCY

CARPAL TUNNEL SYNDROME

The median nerve is compressed in the carpal tunnel under the flexor retinaculum. Pregnant women often complain of tingling pain in the fingers, but median nerve neuropathy is uncommon. The patient complains of pain and numbness in one or both hands, referred along the fingers supplied by the median nerve. It is worst on waking when the fingers feel lifeless. There is reduced pinprick sensation in the affected area, but little else is found on examination. The usual treatment starts with a course of diuretic drugs and goes on to the immobilisation of the wrist by bandages or splinting. If the pain continues to be severe the flexor retinaculum has to be divided.

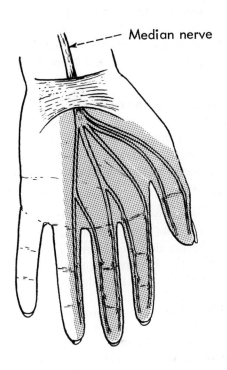

Median nerve

BELL'S PALSY

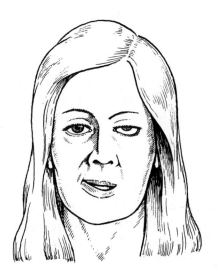

Paralysis of the facial muscles due to compression of the VIIth nerve within the temporal bone. The cause is not known, but a relationship with pregnancy is recognised. Onset is sudden, usually in the third trimester, and there is no pain. The patient finds she cannot frown or raise her eyebrow or whistle, and food tends to lodge in the buccal pouch. Taste buds may be inhibited, but the tongue is painful if bitten. Prednisone 50 mg per day for ten days is said to encourage the return of normal function, but this would be undesirable in pregnancy, and no treatment should be attempted. Recovery takes about three weeks.

VAGINAL DISCHARGE

The increased vascularity of pregnancy induces a fairly copious vaginal discharge, and the moisture and warmth of the vulvo-perineum encourages the growth of organisms. The patient may complain of an offensive smell, but there should be no pruritus, and frequent washing and drying of the vulva should be an adequate treatment.

VAGINAL CANDIDIASIS

The most troublesome complication is infection with Candida albicans which is encouraged by the conditions prevailing in pregnancy.

1. The fungus thrives in the 'tropical micro-climate' of vulva and vagina.
2. Immune defences against C. albicans appear to require adequate iron and folic acid stores which are depleted in pregnancy.
3. The high level of circulating oestrogen supports an increased vaginal glycogen level which is favourable to the fungus.
4. The increase in the level of steroid hormones generally, probably has an immunosuppressive effect.
   (It is not possible to be dogmatic about C.albicans. There is no firm immunological evidence of decreased resistance, and the fungus may be present without symptoms, or apparently absent in the presence of severe irritation.)

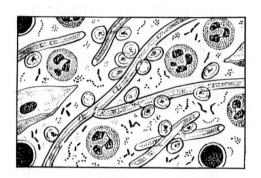

Mycelia and spores of C.albicans.

The complaints are of discharge and constant irritation. A swab should be taken, and the characteristic plaques of yeast may be seen.

Treatment
In acute cases, immediate relief may be achieved by the instillation of 1% gentian violet. Thereafter, nystatin or clotrimazole pessaries are used night and morning for two weeks. Candidiasis may not be eradicated during pregnancy, but treatment is required to relieve the patient and to reduce the chance of infecting the fetus during its passage down the vagina.

TRICHOMONAS VAGINALIS

If this organism is demonstrated in the discharge, treatment should be given. There have been suggestions of embryonic damage by metronidazole (Flagyl), but this has not been confirmed. Miconazole cream or clotrimazole applied locally are claimed to be effective against both C.albicans and T.vaginalis. They are to be preferred in early pregnancy.

X-RAYS IN PREGNANCY

X-rays may be used for the measurement of the actual pelvic diameters and the demonstration of skeletal abnormalities in the fetus. This form of investigation is declining in importance.

1. The risk to the fetus of ionising radiations is now well understood by doctors and patients.
2. Even in the best hands, X-ray pelvimetry was never so accurate in its predictions as to relieve the obstetrician of the need to carry out a trial of labour, unless in the most extreme cases of contraction, which could be identified clinically.
3. Contracted pelvis and skeletal abnormalities are much less common than 50 years ago when X-ray pelvimetry was introduced; and the significance of anomalies such as a straight sacrum, or fused vertebrae or an 'android' pelvis is being questioned. Any woman who achieves a vaginal delivery may be said to have a normal pelvis whatever its shape.

Probably the most useful function of X-ray pelvimetry in modern obstetrics is to provide a postpartum visual record of abnormality.

The **ERECT LATERAL VIEW** allows measurement of the sagittal diameters of the brim, and inspection of the sacrum and lower vertebrae.

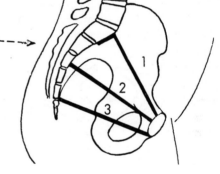

The **ANTEROPOSTERIOR VIEW** allows measurement of the transverse diameter of the brim, and the interspinous diameter. It gives some idea of the pelvic shape.

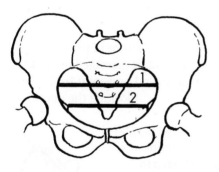

The **OUTLET VIEW** shows the shape of the subpubic arch. Various mensuration techniques were used to predict whether or not the head would emerge safely under the arch, but none were reliable.

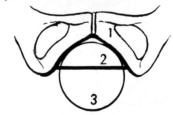

Ultrasound has largely replaced X-ray in the investigation of the fetus but X-rays may still occasionally be used in suspected fetal abnormality or multiple pregnancy in the third trimester.

PARENTCRAFT AND PHYSIOTHERAPY

Most hospitals run classes on these subjects, covering all aspects of pregnancy, labour, delivery and baby care. Apart from their educational role they help to familiarise the mother with the hospital and, hopefully, instil confidence in her attendants. Midwives, physiotherapists, obstetricians, anaesthetists and paediatricians may take part in the classes. The attendance of husbands at appropriate sessions should be encouraged.

Two important physical topics to be covered are **Care of the breasts**, and **Exercise** and **Relaxation**.

CARE OF THE BREASTS

On the assumption that the woman is going to breast-feed, the nipple and areola should be kept clean with soap and water to avoid the formation of crusts of colostrum. Such crusts, if present, may be removed with a little ether.

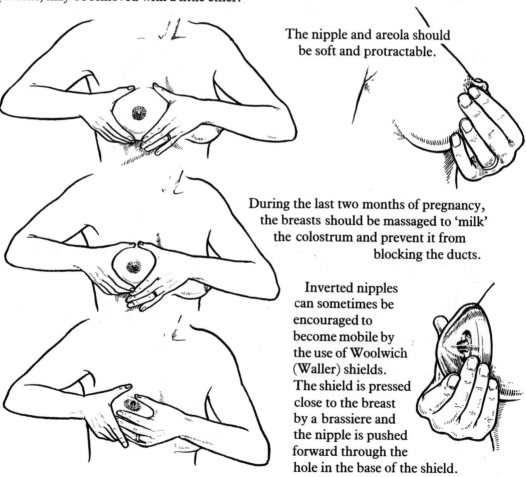

The nipple and areola should be soft and protractable.

During the last two months of pregnancy, the breasts should be massaged to 'milk' the colostrum and prevent it from blocking the ducts.

Inverted nipples can sometimes be encouraged to become mobile by the use of Woolwich (Waller) shields. The shield is pressed close to the breast by a brassiere and the nipple is pushed forward through the hole in the base of the shield.

PARENTCRAFT AND PHYSIOTHERAPY

EXERCISE AND RELAXATION

The fear of labour is universal, and it has long been an article of faith among obstetricians that a frightened woman will have a longer and more difficult labour than one who has confidence in her attendants. Systems of instruction for establishing this confidence come and go in their fashion, but there is general agreement that the patient should be enlightened by lectures on the physiology of pregnancy and labour, and that she should be instructed in achieving muscular relaxation by the principles of physiotherapy.

EXERCISES

Simple exercises should be done every day.

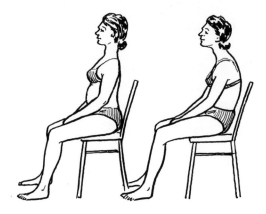

The back is alternately straightened and curved .

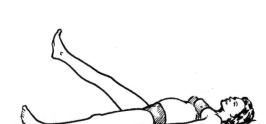

Alternate leg raising improves the tone of the abdominal muscles.

RELAXATION

A position of relaxation is assumed and by deep regular breathing, and conscious relaxation of different groups of muscles, the patient learns with practice to reach a state almost of somnolence, at will. She will make use of this between contractions when in labour.

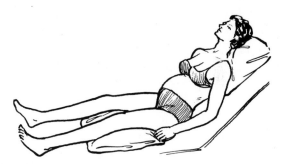

Relaxing with head and shoulders supported .

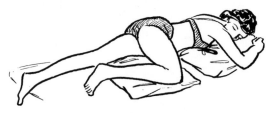

Relaxing in the semi-prone position .

ANTENATAL CARE — SUMMARY

Improvement in the social conditions of the childbearing population is more effective in reducing the mortality and morbidity of pregnancy than any amount of antenatal care. The obstetrician is still obliged, however, to provide close supervision for every pregnant woman by the traditional screening method, employing special tests where indicated. These are discussed in Chapter 6. The system described below may be regarded as offering a minimum standard.

1. Early assessment of the mother and identification of risk factors.
2. Confirmation of maturity by ultrasound.
3. Regular visits shared between the specialist and general practitioner. Defaulting patients should be visited by a health visitor or community midwife.
4. Examinations to detect impaired fetal growth, pregnancy-induced hypertension, anaemia, malpresentation and disproportion.
5. An active educational programme and instruction in relaxation.

CHAPTER 6

ANTE-PARTUM ASSESSMENT OF THE FETUS

This chapter deals with the special tests and techniques available to the clinician to help assess the fetus in the antenatal period. The techniques will be described under four headings:

1. Maturity.   2. Growth   3. Well-being.   4. Abnormality.

In each of these **Ultrasound** plays a vital role. Since the introduction of ultrasound into obstetrics by Donald in Glasgow in the early 1960s, enormous technical advances have taken place. The early static scanners have been replaced by real-time scanning (page 85) which gives a moving picture of the fetus. Modern scanners are small, easily moved about and have greatly improved resolution. Skill in their use is more easily acquired and the quality of the images permits detailed examination of the fetus and placenta.

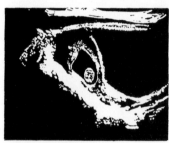
Longitudinal section of early pregnancy.

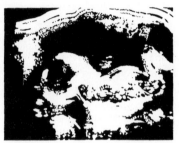
Fetus at 24 weeks.

The following is a summary of the place of ultrasound in modern obstetric practice:

Routine Use: — Confirmation of ongoing intra-uterine pregnancy.
                      Assessment of gestational age (measurement of crown-rump length, biparietal diameter, femur length).
                      Identification of multiple pregnancy.
                      Recognition of major anomalies.

Specific Uses: — Threatened abortion (to confirm fetus alive).
                      Antepartum haemorrhage (placental localisation).
                      Fetal growth studies (head-trunk ratio, estimated fetal weight, liquor volume, placental grade).
                      Assessment of high risk cases (maternal disease, elevated serum alphafetoprotein, history of anomaly).
                      Postpartum (retained products).
                      Pelvic masses.

Adjunct to   — Chorion villus sampling .
Interventional   Amniocentesis.
Procedures: Fetal blood sampling.
                      Intra-uterine therapy e.g. intra-uterine transfusion.

New   — Doppler — blood flow studies.
Developments: Fetal breathing.

FETAL MATURITY

Maturity is traditionally calculated from the date of the LMP and confirmed by a bimanual or abdominal examination (see Chapter 5).

These methods may not be reliable:

1. LMP uncertain or forgotten.   2. Calculation depends on 'normal' 28-day cycle.
3. Widespread use of hormonal contraception — makes ovulation unpredictable.
4. Uterine size difficult to assess — obesity, full bladder, tense or nervous patient.

A. ULTRASOUND

An early ultrasound scan is the best method of determining maturity by measuring the crown-rump length (CRL) or bi-parietal diameter (BPD), depending on gestation. Ideally this should be done routinely, but it is indicated where the LMP is uncertain òr there is a discrepancy between size and dates. Accurate determination of maturity is essential for the assessment of subsequent fetal growth.

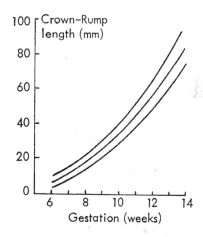

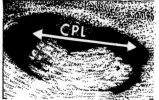

Crown-rump length is the measured length of the fetus excluding the limbs.

Measurement of the bi-parietal diameter gives a reliable indication of maturity in the second and early third trimester. After 28 weeks the variations in skull size and rate of growth considerably lessen the value of BPD measurement.

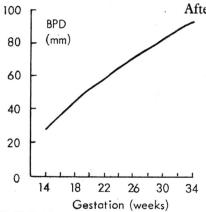

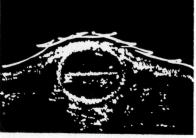

A transverse scan of the abdomen with the fetal head in occipito-transverse.   Note the midline echo, probably the medial sides of the hemispheres.

B. X-RAYS

These may be used in the estimation of maturity when the patient is seen for the first time in the third trimester. Maturity is assessed by identification of centres of ossification:
36 weeks — lower end of femur,   38 weeks — upper end of tibia,   40 weeks — cuboid, *but* the appearance of the ossification centres may be delayed when the fetus is growth-retarded. This may be suspected by a fetal attitude of hyperflexion, due to lack of liquor.

FETAL MATURITY

C. LIQUOR EXAMINATION

Liquor, obtained by amniocentesis, may be examined to assess the functional maturity of fetal lungs, kidneys and skin.

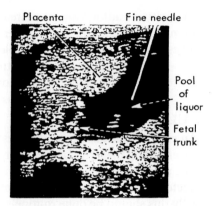

Amniocentesis means the removal of a specimen of liquor by fine needle aspiration under ultrasound guidance. By this means a pool of liquor can be demonstrated and the placental site avoided.

Amniocentesis carries a small risk (approximately 0.5%) of provoking abortion.

1. Lung Maturity: The fetal lung alveoli contribute a fatty secretion to the liquor consisting mainly of lecithin and sphingomyelin, and appearing in gradually increasing quantities. The function of this secretion (called the surfactant) is to lower the surface tension of the alveoli

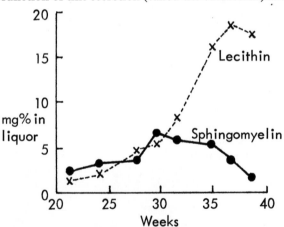

during expiration and prevent their collapse. Failure of this mechanism results in the respiratory distress syndrome (RDS). Before 34 weeks the lecithin/sphingomyelin ratio (LSR) is about 1:1, but thereafter the ratio rises sharply with the rise in the concentration of lecithin. An LSR of 2:1 or more is unlikely to be associated with respiratory distress.

Another phospholipid, phosphatidyl glycerol, has recently been shown to be a sensitive indicator of lung maturity. Its presence in the liquor, even when obtained vaginally, is indicative of mature lungs.

The importance of these tests is diminishing as the paediatric care of premature babies improves.

2. Skin and Kidney Maturity: Assessment of skin maturity by the Nile blue test on cells obtained from the liquor and of renal function, by measuring the concentration of creatinine, have already been noted (Chapter 1). Desquamated skin cells stain orange with Nile blue sulphate. About 10% of cells from the liquor stain orange at 38 weeks while at term the figure has reached 50%. Liquor creatinine levels of 2mg/dl are regarded as indicative of a mature fetus. These tests have little place in practice now.

FETAL GROWTH

The progress of fetal growth is observed by serial abdominal palpation and measurement of the symphysis/fundal height (see Chapter 5). This is one of the traditional 'arts' of the obstetrician, but it is important to acknowledge its limitations. Obesity, abdominal tenseness, the amount of liquor, the lie of the baby and the level of the presenting part can affect observation.

The graph shows the progress of fetal growth. Babies whose weights are below the 10° centile are regarded as 'growth-retarded'. As many as 50% of these babies may be undetected by clinical examination. As the end result of this process may be fetal death, it is essential that the detection of the condition is improved.

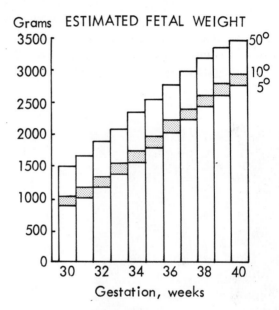

Growth retardation may be associated with some maternal complications in pregnancy or abnormality in the fetus, but many cases are unexplained. At present it is impossible to study all pregnancies in detail but special tests of fetal growth are indicated in the following groups:

> Clinically suspected poor growth.
> Hypertension.
> Ante-partum haemorrhage.
> Diabetes.
> Multiple pregnancy.
> Previous growth-retarded baby.
> Previous perinatal death.

FETAL GROWTH

A. ULTRASOUND

Ultrasound is now the main method of assessing fetal growth. To serial measurements of the biparietal diameter (BPD) have been added measurements of trunk area at liver level, and crown-rump length. Various combinations of these, notably head/trunk ratio and the product of trunk area and crown-rump length, have been used to identify growth-retarded babies.

In late pregnancy the diameters of the fetal abdomen should exceed those of the head because of accumulation of glycogen in the liver. This does not occur in the growth-retarded, starved fetus and the ratio of head to abdominal circumference may be increased.

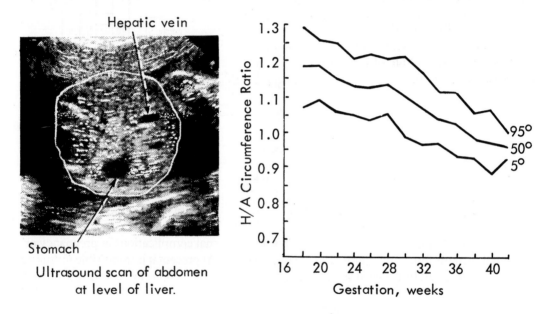

Ultrasound scan of abdomen
at level of liver.

Fetal weight may also be estimated using various formulae. As in clinical estimates, weights at both extremes are least reliable.

FETAL GROWTH

B. BIOCHEMICAL TESTS

Serial estimations of OESTRIOL levels in the mother's urine have been used for years as an indirect test of fetal growth. Levels rise steadily in normal pregnancy and higher levels are found with large babies (and multiple pregnancies) than with small babies.

The placenta is an incomplete endocrine organ, manufacturing oestrogens only when supplied with precursors from maternal and fetal circulations.

Falling oestriol excretion levels imply a failure in both placenta and fetus, the feto-placental unit.

Maternal	Placental	Fetal
Cholesterol →	Pregnenolone →	adrenal enzymes
	↓	↓
	Progesterone	DHA
		↓
	Oestriol ◄———	liver enzymes

The aromatic ring characteristic of oestrogens is substituted in the precursor by *placental* enzymes.

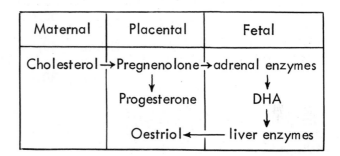

This 16α-hydroxyl group is attached to the precursor by *fetal* enzymes which do not appear in the placenta.

There is wide diurnal variation in the excretion of oestriol and the measurements are therefore carried out on a 24 hour collection of urine, or on a single specimen when the oestriol level is related to that of creatinine, giving an oestriol/creatinine ratio.

FETAL GROWTH

B. BIOCHEMICAL TESTS (continued)

Oestriol levels or oestriol/creatinine ratios may be plotted as shown. Serial estimations may show a clear trend, with a failure to rise indicating a fetus at risk.

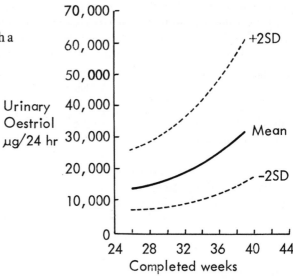

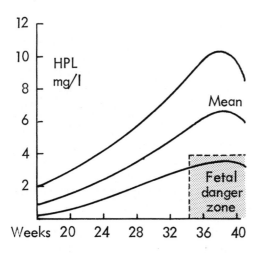

Serial estimations of HUMAN PLACENTAL LACTOGEN (HPL) have been used similarly. HPL is secreted by the syncytiotrophoblast and levels correlate well with placental weight. Estimations are done on blood specimens.

Increasingly these tests are being replaced by biophysical techniques and, in centres with good ultrasound facilities, have disappeared altogether.

FETAL WELL-BEING

The fetus may die in utero from a sudden event such as abruption of the placenta or cord prolapse. These cannot be predicted, but fetal death may come at the end of a process of growth retardation or placental impairment due to hypertension, prolonged pregnancy or other cause. In such circumstances the obstetrician asks and seeks to answer the question "Is the baby at risk of dying?". The tests available are complementary to those used in assessing fetal growth and will often be used in combination with them. They are indicated:

1. Where fetal growth is already under surveillance (see above).
2. Prolonged pregnancy — more than 10 days past the EDD or earlier in older mothers.
3. In any mother who complains of a reduction in fetal movements.

A. FETAL MOVEMENT COUNT

The normal range of fetal activity falls from about 90 movements in 12 hours at 32 weeks to about 50 movements at term. A diminution in this perceptible fetal activity suggests hypoxia.

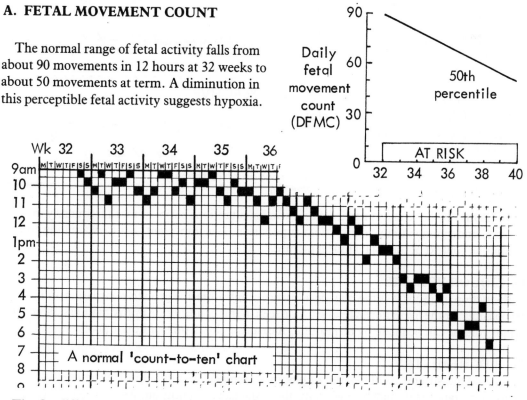

A normal 'count-to-ten' chart

The Cardiff 'count-to-ten' chart is an excellent way of recording the time to feel 10 fetal movements. If the mother has not felt 10 movements within 12 hours, she is asked to record the number of movements felt and contact the hospital. Further investigation by cardiotocography is indicated. This is a simple and physiologically sound method of monitoring, and a normal movement pattern carries a good prognosis. However, its subjective nature lessens its reliability. A certain degree of intelligence is needed and the mother must decide for herself what is or is not a movement. She is far from being an unbiased observer, and some patients will exhibit symptoms of anxiety.

111

FETAL WELL-BEING

B. CARDIOTOCOGRAPHY (CTG)

This is now widely used as a test of fetal well-being and has the great advantage of giving immediate information about the baby's condition.

The fetal heart is recorded continuously by an ultrasound transducer on the mother's abdomen over a period of 20–30 minutes. A tocograph is also applied to record any uterine contractions and the mother is asked to note fetal movements. A normal trace shows base-line variability and accelerations in response to fetal movements or uterine contractions (4 in 20 minutes).

A fetal sleep pattern may also be observed in which there is an absence of movements and accelerations.

Non-reactive traces or the presence of decelerations suggest hypoxia and require further assessment.

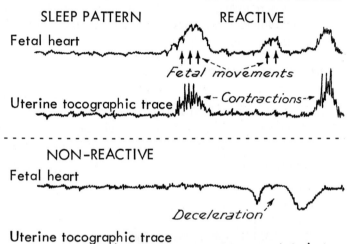

CTGs may be done once or twice weekly on an outpatient basis, or more frequently in patients undergoing intensive in-patient supervision. It is important that they are interpreted within the context of the total clinical picture.

C. LIQUOR VOLUME

Reduction in liquor volume may be a feature of intra-uterine growth retardation and is responsible for the hyperflexed fetal attitude seen in this condition. Approximate assessment of liquor volume can be made by ultrasound, measuring the depths of liquor pools.

D. BIOCHEMISTRY

Isolated measurements of oestriol or placental lactogen are not helpful. When serially measured, static levels may be a warning about the baby's condition. As these tests give less immediate information than cardiotocography however, they are being superseded by this technique.

E. OTHER TECHNIQUES

Ultrasound has also been used to study fetal breathing movements and the progressive maturation of placental architecture. Doppler ultrasound is being used to study blood flow in fetal vessels. None of these procedures is at present established as an indicator of fetal well-being.

FETAL ABNORMALITY

It is now possible to detect a wide range of abnormalities in the fetus in the antenatal period. Some of these are severe enough and detectable at a sufficiently early gestation to allow termination of the pregnancy where the mother so wishes. In other cases termination is not indicated but knowledge of the presence of the defect may allow preparations for its treatment to be made in advance or even allow intra-uterine therapy. The term 'prenatal diagnosis' has become established usage to describe these techniques.

A. MATERNAL SERUM ALPHA-FETOPROTEIN ESTIMATION (MSAFP)

This test is widely used to screen for open neural tube defects. AFP is a major serum protein in the fetus, at its maximum at 13 weeks. There are small quantities in the liquor, and even smaller quantities are detected in the maternal serum.

MSAFP is elevated in:
   Anencephaly,
   Open spina bifida,
   Exomphalos,
   Gastroschisis,
   Placental abnormalities
but also in:
   Threatened abortion,
   Fetal death in utero,
   Multiple pregnancy.

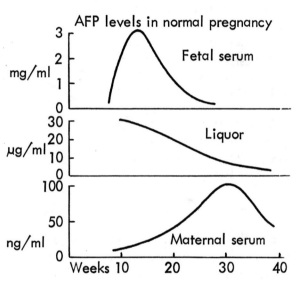

AFP levels in normal pregnancy

The assay must be done between 16 and 20 weeks when the distinction between normal and abnormal levels can be made most reliably. Accurate knowledge of fetal maturity is essential.

FETAL ABNORMALITY

A. MATERNAL SERUM ALPHA-FETOPROTEIN ESTIMATION (continued)

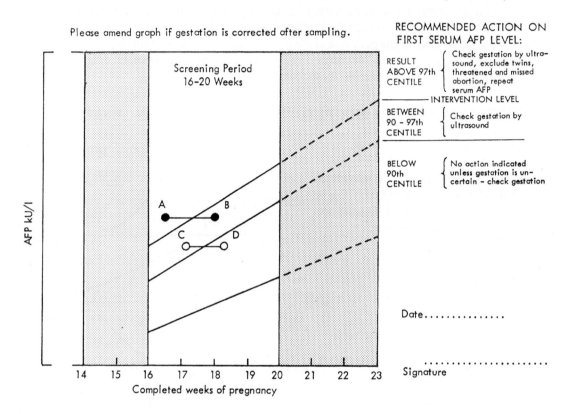

Please amend graph if gestation is corrected after sampling.

Screening Period
16–20 Weeks

AFP kU/l

Completed weeks of pregnancy

RECOMMENDED ACTION ON
FIRST SERUM AFP LEVEL:

RESULT ABOVE 97th CENTILE — Check gestation by ultra-sound, exclude twins, threatened and missed abortion, repeat serum AFP

INTERVENTION LEVEL

BETWEEN 90 – 97th CENTILE — Check gestation by ultrasound

BELOW 90th CENTILE — No action indicated unless gestation is un-certain – check gestation

Date..............

....
Signature

The prediction graph used in the West of Scotland is illustrated. A raised MSAFP is followed by a repeat test and either a detailed ultrasound scan to try and identify the lesion or amniocentesis to measure the liquor AFP. All anencephalics and approximately 85% of open neural tube defects should be detected in this way.

B. ULTRASOUND

Routine ultrasound scanning for fetal abnormalities between 16 and 20 weeks is employed in some centres, especially where routine MSAFP testing is not done. Neural tube and abdominal wall defects should be detected in this way. Detailed scanning can be carried out in special centres to identify a wide range of morphological abnormalities. This may be indicated by a screening technique such as MSAFP, a clinical abnormality such as an excess or deficiency of liquor, or the patient's history. Heart, intestinal, renal and skeletal abnormalities may be detected in this way.

FETAL ABNORMALITY

C. AMNIOCENTESIS

Amniocentesis is widely used in antenatal diagnosis. Biochemical estimations on the fluid or chromosome or enzyme analysis on cultured fetal cells may be done. The cell culture usually takes 2–3 weeks. Estimation of the liquor AFP and chromosome analysis for Down's syndrome are the commonest tests. Fetal sexing and exclusion of many in-born metabolic errors are also possible.

D. CHORION VILLUS SAMPLING (CVS)

Chorionic villi may be obtained either vaginally or transabdominally by an aspirating needle guided by ultrasound or endoscope. This may be used as an alternative to amniocentesis for obtaining a specimen for chromosome analysis by direct examination or to culture cells for DNA or other studies. Its advantage for chromosome analysis is that the test is done early in pregnancy (8–10 weeks), and the result is available within 48 hours. The disadvantage is that at present the risk of abortion with this technique is 2–3 times that of amniocentesis.

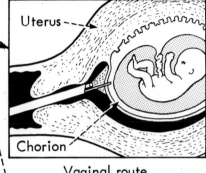

Vaginal route

E. FETOSCOPY and FETAL BLOOD SAMPLING

The fetoscope is a fine fibre-optic telescope which may be passed into the amniotic sac under ultrasound control. It allows direct inspection of the fetus and biopsies of skin or blood samples from the placenta or cord can be obtained.

The main use of the fetoscope has been in fetal blood sampling, but with the advance of ultrasonic technology cord blood sampling (and fetal tranfusion e.g. in Rhesus disease) can be done without fetoscopy.

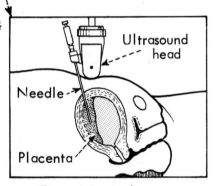

Transabdominal route

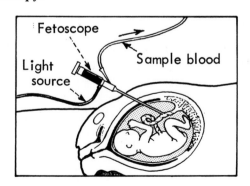

Indications for fetal blood sampling:
Diagnosis of haemoglobinopathy or
bleeding disorder e.g. haemophilia,
Karyotyping,
Blood grouping
Investigation of fetal hydrops.

115

CHAPTER 7

SYSTEMIC DISEASES IN PREGNANCY

CARDIAC DISEASE

Cardiac disease in pregnancy is less common than formerly due to the decline in the incidence of rheumatic heart disease. This is offset to some extent by an increase in cases of congenital heart disease reaching childbearing age because of corrective surgery, and an increase in the diagnosis of congenital valve lesions by echocardiography.

An incidence of about 1% is widely quoted in the UK but the report on maternal deaths for Scotland in 1976–80 quotes an incidence of only 0.26%.

TYPES OF LESION

Formerly rheumatic heart disease was 8–9 times commoner than congenital heart disease. This balance has changed greatly and the incidence now is approximately equal. Mitral stenosis is still much the commonest acquired lesion. Patent ductus arteriosus and septal defects are the commonest congenital lesions and these will usually have been corrected in childhood and be uncomplicated. Patients who have had corrections of major lesions such as Fallot's tetralogy may be encountered.

MATERNAL MORTALITY

The risk of death in pregnancy from heart disease is of the order 0.3–0.5%.

EFFECTS OF PREGNANCY ON HEART DISEASE

The physiological changes in the cardiovascular system have been described in Chapter 2. In summary it can be said that there is an early and sharp rise in cardiac output in the first trimester and a further slower rise to a maximum of 40% above normal in mid-pregnancy. During labour, cardiac output rises even higher during contractions but falls again between contractions. There is a further rise after delivery when blood returns to the circulation from the placental bed and from the pelvis and lower limbs due to the release of pressure by the emptying of the uterus.

Cardiac failure may come on gradually in pregnancy as the demand for a rise in cardiac output accompanies the increasing blood volume. Acute failure in the form of pulmonary oedema may occur early in pregnancy when the blood volume begins to increase or when it is approaching its maximum. More commonly however, acute failure is precipitated by some other incidental change. Usually it is some circumstance which causes tachycardia in excess of 110 per minute thus reducing the diastolic period, the filling of the left ventricle and the cardiac output. This in turn leads to obstruction of the pulmonary blood flow and to oedema of the lungs.

ANY FEBRILE ILLNESS

118

CARDIAC DISEASE

Common aggravating factors are:-

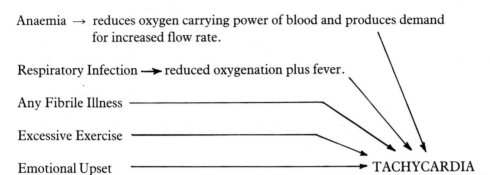

Anaemia → reduces oxygen carrying power of blood and produces demand for increased flow rate.

Respiratory Infection → reduced oxygenation plus fever.

Any Fibrile Illness ——————————

Excessive Exercise ——————————

Emotional Upset ——————————————→ TACHYCARDIA

In mitral stenosis acute failure may also occur immediately after the third stage of delivery due to the sudden increase in the circulating volume, which may exceed the capacity of the mitral valve to pass blood.

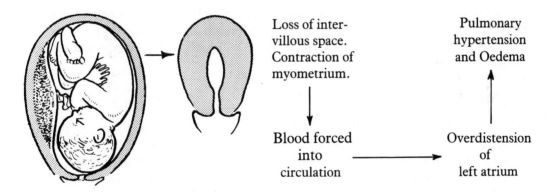

Loss of inter-villous space. Contraction of myometrium.

↓

Blood forced into circulation ——————————→ Overdistension of left atrium

↑

Pulmonary hypertension and Oedema

Infective endocarditis is a further worrying risk. It may follow any infection complicating pregnancy or arise from the normal bacteraemia associated with labour .

EFFECT OF HEART DISEASE ON PREGNANCY

An increased risk of premature labour and intra-uterine growth retardation has been described.

CARDIAC DISEASE

PRE-PREGNANCY AND EARLY PREGNANCY ASSESSMENT

(a) Pre-pregnancy counselling is important for women with known heart disease. It allows a full assessment of their cardiac status and the likely effect on it of pregnancy. Pregnancy may be contraindicated as for example in Eisenmenger's syndrome or Fallot's tetralogy.

(b) A heart murmur may be detected for the first time at the booking ante-natal visit. Haemic, systolic murmurs are common in pregnancy and it may be difficult to be certain whether or not a given murmur is organic. Careful enquiry should be made for any history which might suggest organic disease and assessment by a cardiologist should be requested.

(c) Patients with known heart lesions should be supervised throughout the pregnancy jointly by obstetrician and cardiologist.

TERMINATION OF PREGNANCY AND SURGICAL TREATMENT

Termination of pregnancy is not usually indicated on grounds of cardiac disease alone. Exceptions to this may be lesions such as Eisenmenger's syndrome (mortality 30–50%) and Fallot's tetralogy (mortality 4–20%), even if the latter has been corrected. After 12 weeks the risks of termination are as great as those of continuing the pregnancy.

The decline in rheumatic heart disease means that mitral valvotomy in pregnancy is now very rare. Furthermore, surgeons tend to prefer an open approach to valvotomy which is undesirable in pregnancy. For the same reason congenital lesions will rarely justify surgical treatment in pregnancy.

ANTE-NATAL CARE

This is shared between the obstetrician and cardiologist. The principles are simple: Plenty of rest and avoidance of the aggravating factors mentioned on page 119.

(1) Most cardiac patients will spend their pregnancies outwith hospital but admission for rest and treatment should be available at any time. Any change or deterioration in the cardiac state is an indication for admission and expert cardiological opinion.

(2) The patient should not smoke and any respiratory infection should be treated vigorously.

(3) Avoid anaemia.

(4) Good dental care is essential and treatment should be covered with antibiotics.

(5) Patients with prosthetic valves, previous corrective surgery or in atrial fibrillation may be receiving anti-coagulant therapy. The risks of this to the pregnancy have to be accepted. Warfarin is usually the drug of choice and must be discontinued at 37 weeks. It is then replaced by intravenous Heparin. Subcutaneous Heparin is not adequate where there is a risk of systemic embolus.

CARDIAC DISEASE

LABOUR AND DELIVERY

Most cardiac patients may be allowed to labour. If, however, obstetric factors make the outcome of labour more speculative than normal, planned Caesarean section may be the safest choice.

The aim should be to make the labour as easy and non-stressful as possible. Prolonged labour is physically and emotionally exhausting and carries an increased risk of infection.

(1) Position

The patient should labour in a propped-up, comfortable position. She may maintain this position for delivery, even when this has to be assisted. The lithotomy position is best avoided because of the sudden surge of blood returning to the heart from the lower limbs when they are taken out of the stirrups.

(2) Analgesia

Good analgesia is essential. It avoids the tachycardia which anxiety and pain can induce. An epidural block is the method of choice provided hypotension is avoided. It also allows operative delivery, abdominal or vaginal, should this become necessary. If epidural anaesthesia is unavailable the traditional Morphine 15mg has much to commend it.

(3) Antibiotics

Opinion is divided on the routine use of antibiotics to cover the bacteraemia associated with labour and delivery. Most favour their use to try to lessen the risk of endocarditis. A combination such as Ampicillin and Gentamicin given intramuscularly is recommended.

(4) Second Stage

If the second stage proceeds easily and quickly normal delivery is allowed, facilitated by episiotomy. The patient should not however be asked to make substantial expulsive efforts and forceps or vacuum extractor should be used readily. The latter is often excellent and allows delivery in the upright position.

(5) Third Stage

There should be no hurry at this point. Time should be allowed for circulatory adjustment as blood enters the circulation from the placental site as the uterus retracts. There is also increased flow from the lower limbs due to the emptying of the uterus. If the placenta is allowed to separate spontaneously, an oxytocic can then be given after physiological retraction has occurred to prevent atonic bleeding. Synthetic Oxytocin is the drug of choice (10 units IM) given then or during the delivery as in normal cases. It is preferred here to Ergometrine because of the vasopressor effects of the latter especially if given intravenously.

The period after the third stage is the most dangerous in pregnancy from the point of developing pulmonary oedema.

CARDIAC DISEASE

ACUTE PULMONARY OEDEMA

The patient becomes quickly breathless and may have frothy sputum and/or haemoptysis. She should be propped up and given oxygen by face mask. Morphine (10–15mg), Frusemide (40mg) and Aminophylline (250mg) may be given intravenously. Occasionally it is necessary to reduce venous return by the application of inflatable cuffs to the limbs. If time allows, a cardiologist should be consulted about digitalisation.

PUERPERIUM

Early ambulation but plenty of rest are advised. There should be careful scrutiny for evidence of infection and any pyrexia merits blood culture. Careful counselling about future pregnancies should take place.

RESPIRATORY DISEASES

ASTHMA

The effect of pregnancy is very variable. In most cases the condition is unaffected. The patient will normally continue with her existing medication. Broncho-dilators such as Salbutamol can be used safely and if the patient should require steroids Prednisone or Prednisolone are to be preferred because of their slow transfer across the placenta.

TUBERCULOSIS

This is now an uncommon condition in the UK and routine chest X-ray is not done. It should, however, be performed, with appropriate precautions, if there has been recent contact or family history of tuberculosis. Medication is as in non-pregnant patients, avoiding Streptomycin which is now rarely used anyway. Isoniazid, Para-aminosalicylic acid and Ethambutol may be employed. The teratogenicity of Rifampicin is unconfirmed but it should be avoided in the first trimester.

After delivery special precautions are necessary if the mother has active (sputum positive) tuberculosis. Mother and baby can be kept together while both are treated. Isoniazid-resistant BCG is available and should be given to the baby together with Isoniazid therapy. A Mantoux test should be done at 6–8 weeks and Isoniazid therapy should continue until the baby is Mantoux positive and the mother's sputum is negative.

VENOUS THROMBO-EMBOLISM

Venous thrombosis is not common in pregnancy or the puerperium but it attracts much attention because of its disabling effects and because thrombo-embolism is a continuing cause of maternal death. It is said to be about 5 times commoner in pregnancy and the puerperium than in non-pregnant women of similar age.

Causes

1. Changes in the composition of the blood.
2. Changes in the rate of blood flow.
3. Lesions of the vascular intima.

These changes are called 'Virchow's Triad'

Changes in the composition of the blood

These have been described in Chapter 2 and induce a hyper-coagulable state of the blood.

Changes in rate of flow

The rate of flow in the leg veins is much reduced in the later weeks partly from pressure in the pelvis by the gravid uterus, and also from the reduced activity of the woman advanced in pregnancy. Bed-rest in pregnancy for any reason will increase this risk. Early mobilisation after delivery is now invariable.

Changes in the vascular intima

These can result from hypertensive disease, surgery and local or blood-borne infection which can follow any delivery, spontaneous or operative. The risk of thrombo-embolism after section is 5 times higher than after vaginal delivery.

Sites of thrombosis formation

1. Calf veins (often extending to the popliteal vein).

2. Common femoral vein.

3. Iliofemoral (perhaps extending to the vena cava).

4. Saphenous vein at or above the knee.

5. Superficial thrombosis in varices.

Emboli may come from any of these sites except the last. However in many cases of pulmonary embolism there are no preceding signs of venous thrombosis; and clinical diagnosis of thrombosis is often made when more sophisticated tests show the veins to be patent.

123

VENOUS THROMBO-EMBOLISM

SUPERFICIAL THROMBO-PHLEBITIS

This is easily diagnosed. There is a reddened, tender superficial vein with a surrounding area of inflammation and oedema. It may be accompanied by a mild pyrexia. As long as the condition remains superficial there is no risk of thrombo-embolism. The traditional remedy of a Kaolin poultice with a supporting bandage will give comfort. Occasionally analgesics are necessary and activity should be encouraged.

DEEP VEIN THROMBOSIS

1. **Clinical Features** There may be no complaint, but examination of the legs either as a routine or in search of mild pyrexia may reveal signs.

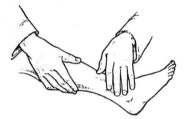

Palpation of the calf demonstrates tenderness and oedema.

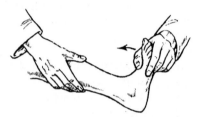

Homan's Sign (calf pain on dorsiflexion of the foot) may be positive.

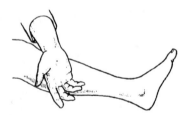

The affected leg may feel warmer to the back of the hand.

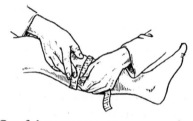

Careful measurement may reveal some swelling compared with the other leg.

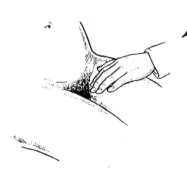

The femoral vein must also be palpated in the groin. It may be palpable in the condition known as *Phlegmasia Alba Dolens* - - - - ➤ (painful white inflammation). This is an old name for an extreme degree of thrombosis which completely blocks the femoral vein, causing a solid oedema which does not pit on pressure. The superficial veins give a marbled appearance, but arterial supply is not affected. The condition is very painful and gives rise to what is now called the post-phlebitic syndrome.

VENOUS THROMBO-EMBOLISM

DEEP VEIN THROMBOSIS (continued)

2. **Complications of thrombosis**
  (a) Pulmonary embolism — This can be mild or severe, isolated or recurrent, and in more than 50% of cases is not preceded by clinical signs of thrombosis.
  (b) Post Phlebitic syndrome — A result of the damage sustained by the vein, in particular the loss of functioning valves. It includes swelling, varicose veins, eczema, ulceration, and is much more severe if the acute condition is not energetically treated.

3. **Diagnosis**
  This is not always easy as the clinical signs are unreliable. Because of the dangers of the condition, the risks of the treatment and the implications for the future it is important to try to establish the diagnosis accurately.
  (a) *Venography*, using radio-opaque dye injected into the foot, is the method of choice taking precautions to protect the fetus.
  (b) *Ultrasound* — This technique makes use of the Doppler flowmeter, an apparatus developed for the purpose of fetal heart auscultation in obstetrics. It is non-invasive but less accurate than venography.

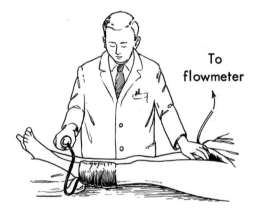

To flowmeter

   The flowing movements of blood in a vein produce characteristic sounds when picked up by a transducer held over the vessel. If the flow is accelerated the frequency and amplitude of the sounds are increased. The transducer is placed over the groin and the thigh or calf squeezed with an inflatable cuff. The increased sound is easily heard, and its absence suggests that the blood flow is being impeded by a thrombus.

  (c) *Isotope* — This, although a ward technique, requires special apparatus and the use of isotopes is controlled by strict regulations. This is not applicable ante-natally or in lactating mothers.

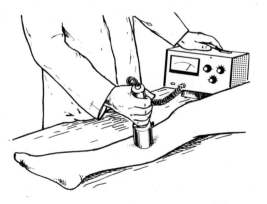

   A small amount of ^{125}I-labelled fibrinogen is injected after the thyroid has been blocked with sodium iodide to prevent uptake of the isotope. A scintillation counter is applied to the legs and an increase in radioactivity suggests thrombus formation.

VENOUS THROMBO-EMBOLISM

DEEP VEIN THROMBOSIS (continued)

4. **Treatment**

The aim is to prevent extension of the thrombus and reduce the risk of embolus. Treatment has to be continued for the rest of the pregnancy and into the puerperium.

In the acute phase intravenous Heparin 40,000 units/day is given until the clinical signs have resolved. Maintenance therapy is either by subcutaneous Heparin or Warfarin. Ante-natally subcutaneous Heparin is usually preferred. Initially 7,500 units are given 12 hourly and therapy is monitored by plasma Heparin levels. Treatment can be suspended at the onset of labour but is resumed or replaced by Warfarin after delivery and continued for 6 weeks post-partum.

Heparin does not cross the placenta but is not free from risk. Demineralisation of bone has been reported.

Warfarin is the drug of choice for long-term treatment of puerperal thrombosis and may be used ante-natally after the first trimester. It has been reported as a cause of central nervous system abnormalities due to repeated small episodes of intracranial bleeding. If used it should be discontinued at 37 weeks and replaced by Heparin.

5. **Prophylaxis**
  (a) *Preventing stasis*

    Patients with varicose veins should wear full thigh and lower leg elastic stockings. Bed-rest should be discouraged before and after delivery and the physiotherapist should attend all puerperal patients. As short as possible a stay in the post-natal ward is beneficial.
  (b) *Dextran Infusions*

    Dextrans are polysaccharides of varying molecular weights. Thus Dextran-40 has an average MW of 40,000. Dextrans have an antithrombotic effect and have been found to reduce the incidence of thrombosis if given at the same time as an operation. Thus half a litre of Dextran-40 might be given during a section, and another half-litre 48 hours later. They may be used to cover surgery in a high-risk patient or in one who has been on anticoagulants prior to delivery.

SYSTEMIC SPREAD OF THROMBOSIS

PULMONARY EMBOLISM

A large embolus lodging in the pulmonary artery produces signs of shock and circulatory failure, and death often occurs within 15 minutes. Smaller emboli are more difficult to diagnose and cause dyspnoea, pleuritic pain, fever and some malaise. In at least 50% of cases of embolism there is no clinical evidence of thrombosis elsewhere.

Diagnosis

Chest X-ray may be helpful but is not invariably so. ECG changes may be present in large emboli. Pulmonary angiography is diagnostic but is an invasive and highly specialised technique. Help from a specialist in pulmonary diseases is advisable.

Treatment

Continuous intravenous Heparin, as described above, is employed. Where there has been a major embolism treatment is best supervised in an intensive care unit.

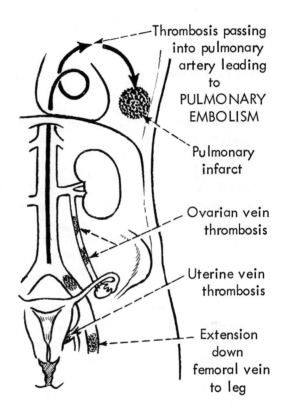

Thrombosis passing into pulmonary artery leading to PULMONARY EMBOLISM

Pulmonary infarct

Ovarian vein thrombosis

Uterine vein thrombosis

Extension down femoral vein to leg

ANAEMIA

Pregnancy makes considerable nutritional demands on the mother. It is not surprising therefore that anaemia is a common complication.

The main nutritional factors involved are iron, folic acid and other vitamins of the B group, and protein.

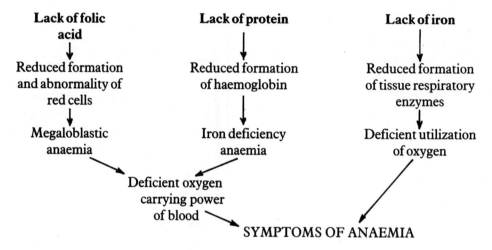

Although there are two distinct anaemic conditions each apparently due to deficiency of a single factor (iron deficiency anaemia and megaloblastic anaemia due to folic acid deficiency) it should be remembered that a single deficiency is almost an impossibility.

The deficiency of any substance may be due to:-

        1. Diminished intake.
        2. Abnormal absorption.
        3. Reduced storage.
        4. Abnormal utilization.
        5. Abnormal demand.

The aetiology of anaemia must be considered in relation to these principles.

The presence of anaemia increases morbidity in pregnancy and makes the mother more vulnerable to infection and the dangers of blood loss at delivery.

IRON DEFICIENCY ANAEMIA

The average UK diet just meets daily requirements in respect of iron during menstrual life. Additional loss (e.g. menorrhagia) or the need to provide extra iron in pregnancy can quickly lead to anaemia. During pregnancy there is an increased demand for iron amounting to approximately 1,230mg. There is however a saving of 220mg due to 9 months amenorrhoea. The total amount of extra iron required will be 1,010mg.

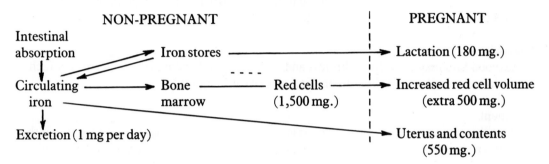

The main factors in this anaemia appear to be:-

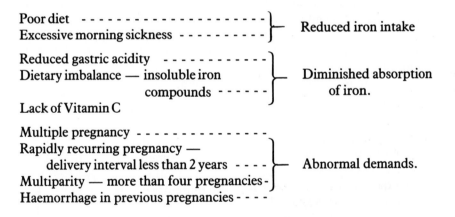

Symptoms: The majority of patients make no complaint even if the anaemia is moderately severe. Subjective feelings are accepted as part of the 'burden of pregnancy'.

Equally, due to the peripheral vasodilatation of pregnancy (heat loss mechanism) pallor is not necessarily a feature. The haemoglobin level should be checked regularly throughout pregnancy.

Close questioning may reveal the same symptoms as in non-pregnant anaemic subjects.

IRON DEFICIENCY ANAEMIA

Blood Changes

These have been noted in Chapter 2. The progressive haemo-dilution in pregnancy makes it impossible to set a single point on the haemoglobin scale which will divide anaemic from non-anaemic subjects. In healthy non-pregnant individuals the haemoglobin reading is usually 12.6g/dl or over. This value declines in pregnancy as the plasma volume increase exceeds the rise in the red cell mass. The aim should be to have the patient's haemoglobin value at 11g or over at term.

Diagnosis

The blood film may show hypochromia and microcytosis. Serum iron and ferritin (which reflects storage) are low and the iron binding capacity is increased.

Treatment

This will vary with the severity of anaemia and the duration of the pregnancy. Oral iron is the treatment of choice and in many UK centres it is given prophylactically throughout pregnancy to all women. A preparation containing 100mg of elemental iron (preferably in a single tablet) should be given. Lack of response is generally due to failure to take the treatment which in turn may sometimes be due to sickness caused by the iron. If there is no response and the patient is known to have taken the tablets, a more complete haematological investigation should be undertaken.

Where there is failure to respond to oral therapy or non-compliance iron may be given parenterally. This may be done in two ways:

        1. Repeated intramuscular injection.
        2. Total dose infusion.

1. *Repeated intramuscular injection*

    250mg of iron raises haemoglobin by 1g per dl. Injections are given every other day. Iron-sorbitol, which is a smaller, more easily absorbed molecule, may be used instead of iron-dextran. There is less likelihood of staining.

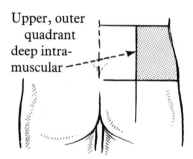

Upper, outer quadrant deep intra-muscular

IRON DEFICIENCY ANAEMIA

Iron Administration (continued)

2.   *Total Dose Infusion* The total iron deficiency is corrected by an intravenous infusion of iron-dextran in 10dl saline given slowly over several hours.

The deficiency in haemoglobin in g x 250 = mg of iron to be given. To allow for depleted iron stores, blood loss at delivery and fetal demands, this figure is increased by 50 per cent.

Example:-

Haemoglobin reading of patient = 8 g per dl
Haemoglobin reading desired = 12 g per dl
Haemoglobin deficit = 4 g per dl
Iron required for maternal haemoglobin = 4 x 250 = 1,000 mg
Iron required for storage, fetus and delivery = 500 mg
Total dose for infusion = 1,500 mg

Anaphylactoid reactions can be severe and are not infrequent. This method is never used in patients with any history of hypersensitivity.

Oral antihistamine is given 30 minutes before infusion. Iron solution is given at the rate of 10 drops per minute for 30 minutes. If there is no reaction the rate is increased to 45 drops per minute. A syringe containing 1/1000 adrenalin should be available.

Severe anaemia near Time of Delivery

Up to the 35th week parenteral iron may be given. Beyond this time, in view of the usual uncertainty of the time of delivery and the possibility of premature labour, a transfusion of packed red cells may be given. This is an emergency treatment and should only be used if the patient's haemoglobin is below 9g per dl. It must be realised that while the haemoglobin and therefore the oxygen carrying power of the blood will be increased the respiratory enzymes (iron containing) of the tissues will be unaffected. The tissues are unhealthy, particularly the myocardium. The transfusion must be given very slowly and preferably in two or more stages to avoid cardiac failure. One pint of blood raises the haemoglobin value by approximately 0.7g per dl.

The main reason for blood transfusion in this condition is not primarily correction of anaemia but that any further blood loss at delivery may be dangerous.

131

IRON DEFICIENCY ANAEMIA

REFRACTORY ANAEMIAS

In most cases seemingly refractory anaemia is due to failure to take the prescribed treatment. If however the anaemia truly fails to respond to treatment remember that nutritional deficiencies are rarely single. Folic acid deficiency should be suspected and looked for. If the haemoglobin still fails to rise further investigation is required to eliminate the possibility of a rarer blood disease.

To summarise:

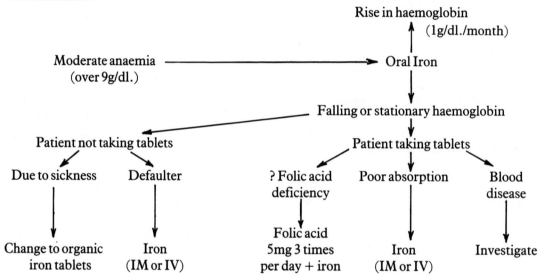

FOLIC ACID DEFICIENCY

Folic acid is necessary for the formation of nucleic acids and therefore nuclei. Its absence leads to reduction of cell proliferation. Where the deficiency is partial those tissues, such as bone marrow, which are constantly proliferating, show the main effects.

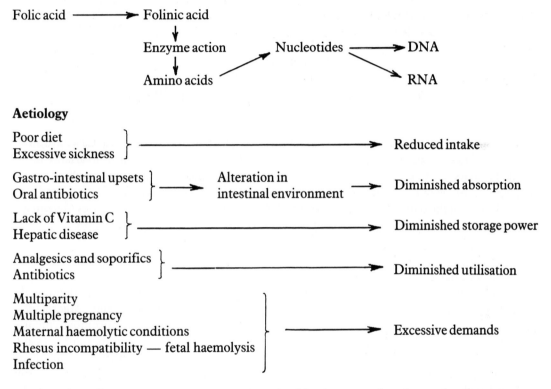

Aetiology

The main factors are poor intake coupled with the excessive demands of pregnancy. Malabsorption may also be important and haemolysis, as in the haemoglobinopathies, will lead to folic acid deficiency.

Clinical findings

These depend on the severity of the deficiency. In the early stages the patient may have no symptoms and no apparent signs apart from a moderately low haemoglobin value. The diagnosis is frequently made when, despite continued iron therapy, the haemoglobin value first increases and then remains static. The deficiency in these cases is a double one and may be visualised as follows:-

FOLIC ACID DEFICIENCY

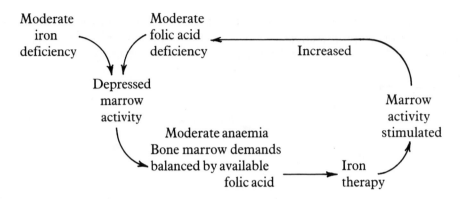

In its severe form this deficiency is characterised by a megaloblastic anaemia. Cases are most often seen among patients with haemoglobin values below 8g per dl. Almost invariably these patients have symptoms of anaemia — breathlessness, giddiness, palpitations, swelling of feet and ankles. Signs of nutritional deficiency may be present — glossitis, oral fissures, and irregularities of the nails. The spleen is commonly enlarged and in very severe cases there may be vomiting, diarrhoea and pyrexia and even a purpuric rash.

Laboratory Diagnosis

In almost all cases the diagnosis can be made by examination of the peripheral blood, and apart from the low haemoglobin value most of the changes are seen in a blood film. Macrocytes are seen which are usually normochromic but may be hypochromic due to accompanying iron deficiency. Giant multi-segmented polymorphs are seen and in severe cases megaloblasts are present but may only be found by examination of a film made from the buffy coat. Blood and red cell folate levels may be examined for confirmation and laboratories invariably do a serum B_{12} level at the same time. Treatment by folic acid need not await this result as patients with Addisonian pernicious anaemia are invariably infertile.

Treatment

Prophylactic folic acid therapy (350 micrograms daily) is commonly combined with oral iron. The treatment of established deficiency is folic acid 5mg tid orally. Treatment should be given throughout pregnancy.

HAEMOGLOBINOPATHIES

The haemoglobinopathies are defects in globin structure or synthesis leading to haemolytic anaemia in homozygotes i.e. those who have inherited the abnormal globin chain from both parents. Heterozygotes are not anaemic but are carriers of the defect.

Sickle-cell disease and the thalassaemias (alpha and beta) are seen increasingly in the UK among the immigrant population, the former in negroes and the latter in those of Mediterranean or Far Eastern origin. Definitive diagnosis depends on electrophoresis but there is a screening test for haemoglobin S which should be carried out on all black patients.

In homozygous sickle-cell disease there is chronic anaemia and an increased risk of haemolytic crises in pregnancy. Homozygous alpha-thalassaemia causes fetal hydrops and still-birth.

Beta-thalassaemia is the commonest form seen in the UK. The heterozygous form (thalassaemia minor) causes chronic anaemia but homozygous beta-thalassaemia causes severe anaemia and commonly leads to death in childhood.

If a woman is found to be a carrier of thalassaemia or sickle-cell disease her husband should be tested. If he too is a carrier pre-natal diagnosis can be carried out by fetoscopic blood examination or chorion villus sampling for DNA analysis.

IDIOPATHIC THROMBOCYTOPENIC PURPURA (ITP)

This is now recognised as an auto-immune disease and the presence of antiplatelet antibody (IgG) can be demonstrated. This can cross the placenta and cause fetal disease. The baby may still be at risk even if the mother has had a splenectomy. The main risk is of intra-cranial haemorrhage. If non-fatal these can produce cerebral damage. Thrombocytopenia in the mother is treated by steroids and platelets should be available for transfusion at the time of delivery. Caesarean section in the baby's interest to avoid trauma has been advocated.

135

DIABETES

Pregnancy is a diabetogenic state.

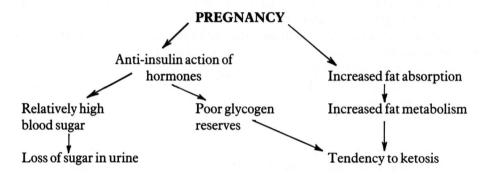

These effects will aggravate established clinical diabetes and may reveal impaired glucose tolerance.

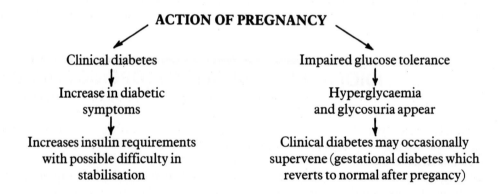

The World Health Organisation has laid down criteria for the diagnosis of diabetes and impaired glucose tolerance using a 75g oral glucose tolerance test.

	Venous Plasma Glucose (mmol/l)	
	Fasting	2hr post-glucose
Normal	<6.0	< 8.0
Impaired glucose tolerance	<8.0	⩽ 8.0 to <11.0
Diabetes	⩾8.0	⩾11.0

DIABETES

Because of the potential implications of impaired glucose tolerance some authorities recommend random plasma glucose estimation at booking and again at 28 weeks. This may identify patients in whom a full glucose tolerance test should be performed. The majority of obstetricians carry out glucose tolerance tests in certain high-risk groups. The widely accepted list of indications is:

1. Glycosuria on routine testing (twice or more).
2. Diabetes in first degree relative.
3. Maternal weight greater than 85kg.
4. Previous baby weight 4.5kg or more.
5. Previous unexplained still-birth or neo-natal death.
6. Previous congenital abnormality.
7. Polyhydramnios.

Effect of pregnancy on diabetes

1. Control is more difficult with rise in insulin requirements and increased loss of glucose in urine. Complications of pregnancy are more frequent if control not achieved.
2. Diabetic lesions such as retinopathy and nephropathy require careful assessment. A more optimistic attitude exists now than formerly to them and there does not appear to be an inevitable deterioration.

Effect of diabetes on pregnancy

1. Increased abortion rate.
2. Increased peri-natal loss. The risk of intra-uterine death in the last weeks of pregnancy has long dictated intervention to deliver at 36–37 weeks. The cause of these deaths is probably metabolic rather than due to placental insufficiency. Fetal abnormality contributes to the peri-natal loss and it appears that this relates to poor diabetic control at the time of organogenesis.
3. Macrosomia — babies tend to be big and their weight may be increased by oedema. This carries a risk of dystocia.
4. Fetal lung maturation may be delayed.
5. Increased risk of pregnancy complications:
    Urinary tract infection
    Thrush infection
    Pre-eclampsia
    Polyhydramnios

ALL these risks are reduced by good diabetic **CONTROL** from conception onwards.

DIABETES

MANAGEMENT OF PREGNANCY

1. **Pre-pregnancy**

   There is much to be gained by the diabetic woman receiving advice and assessment before she conceives. The importance of control can be emphasised and checked by haemoglobin A_{1c} estimations. Glycosylated HbA_{1c} levels reflect control in the 8–10 weeks previously. They can be used to check control throughout pregnancy. Renal function and the state of the optic fundi can be assessed and the patient, if on an oral agent, can be changed to insulin therapy.

2. **Pregnancy**

   Supervision must be shared between the obstetrician and a specialist diabetic physician.

   (a) Early admission for the above assessment if not already done. A 24 hour blood sugar profile is started (fasting, pre-lunch, pre-supper and 21.30 hours) and control aims to keep the blood sugar at less than 8mmol/l. A mixture of short and medium acting insulins is usually given. The patient is instructed in home glucose monitoring and provided with an instrument.

   Routine early pregnancy assessments are performed, especially an ultrasound scan for maturity.

   (b) Subsequent attendances will usually be fortnightly to the combined clinic. Routine ante-natal examinations are carried out together with tests for fetal abnormality. Fetal growth is followed by serial ultrasound. The mother does twice weekly blood sugar profiles and these results are examined. Control can be checked by HbA_{1c} estimation.

   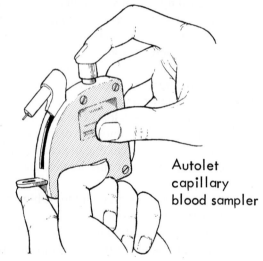

   Autolet
   capillary
   blood sampler

   (c) After 32 weeks, supervision is carried out weekly or the patient may be admitted to hospital.

   (d) At 36 weeks the patient is admitted if not already in hospital. Blood sugar profiles continue and fetal growth and well-being monitored by ultrasound and cardiotocography.

DIABETES

LABOUR AND DELIVERY

With good control and in the absence of other abnormality, pregnancies in diabetic mothers are increasingly stretching beyond 37 weeks. Delivery at 38–40 weeks is now common practice in centres with special experience. If the maturity is certain, tests for lung maturity can be omitted.

In the absence of obstetric indications vaginal delivery is planned. On the day of induction the morning dose of insulin is omitted. A Dextrose infusion with 5 units of insulin/5dl is set up. Artificial rupture of the membranes is performed and an infusion of Syntocinon is given if required. The blood sugar level is checked 2-hourly and the Dextrose/Insulin infusion changed accordingly.

Caesarean section will be carried out for obstetric reasons arising in labour or for failure to progress. An arbitrary time limit of say 8–10 hours may be set. Section, if required, is best done under epidural anaesthesia which allows an early return to normal diet. Insulin rquirements fall immediately after delivery and the patient should return to her pre-pregnancy insulin dosage.

BABY

With good control the baby will be normal. Poor control results in large babies subject to respiratory distress and poor temperature control. Hypoglycaemia, due to over-activity of the fetal pancreatic islets in response to high maternal blood sugar, is a risk and blood sugar levels should be checked 2–hourly in the first day. Breast feeding is not contra-indicated.

URINARY TRACT INFECTION

Pregnant women are particularly liable to this condition, especially if there is a history of urinary tract infection. The main predisposing causes are stasis of urine, and an increased susceptibilty to ascending infection.

Stasis

Progesterone normally produces atony of the muscles of the renal pelvis and ureters, and in the days when pyelography was frequently done in pregnancy, it was usual to observe some dilation and kinking of the ureters. To this is added the mechanical effect of the uterus pressing on the ureters as they cross the pelvic brim. This effect is probably maximum at 20–24 weeks. As a result the rate of flow of urine is reduced and bacterial growth encouraged.

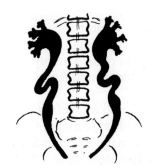

Pyelogram in pregnancy

Increased susceptibility to ascending infection

There is a much higher incidence of urinary infection among women compared with men, presumably because of the ease with which bacteria can gain access to the bladder through the short female urethra. During pregnancy there is a great increase in the moistness and in the bacterial population of the vestibule and vagina, and reflux from the bladder into the ureters occurs.

Sites of Infection

When the urine is infected there is always the likelihood that the renal parenchyma is involved. In pregnancy it must be assumed that this is so and that the disease is a pyelonephritis and not just a pyelitis or cystitis.

Organisms

By far the commonest is E. coli. Other organisms sometimes found include B. proteus, Strept. faecalis and sometimes Pseudomonas aeruginosa.

URINARY TRACT INFECTION

Bacterial counts in urine

A midstream specimen of urine (MSU) always contains some contaminating organisms from the vulva; but a bacterial population in excess of contaminants can be identified by the following means.

1. Freshly voided urine is used, after a standardised amount of vulval cleansing (e.g. no antiseptics).
2. It is cultured at once (or kept at 4°C until this can be done).
3. A count is made of the colonies which are grown overnight. This gives an approximation of the number of bacteria per ml in the specimen.
4. A normal urine contains less than 10,000 bacteria/ml. Over 100,000 indicates infection. 30,000 or over is suspicious.

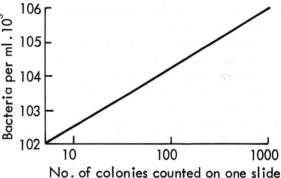

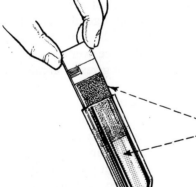

Techniques of counting

Various methods are used to provide a simple screening test. The 'Uricult' system uses a slide coated with agar which is dipped into the fresh urine, cultured overnight and read the next day.

Asymptomatic bacteriuria

About 6–7% of women attending a booking ante-natal clinic have an infected urine according to bacterial count. Such women have a greatly increased risk of developing clinical pyelonephritis during pregnancy. By identifying them and treating any infection it is hoped to prevent this complication. In addition some of these women (approximately 10%) will have a renal tract abnormality on intravenous pyelography.

URINARY TRACT INFECTION

Clinical features   These are variable and often vague.

1. Dysuria. The patient says that the urine 'felt hot' or that it was 'like passing needles'.
2. Fever. Temperature may be raised to 39°C and pulse rate is also elevated.
3. Loin Pain. This sign is diagnostic. Tenderness may be elicited over one or both kidneys.
4. Abdominal Pain. This is usually referred to the lower quadrants and is presumably related to the inflammatory process in the ureters and bladder.
5. There may be nausea and vomiting. This may be severe and lead to dehydration.
6. A positive urine culture may be obtained.

Laboratory investigations

A mid-stream specimen of urine must be collected and swabs from the throat and vagina should be sent at the same time.

Differential diagnosis

Both patient and doctor often mistake the condition for the onset of premature labour. Loin tenderness should be diagnostic. Appendicitis is much less common, and the urine should be normal. Concealed accidental haemorrhage may in the early stages cause confusion, but there is no pyrexia, and again the urine should be sterile although protein will be present.

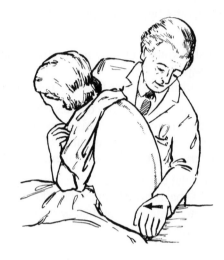

To elicit loin tenderness, first palpate the spine gently to accustom the patient to the touch, then tap gently with the thenar eminence over the loin. If positive, the patient gives an unmistakable wince.

Treatment

The patient is put to bed, given mild analgesics and encouraged to drink. A 'holding antibiotic' such as sulphadimidine or nitrofurantoin should be given until the sensitivity is reported. Antibiotic treatment is maintained for 10 days and the urine should be sterile on completion. The patient may however be acutely ill and require rehydration and intravenous therapy together with strong analgesics.

URINARY TRACT INFECTION

Prognosis

An apparently isolated attack of urinary tract infection may be the acute phase in an undiagnosed so far 'silent' pyelonephritis, or at least another stage towards the development of that disease.

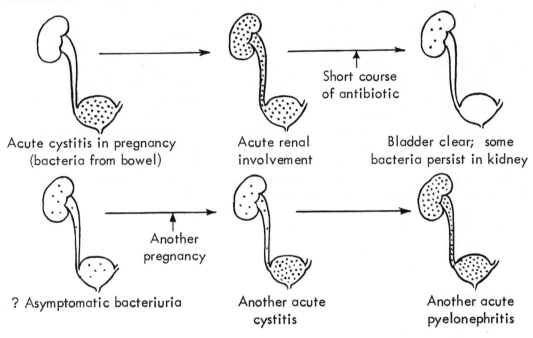

Acute cystitis in pregnancy
(bacteria from bowel)

Acute renal
involvement

Short course
of antibiotic

Bladder clear; some
bacteria persist in kidney

? Asymptomatic bacteriuria

Another
pregnancy

Another acute
cystitis

Another acute
pyelonephritis

The infection is quite likely to recur later on in pregnancy and especially during the puerperium. Where this occurs, long-term maintenance therapy for the remainder of the pregnancy and puerperium is justified. A full renal tract investigation should be carried out once the pregnancy is over, waiting at least 3 months for the changes of pregnancy to regress.

CHRONIC RENAL DISEASE

When chronic renal failure develops it adds a serious complication to pregnancy whatever may be its aetiology. There is argument as to whether the pregnancy has a permanently damaging effect on diseased kidneys; but there is no doubt about the effect of renal disease on pregnancy. Hypertension, if not already present, nearly always occurs and placental function is affected. The fetal prognosis is poor; and if renal impairment is severe the added stress of pregnancy may be fatal for the mother. If the patient has severe nephritis it is best to advise termination.

In less severe cases, and when termination is refused, renal function must be observed closely in addition to the usual intensive antenatal supervision, and treatment modified to suit the circumstances. A physician specialising in renal disease should be asked to share the management, and if renal function is deteriorating, the pregnancy should be terminated by section as soon as the fetus is judged mature enough to survive.

143

EPILEPSY

In this condition there is again a strong case for pre-pregnancy counselling. The available anti-convulsant drugs are teratogenic and if the patient has had no fits for 2–3 years it may be possible to withdraw them slowly before conception occurs. The overall incidence of malformation in the children of mothers taking anti-convulsant drugs is about 6%, that is to say about twice the risk of the general population.

If it is not possible to withdraw medication the dosage of drugs should be minimised but this needs to be checked by serum or saliva concentrations because of changes in absorption, distribution, protein-binding and clearance of the drugs during pregnancy. Of the drugs in use Phenytoin has been associated with cleft palate and heart lesions. Sodium Valproate is particularly likely to result in neural tube defects and Carbamazepine has been associated with microcephaly and intra-uterine growth retardation. Anti-convulsants have also been associated with lowered serum folate concentrations and alterations in vitamin K metabolism increasing the risk of neo-natal haemorrhage. Folate and vitamin K supplements may therefore be given to the mother and all neo-nates of treated mothers should receive intramuscular vitamin K.

Pregnancy does not seem to have any constant effect on the disease itself and the risk of an epileptic mother having an epileptic child is about 1 in 40.

JAUNDICE

Jaundice is uncommon in pregnancy. The incidence is 1 in 1,500 pregnancies.

Aetiology

A. **Pregnancy jaundice**
   1. Acute fatty liver
   2. Cholestatic jaundice.
   3. Complicating pre-eclampsia and eclampsia.

B. **Intercurrent jaundice**
   1. Viral hepatitis.
   2. Obstructive jaundice due to gall stones.

C. **Iatrogenic jaundice**
   1. Hepatotoxic drugs.
   2. Drugs interfering with conjugation of bilirubin.
   3. Drugs causing haemolytic conditions.

The most common causes of jaundice in pregnancy are:-
1. Viral hepatitis: 41%
2. Cholestatic jaundice: 21%
3. Obstructive jaundice: less than 6%

VIRAL HEPATITIS

In epidemics the incidence is the same in pregnant and non-pregnant, but sporadic cases are more frequent in pregnancy.

Two types exist:- Hepatitis A virus, the cause of so-called catarrhal jaundice, is usually a mild condition; Hepatitis B virus (Australia antigen) is more serious and may be fatal. Hepatitis A is passed via faeces, water, milk, and is relatively uncommon in this country. Hepatitis B (serum jaundice) is spread by blood and blood products. Increasing use of these makes it a danger not only to the patient but also the the attendant staff. Laboratory specimens from an infected patient are dangerous and, at delivery, her blood will contaminate dressings and instruments. Folic acid deficiency is likely to develop in such a patient since the damaged liver is unable to store the vitamin. Spontaneous abortion and premature birth are said to be common.

RECURRENT CHOLESTATIC JAUNDICE OF PREGNANCY

This is a mild jaundice of unknown aetiology occurring in the last trimester. Jaundice may be absent and pruritus the only feature. The urine is usually dark and the stools pale. It recurs with each pregnancy.

This jaundice may be related to the high blood steroid level in pregnancy. A recurrent jaundice occurs in some patients given oral contraceptives, and these drugs should not be prescribed for any patient who has suffered from cholestatic jaundice in pregnancy.

JAUNDICE

ACUTE FATTY LIVER OF PREGNANCY   (Acute Yellow Atrophy of Pregnancy)

This is a rare but fatal disease occurring in the last trimester of pregnancy, characterised by a liver in which the cells are filled by small vacuoles of lipid surrounding a central nucleus.

The patient has severe nausea and vomiting, abdominal pain, haematemesis and becomes jaundiced. Headaches are severe and convulsions may occur. She becomes stuporose, lapses into coma; and death commonly takes place several days after delivery. The course is the same as in fulminating viral hepatitis. Acute pyelonephritis is frequently present and the patient is undernourished. Azotaemia, hyperuricaemia and acidosis occur.

Treatment is largely symptomatic. Vitamins such as B_{12} and folic acid plus lipotrophic substances like choline may be given but their efficiency is doubtful. The prognosis is extremely poor. The mother usually dies and the fetus is still-born.

PRE-ECLAMPSIA-ECLAMPSIA

In this condition the serum transaminase and alkaline phosphatase are commonly raised but jaundice is infrequent. When it does occur it is of haemolytic type and is usually a terminal event. It is related to haemorrhage in the liver.

GALL-STONES

These are associated with obesity and parity but not necessarily with multiparity. Jaundice due to gall-stones is uncommon in pregnancy. The management is the same as in the non-pregnant patient.

	Serum bilrubin	Serum Transaminase	Alkaline phosphatase
Viral hepatitis	Increased	Very high	Slightly increased
Recurrent Cholestatic Jaundice	Increase of conjugated bilirubin	Normal. Occasionally high	Increased
Acute fatty Liver	Increased	Moderate increase	Moderate increase
Gall-stones	Increase of conjugated bilirubin	Normal	Increased

JAUNDICE

OTHERS

Jaundice can be a terminal event in severe hyperemesis but this is a rare occurrence. Milder jaundice may be caused by haemolytic blood diseases e.g. acholuric jaundice, sickle-cell anaemia, haemoglobinopathies.

DRUGS AND JAUNDICE

Tetracycline, in large doses, can cause acute fatty liver.

Chlorpromazine, phenothiazine, chlorpropamide and anabolic steroids can cause a mild cholestatic jaundice.

Sulphonamides tend to displace bilirubin from its sites of conjugation and novobiocin inhibits conjugation of bilirubin in the liver. They should therefore be avoided in the newborn since they may lead to jaundice and kernicterus.

Glucose 6-phosphate dehydrogenase deficiency occurs in Mediterranean races. Phenacetin given to a mother bearing a child with such a deficiency may precipitate jaundice in the baby. Isoniazid and P.A.S. can cause a severe jaundice resembling viral jaundice. Serum transaminase rises before jaundice appears.

THYROID DISEASE

Overt thyroid disease is uncommon in pregnancy since abnormal thyroid function affects fertility, but hyper- or hypothyroidism may declare themselves.

Physiology of the Thyroid Gland

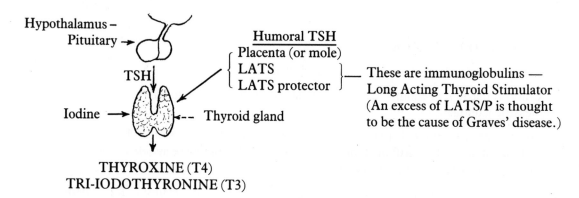

HYPERTHYROIDISM

Diagnosis

This is difficult in pregnancy because many of the signs and symptoms — anxiety, peripheral vasodilatation, weight loss, tachycardia, goitre — are all likely to appear to some degree in normal women. Diagnosis depends on the demonstration of a raised serum-free thyroxine.

Treatment

The thionamides (Carbimazole and Propylthiouracil) are the mainstay of treatment. Propylthiouracil is less readily transferred across the placenta or into breast milk and is probably the drug of choice. Biochemical control is essential and the aim is to keep the serum-free throxine in the high normal range. There is still a risk of fetal goitre due to fetal TSH secretion being suppressed. The newborn may suffer from transient goitre or hypothyroidism but death from tracheal compression and cretinism has been described.

Partial thryroidectomy is sometimes practised but fine judgement is required to avoid hypothyroidism after pregnancy.

THYROID DISEASE

The baby should be examined carefully after birth.

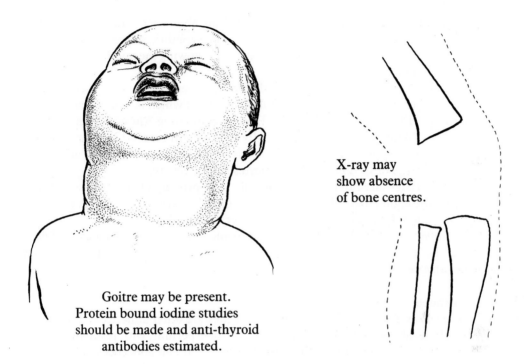

X-ray may
show absence
of bone centres.

Goitre may be present.
Protein bound iodine studies
should be made and anti-thyroid
antibodies estimated.

HYPOTHYROIDISM

Hypothyroidism causes reduced fertility but under treatment with thyroid substitutes fertility may be restored.

Thyroxine may be needed throughout pregnancy in varying dosage because of the altering demands as pregnancy advances. In some cases the thyroid gland hypertrophies and increases its function so that the thyroid substitution therapy can be reduced or stopped.

INFECTIONS

1. SEXUALLY TRANSMITTED DISEASES

(a) **Syphilis**

The fetus can be infected in utero with resulting abortion or still birth, and the liveborn baby may be congenitally syphilitic. The syphilitic placenta is a large pale organ very like the placenta in hydrops fetalis, and showing the microscopic changes of endarteritis and fibrosis.

Serological Tests — Every patient should be screened. The tests used are the VDRL (Venereal Disease Reference Laboratory) test which is non-specific together with the TPHA (Treponema Pallidum Haemagglutinating Antibody) test and the FTA–ABS (Fluorescent Treponema Antibody Absorption) test. The last is the most sensitive test for syphilis and becomes positive early in primary syphilis and remains so. The presence of IgM in this test indicates recent infection.

Clinical Signs are rarely seen antenatally. The primary chancre is usually on the labia and the inguinal glands enlarged. Signs of secondary syphilis include condylomata lata, mucous patches and a generalised rash.

Treatment — 600,000 units of procaine penicillin G given daily for a fortnight will protect the fetus and cure it if already infected. Both mother and child will require follow-up examination after delivery.

(b) **Gonorrhoea**

Symptoms in the female are so slight that they are often unnoticed. The patient may then develop a salpingitis especially in the puerperium, with resultant sterility. The infection is transmitted to the baby during labour and gonococcal ophthalmia appears about the 4th day. It is a serious condition which will lead to blindness if not treated.

Diagnosis — Smears should be taken from the urethral meatus and cervix, and the presence of intra-cellular Gram negative diplococci is highly suggestive. Material for culture must be sent off in a transport medium.

Treatment — A course of penicillin or erythromycin is given. When infection is or has been present, a smear for culture should be taken from the baby's eyes at birth and prophylactic antibiotic treatment given.

The patient's sexual partner or partners must also be investigated, and referral to a venereological clinic is the best way of doing this. The obstetrician's immediate responsibility is to ensure that the woman is adequately treated and that the fetus is protected.

INFECTIONS

SEXUALLY TRANSMITTED DISEASES (continued)

(c) **Acquired Immune-Deficiency Syndrome (AIDS)**
This condition is due to infection by a virus which has come to be known as Human Immunovirus (HIV). At the time of writing, knowledge about the effects of this virus on pregnancy is still scanty but the effects appear to be dire. Pregnancy appears to increase the risk of HIV carriers developing the full clinical syndrome. In addition, the babies of such infected mothers have a greater than 50% risk of being born with the disease and dying within 2 years. Current opinion favours offering these women termination of pregnancy. The issue of screening all pregnant women considered to be at risk is currently under debate.

2. 'TORCH' INFECTIONS

This acronym has been coined to describe a group of viral and protozoan infections producing similar fetal damage as a result of intra-uterine infection.

TO — Toxoplasmosis   R — Rubella
C — Cytomegalovirus   H — Herpes

(a) **Toxoplasmosis** — This is a protozoan parasite in which cats act as a host. Infection may occur from the ingestion of raw or partially cooked meat or any food contaminated by cat faeces. In communities where meat prepared in this way is commonly eaten antibodies will be detected in a high proportion of the population. Infection in the mother may be symptomless but it produces severe fetal effects. It can cause abortion and still-birth and neurological disorders such as microcephaly, hydrocephaly and cerebral calcification.

(b) **Rubella** — The dangers of Rubella infection in pregnancy are now well recognised. Cardiovascular lesions, cataract and deafness are the main lesions resulting from infection in early pregnancy. The risk of damage is greatest at this time and is over 30% when infection occurs within the first 4 weeks of pregnancy. Although much less common, mid-trimester infection can also produce damage, usually psychomotor defects leading to spasticity and mental retardation. All pregnant women are screened for Rubella immunity and about 85% of them will prove to be immune. Those who are not immune should be offered vaccination following pregnancy. It is also recommended that schoolgirls should be vaccinated routinely in the early 'teen years. Where there has been contact with Rubella in early pregnancy the mother may be reassured by the knowledge that she is immune. If there is a clinical suspicion of the disease serial testing may confirm or refute the diagnosis. Termination is commonly offered where infection is confirmed.

INFECTIONS

'TORCH' INFECTIONS (continued)

(c) **Cytomegalovirus** — This is a common infection which is usually subclinical in the mother. Congenital infection can occur from primary or re-infection of the mother. Abortion, still-birth, growth retardation, microcephaly and cerebral palsy can result. Intra-uterine infection occurs via the placenta but the baby may also be infected from the cervix at delivery or via breast milk. There is no way of confirming fetal infection and no treatment is available.

(d) **Herpes** — This is a common infection in the female genital tract, usually due to HSV type II. This can be identified by culture or by careful cytological examination. Infection of the fetus can be via the placenta or more commonly during vaginal delivery. If there is evidence of active infection Caesarean section is advisable. Infection via the placenta may result in abortion, growth retardation or neurological damage. In the neo-nate surface lesions may be present or the baby may die from widespread systemic infection. Local, external lesions on the mother may be treated with Acyclovir.

ACUTE ABDOMINAL CONDITIONS IN PREGNANCY

BOWEL OBSTRUCTION

Usually caused by adhesion bands altering in position with the rising uterus, but volvulus is sometimes found. Colic, distension, vomiting, diminished or absent bowel sounds are signs that laparotomy is required.

APPENDICITIS

The point of maximum tenderness is higher in pregnancy, and the high steroid levels will reduce the usual response to inflammation. There is usually sickness; and if doubt persists after a period of observation, laparotomy should be carried out. If pus is present, wound drainage should be continued for at least a week. Acute pyelonephritis may present much the same clinical picture, but loin tenderness and urine findings help in diagnosis.

URINARY CALCULUS

This causes acute pain radiating to the groin and haematuria is present. Treatment is conservative unless hydronephrosis develops and ureteric drainage is required.

DEGENERATING FIBROIDS

Necrobiosis causes pain, vomiting, tenderness and pyrexia, and diagnosis is difficult. The condition should settle with rest and sedation, and operation is only likely to be indicated when there is torsion of the pedicle of a fibroid.

PERFORATION OF ACUTE PEPTIC ULCER

This is very rare in pregnancy because of the high steroid level. The clinical appearances in the early months are unmistakably of perforation, but are less clear in the 3rd trimester. There is little rigidity, but shock is marked and air may be palpated or shown by X-ray, under the diaphragm.

OVARIAN CYST

Torsion of the pedicle causes acute pain, tenderness, vomiting and often pyrexia. Under anaesthesia a mass separate from the uterus may be distinguished, and laparotomy must be performed.

Laporotomy for these conditions often brings on labour or abortion, although removal of an untwisted ovarian cyst is usually safe enough. Section is not advisable in the presence of intra-abdominal infection.

CHAPTER 8

DISEASES OF PREGNANCY

VOMITING IN PREGNANCY

This is common and causes much misery. Nausea and morning sickness have been mentioned under Antenatal Care but vomiting can occur at any time.

It is associated with a long interval between meals and frequent, small carbohydrate meals help. Drug treatment may sometimes be necessary. Antihistamines such as Meclozine and Cyclizine are the drugs of choice.

Morning sickness usually stops spontaneously at 14–16 weeks.

HYPEREMESIS GRAVIDARUM or PERNICIOUS VOMITING OF PREGNANCY.

This is a progression from morning sickness to vomiting all food and drink.

This leads to dehydration and starvation with ketosis, multiple neuropathies, liver damage, jaundice, Wernicke's encephalopathy and ultimately to death.

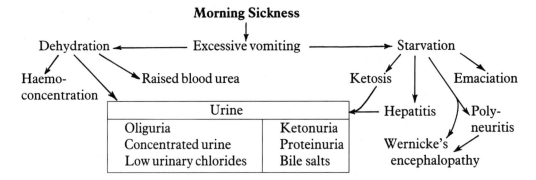

The progress from mild sickness to excessive vomiting is often insidious and accompanied by short lived improvements.

Removal to hospital usually gives marked improvement or cure and stimulates the belief that the illness is of the psyche.

Sickness may be severe and dangerous before a period has been missed. This supports the humoral theory; one in five have severe vomiting prior to the missed period.

Oestrogens, progesterones and chorionic gonadotrophins all have been blamed but no consistent proven relationship established.

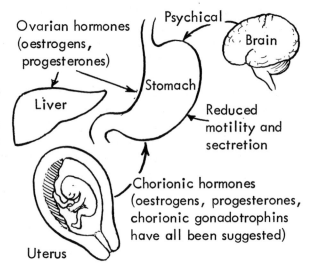

VOMITING IN PREGNANCY

The condition is aggravated by multiple pregnancy and hydatidiform mole and relieved by abortion.

Immune reactions have been postulated.

Rejection of the pregnancy, or of the husband or a demand for more attention have all been suggested as psychological causes.

Treatment

1. Admit to hospital.
2. Check blood for haemoglobin, full blood count, urea, sugar, electrolytes and liver function tests.
3. Intravenous fluids, salts and sugars are given unless the general condition is satisfactory when oral fluids may be used.
4. Insulin may be given to stimulate appetite and metabolism of carbohydrates. Intravenous amino acids and vitamins may be used.
5. When dehydration is overcome, oral foods are given, preferably without, or with very little, liquid accompaniment. Fluids should be taken separately. Any food notions of the patient within reason should be followed.
6. A normal diet should be tried.
7. Return to home but if sickness recurs then re-admit to hospital.
8. In intractable cases total parenteral nutrition may be employed to allow the pregnancy to continue.
9. Occasionally an otherwise normal pregnancy has to be terminated if there is deterioration despite treatment, and if polyneuritis or psychosis develops.
10. A pathological conceptus should be evacuated when the patient is fit.

Other causes of vomiting besides pregnancy should be considered at any period of gestation. The diagnosis of pregnancy should be established.

Appendicitis, bowel obstruction and volvulus can occur and be difficult to recognise.

Abdominal tumours such as twisting cysts or fibroids can cause vomiting.

Hepatic disorders, cerebral tumours and uraemia may be present and cause sickness in pregnancy.

Urinary infection often presents as sickness in mid and late pregnancy. A mid stream specimen of urine should be examined.

Hiatus hernia may give much misery with regurgitation and sickness in mid and late pregnancy. Treatment is by posture, antacids and small frequent meals.

Acute hydramnios and pre-eclamptic toxaemia can cause vomiting.

Acute fatty liver of pregnancy may present with sickness (see **JAUNDICE** — Chapter 7).

RHESUS INCOMPATIBILITY

Haemolytic disease of the newborn occurs when antibodies formed in the mother, in response to the introduction into her circulation of foreign antigen, cross the placenta and destroy fetal cells bearing the foreign antigen.Rhesus incompatibility is the commonest cause of haemolytic disease but it can be caused by ABO incompatibility when small molecule alpha and beta haemolysins are present, or by the presence of other antibodies such as anti-Duffy and anti-Kell.

Pregnancy is the time when a woman is most likely to be exposed to the stimulating antigen by the escape of fetal cells into the maternal circulation. This occurs at times of placental separation, notably the third stage of labour. It may also occur however with abortion or ante-partum haemorrhage or due to surgical procedures such as amniocentesis or external version. Inappropriate blood transfusion should no longer be a cause of Rhesus sensitation.

FISHER CLASSIFICATION OF RHESUS FACTOR

In each individual Rhesus genes are carried on two chromosomes either of which may be handed on to the succeeding generation. There are six main Rhesus genes, three carried on each chromosome. Of the six, three are dominant C, D and E and three, their alleles, c, d, e are recessive. Each chromosome has a C locus, a D locus and an E locus which may be occupied by a dominant or recessive gene of the particular type.

The most important gene in Rhesus incompatibility is the dominant D gene. Persons possessing this gene are commonly termed Rhesus positive. When it is absent from both chromosomes and its place is occupied by the recessive d allele, the individual is termed Rhesus negative. The term genotype means the mixture of genes on two chromosomes.

For example:
CDe/cDE — Homozygously Rhesus positive
CDe/cde — Heterozygously Rhesus positive
cde/cde — Rhesus negative.

83% of the UK population are Rhesus positive i.e. possess at least one dominant D gene.

17% of the UK population are Rhesus negative i.e. do not possess a dominant D gene, but have two recessive d genes.

It follows that of the men that a Rhesus negative woman might marry, 83% will be Rhesus positive. Of these 35% are homozygously positive and 48% heterozygously positive.

158

RHESUS INCOMPATIBILITY

The genetic make-up of the father is most important. Examine the following diagrams representing two families.

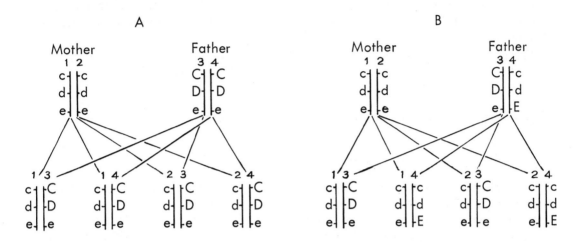

In family A where both mother and father are homozygous the Rhesus genetic make-up of their offspring will always be the same $\begin{array}{c} c \\ d \\ e \end{array} \bigg| \begin{array}{c} C \\ D \\ e \end{array}$. If, as is likely, the mother forms antibodies, every child will be affected and the outcome of each succeeding pregnancy will tend to be more hazardous than the previous.

In family B the outcome of a pregnancy will depend on which chromosome is handed on by the father. If chromosome 3, $\begin{array}{c} C \\ D \\ e \end{array}$ is transmitted to the fetus then antibody formation will result. On the other hand chromosome 4, $\begin{array}{c} c \\ d \\ E \end{array}$ is unlikely to stimulate antibody formation. In circumstances such as these, the disease may only affect every other child in the family.

In practice, the capacity of the various Rhesus genes to stimulate antibody formation varies. D is the strongest antigen and d is the weakest. Formerly more than 95% of cases of Rhesus incompatibilty were due to the dominant D but with the introduction of anti-D prophylaxis haemolytic disease due to antibodies other than D is relatively more important. Anti-c and anti-E are the commonest antibodies implicated.

RHESUS INCOMPATIBILITY

The other factor which determines whether the process of immunisation is initiated in the mother or not, is the ABO blood group of the mother and fetus. The immunisation of the mother is brought about by the escape of fetal red cells into the maternal circulation. If the fetal cells are ABO compatible with those of the mother they will persist in her circulation and will stimulate antibody formation. If they are ABO incompatible they will be destroyed rapidly and no immunisation will occur.

The circumstances might be as follows.

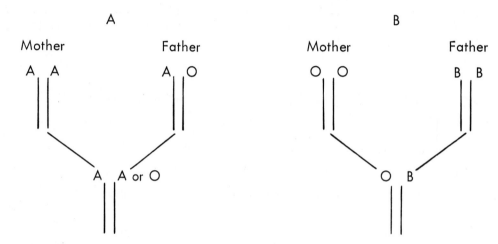

In family A the fetal blood is compatible with the maternal, and fetal cells will continue to live after escape into the maternal circulation. If the mother is Rhesus negative and the fetus Rhesus positive antibodies will form. The fetal cells in example B are incompatible with the maternal blood and will be rapidly destroyed on entry into the maternal circulation. No antibodies are likely to form even if there is Rhesus incompatibility.

Before Rhesus immunisation is likely to occur the red cells of the fetus must have a blood group either the same as the mother or group O, and must possess a Rhesus gene not found in the mother.

RHESUS INCOMPATIBILITY

ANTIBODY FORMATON AND DETECTION

When fetal cells enter and persist in the mother's circulation two antibodies are formed. The first, the Saline Antibody (IgM), generally appears seven days after stimulation. It agglutinates Rhesus positive cells suspended in saline. It is a large molecule and does not cross the placenta.

Twenty-one days after stimulation the Albumin Antibody (IgG) appears in the maternal blood. It is a small molecule and crosses the placenta easily and attacks the Rhesus positive red cells of the baby. It generally agglutinates Rhesus positive cells provided they are suspended in plasma, serum or albumin. Frequently, however, it is difficult to read tests for the antibody formed in this way and its detection is made easier if the Rhesus positive cells are first treated with enzymes such as papain.

Kleihauer Test

The presence of fetal cells in the mother's circulation can be demonstrated by this test. It depends on the fact that fetal haemoglobin is more resistant than adult to acid elution. When a blood film is stained following elution the fetal cells will stand out against the adult 'ghost' cells. It is roughly quantitative by counting the number of fetal cells per 50 low power fields. 5 cells per 50 fields = a bleed of 0.5ml.

Fetal cell

Adult 'ghost' cell

Coombs' Test

This test depends on the fact that antibodies are globulins. If these globulins are injected into an animal antibodies to them will be formed. These antibodies can in turn be used to detect the presence of the original antibodies. The Coombs' reagent therefore is immune anti-globulin.

The **DIRECT** test is used to detect an affected fetus at birth. Cells from cord blood are suspended with the reagent and if the baby is affected (has maternal antibody attached) agglutination will occur.

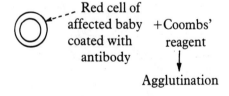

Red cell of affected baby coated with antibody +Coombs' reagent

↓

Agglutination

The **INDIRECT** test (IAGT) is used to detect and measure antibody in the mother's serum. This is suspended with test cells. Antibody in the serum will coat the cells and agglutination will occur when the Coombs' reagent is added. By using dilutions of the mother's serum a measure of the amount of antibody (titre) is obtained.

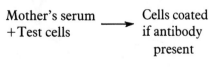

Mother's serum + Test cells → Cells coated if antibody present

Now add Coombs' reagent

↓

Agglutination

161

RHESUS INCOMPATIBILITY

EFFECTS ON FETUS AND NEO-NATE

The basis of the disease is a haemolytic anaemia brought about by the action of maternal anti-Rhesus albumin antibody. Levels of unconjugated bilirubin rise and there is a compensating erythropoesis.

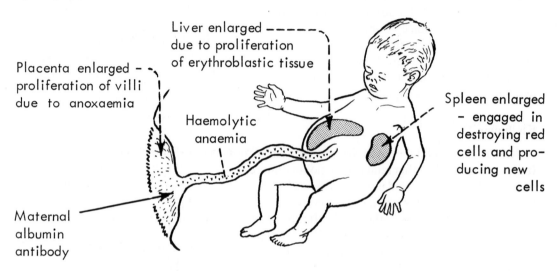

In its most severe form the process produces Fetal Hydrops which is invariably fatal either in utero or shortly after birth. Here the severity of the anaemia has resulted in cardiac failure with widespread oedema. Ante-natally the diagnosis may be made by ultrasound or X-ray.

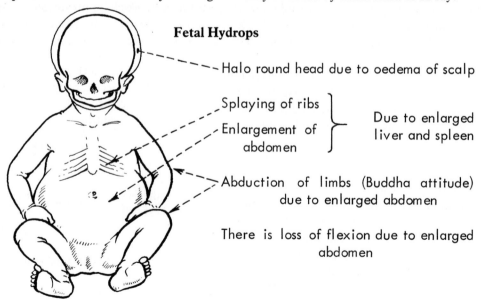

Fetal Hydrops

Halo round head due to oedema of scalp

Splaying of ribs
Enlargement of abdomen
} Due to enlarged liver and spleen

Abduction of limbs (Buddha attitude) due to enlarged abdomen

There is loss of flexion due to enlarged abdomen

RHESUS INCOMPATIBILITY

Effects on Fetus and Neo-Nate (continued)

Less severe degrees of the condition in the neo-nate are known as Icterus Gravis or congenital anaemia of the newborn.

CONGENITAL ANAEMIA OF NEWBORN

A mild haemolytic condition

Child : Pale
Liver : Slightly enlarged
Spleen : Slightly enlarged
Blood : Mild anaemia. Hb 13–15g
          per dl.
          Few reticulocytes.
          Bilirubin scarcely increased.
Urine : Negative test for bile.

ICTERUS GRAVIS

Severe haemolytic condition.
Child : Golden yellow jaundice appears
          within minutes of birth.
Liver : Greatly enlarged.
Spleen : Much enlarged.
Blood : Rapidly increasing anaemia.
          Numerous reticulocytes,
          erythroblasts, normoblasts,
          and early white cells.
          Indirect and direct bilirubin
          increased and rising.
Urine : Positive test for bile.

KERNICTERUS is a condition which may arise in any form of neo-natal jaundice when the unconjugated bilirubin level rises above 340μmol/litre. Rhesus incompatibility is the main cause. Bilirubin enters the fetal brain tissue causing necrosis of neurones especially in the basal ganglia. The infant becomes lethargic and refuses to suck. Convulsions, rolling of eyes and head retraction develop. Death may occur. If the infant survives, permanent mental and physical disabilities develop.

RHESUS INCOMPATIBILITY

PREVENTION OF RHESUS HAEMOLYTIC DISEASE

The initiation of antibody formation starts in the first Rhesus incompatible pregnancy. Many women have antibodies in their blood in the late puerperium. Although small numbers of fetal red cells escape into the maternal circulation during pregnancy, the important immunising dose is usually received by the mother at the time of delivery when the placenta is compressed and separated. It is for this reason that Rhesus sensitisation is uncommon in first pregnancies.

If the fetus is Rh +ve these red cells will stimulate antibody formation.

D antigen on surface of rbc ⟶ Specific IgM and IgG formation stimulated

The problem is to 'hide' the D antigen so that the maternal immune mechanism does not recognise the cells as 'foreign' and antibodies will not then be formed. This is done by giving the mother anti-D which attaches itself to the D antigens of the fetal red cells making them unrecognisable by the immune mechanism and therefore incapable of stimulating antibody formation.

D antigens + injected anti-D ⟶ Shell of anti-D 'hiding' D antigens ⟶ Accepted as compatible by mother — No stimulation of immune mechanism

Procedure

Tests are carried out as in the flow diagram. All Rh -ve women, without antibodies, giving birth to Rh +ve babies are given an injection of anti-D globulin. A rough estimate of the amount of fetal blood escaping into the maternal circulation is made by means of the Kleihauer test and the dose of globulin adjusted. The giving of anti-D is not however dependent on a positive Kleihauer test. The standard dose is 500 I.U., given within 72 hours of delivery. This treatment has greatly reduced the incidence of problems arising from Rhesus incompatibility in pregnancy. It has to be repeated in each pregnancy.

Where pregnancy ends before 20 weeks (the blood group of the fetus will not usually be known), 250 I.U. of anti-D should be given.

Cord blood
↓
Test Rhesus groups

Rhesus +ve
↓
Keihauer test on maternal blood
↓
If less than 4ml fetal rbc
↓
Standard dose of anti-D to mother

Rhesus −ve
↓
No action necessary

If more than 4ml fetal rbc
↓
Increase dose of anti-D to mother accordingly

Similarly when invasive procedures such as amniocentesis or external version are carried out anti-D is given. Other episodes of placental separation such as abortion and ante-partum haemorrhage should be covered by anti-D administation, the dosage being determined by the stage of pregnancy and the estimated volume of the bleed.

RHESUS INCOMPATIBILITY

MANAGEMENT OF PREGNANCY

1. **Rhesus negative without antibodies**
   (a) First visit — Rhesus group and screening test for immune antibodies.
   (b) Repeat antibody check monthly after 20 weeks.
   (c) Give anti-D immunoglobulin for complications as above.
   (d) Delivery: Mother's blood — antibody check and Kleihauer.

   Cord blood — ABO and Rhesus group,

   Haemoglobin,

   Coombs',

   Bilirubin.
   (e) Give anti-D if blood negative for antibodies and baby Rhesus positive. If Kleihauer suggests bleed more than 4ml, further anti-D given.

2. **Rhesus negative with antibodies**
   (a) *First visit* — antibody identified and measured by IAGT and/or direct quantitation.
   (b) *Antibody test* repeated monthly or until management decided on by other investigations e.g. amniocentesis.
   (c) *Rhesus genotyping of partner* — if heterozygously Rhesus positive the possibility of an unaffected child exists.
   (d) *Amniocentesis* — the bilirubin level in the liquor is a useful prognostic index. The amount of bilirubin excreted into the liquor by the baby reflects the degree of haemolysis. The fluid obtained is examined in a spectrophotometer and the optical density measured with light of wavelengths varying from 400mμ to 700mμ. In normal pregnancy the density values at these various wavelengths form a straight line graph. In pregnancy affected by Rhesus incompatibility the fluid contains bile pigments and these cause a peak at 450mμ. The difference in optical density between the normal and the abnormal at this wavelength is an indication of the severity of the disease. Whitfield's modification of Liley's prediction graph with its useful 'Action Line' is widely used (see following page).

RHESUS INCOMPATIBILITY

(d) *Amniocentesis* (continued)
Whitfield's modification of Liley's prediction graph:

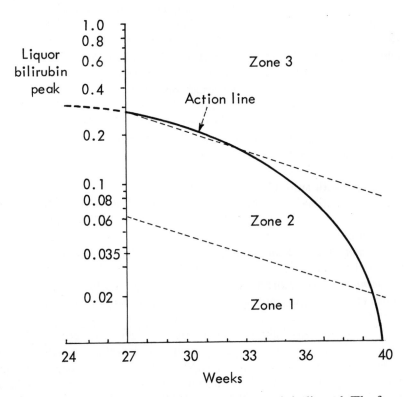

When the bilirubin level crosses the action line treatment is indicated. The form of the treatment depends on the maturity of the pregnancy.

Amniocentesis is indicated in all patients with a history of a significantly affected baby or, in the absence of such history, in all patients with an antibody level of 2.5 I.U./ml or more, or an IAGT titre of 1/8.

The timing of the first amniocentesis is crucial. A rough guide is to perform it 10 weeks before the time of the earliest previous death or delivery of a severely affected baby. If there is no such history the first test should be performed at 28–30 weeks. The test will usually be repeated to establish the trend in 2–3 weeks but may be done sooner in severe cases.

(e) *Ultrasound* — ultrasound can now detect fetal ascites and scalp oedema indicating a severely affected fetus. This may point to the need for intervention in some cases before the results of amniocentesis and is especially valuable in very early cases where fetal transfusion may be contemplated.

RHESUS INCOMPATIBILITY

TREATMENT

1. Delivery

Delivery of the baby, prematurely if necessary, followed by assessment of its condition and exchange transfusion if necessary is the traditional treatment of Rhesus sensitised patients. Those with very low levels of antibody (less than 2.5 I.U./ml) may be safely allowed to proceed to term when they should be induced. The timing of intervention in other cases depends on the patient's history, amniocentesis results and ultrasound surveillance. Where early intervention (under 32–33 weeks) is indicated, the demonstration of fetal lung maturity may determine whether labour should be induced or an attempt made to prolong the pregnancy by fetal transfusion.

After birth the cord blood is examined:

       a. Coombs' test.
       b. Blood grouping and Rhesus typing.
       c. Haemoglobin estimation.
       d. Serum bilirubin.

A positive Coombs' test indicates an affected baby.

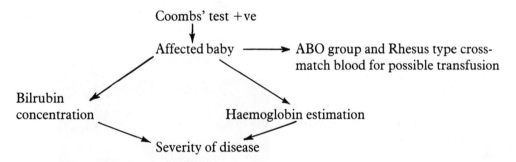

Mild degrees of anaemia (not below 12g/dl) may not require treatment and mild degrees of jaundice may respond to phototherapy. More seriously affected babies will require an EXCHANGE TRANSFUSION. This means the withdrawal of blood through the umbilical vein and its replacement with healthy compatible blood. It thus corrects anaemia and reduces high levels of circulating bilirubin which would cause kernicterus and washes out any free circulating antibodies. The decision to perform transfusion is not based simply on cord blood findings. The patient's history, the maturity of the baby and the rate of increase in the bilirubin level in the baby are all critical.

RHESUS INCOMPATIBILITY

Treatment (continued)

2. Fetal Transfusion

Intraperitoneal fetal transfusion has been used to treat severely affected babies, expected to die, at a gestation when delivery and exchange transfusion would not be possible.

Packed cells, usually O negative, are injected into the fetal peritoneal cavity and are readily absorbed into the circulation. As much as 120ml can be absorbed in a few days.

When first introduced the technique was carried out under X-ray guidance but nowadays real-time ultrasound will often be preferred.

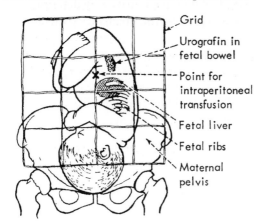

- Grid
- Urografin in fetal bowel
- Point for intraperitoneal transfusion
- Fetal liver
- Fetal ribs
- Maternal pelvis

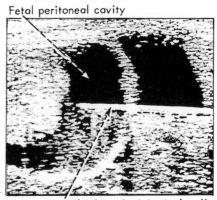

Fetal peritoneal cavity

Needle through abdominal wall

The procedure may be repeated as required at intervals of about 2 weeks.

Direct intravascular transfusion at very early stages of gestation (less than 23 weeks) has been employed in recent years. Injections can be made directly into the cord, guided either by fetoscopy or ultrasound.

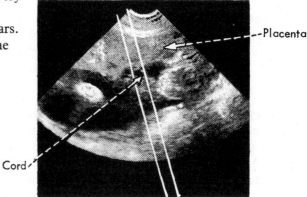

Placenta

Cord

3. Plasmaphoresis

Reduction of high antibody levels has been achieved by the use of a continuous flow cell separator. In some cases intraperitoneal transfusion has thus been avoided or postponed. The need for such therapy has however been reduced by improvements in the technique of fetal transfusion and standards of neo-natal care.

HYPERTENSION IN PREGNANCY

Raised blood pressure in pregnancy is a common and potentially dangerous complication associated with increased mortality and morbidity, both maternal and fetal.

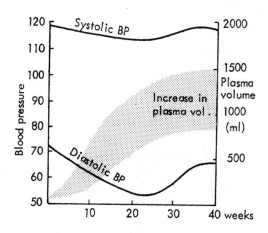

The normal resting blood pressure is virtually never above 120/80, and since the plasma volume increase averages 12 dl, there must be some vasodilatation to allow the peripheral pressure to remain low. If this vasodilatation is counteracted by arteriolar spasm, hypertension results, and there is a reduction in the perfusion of all organs, including the uterus and thus the placental site.

Blood pressure readings of > 140/90mmHg or where the diastolic pressure has risen by more than 20mmHg are considered abnormal.

The reported overall incidence varies widely and usually lies between 12 and 25% of all pregnancies.

Hypertension is conveniently divided into:

(a) *Pregnancy Induced or Gestational*, where the blood pressure rises after 20 weeks in a previously normotensive woman. This group will include patients in whom hypertension is the first sign of developing pre-eclampsia and some patients with latent essential hypertension.

(b) *Pre-existing* hypertension, where there is an elevated blood prssure before pregnancy or in the first 20 weeks. This may be due to essential hypertension, renal or adrenal disorders, connective tissue disorders, drug therapy or coarctation of the aorta.

The term **Pre-eclampsia** is increasingly confined to patients with hypertension and proteinuria developing in the second half of pregnancy. Exceptions to this may be hydatidiform mole or multiple pregnancy and severe Rhesus disease.

Two other physical signs, proteinuria and oedema, are commonly associated with hypertension.

Proteinuria is a serious complication of hypertension. It indicates renal impairment and it is inferred that placental function is similarly affected with consequent threat to the baby. A small amount of proteinuria is normal in pregnancy but the level should be < 300mg/vol in a 24 hour collection.

Other causes of proteinuria: Contamination, Urinary tract infection, Renal disease, Connective tissue disorders, Orthostatic — 'lordotic proteinuria'

Oedema in pregnancy, even when generalised, is so common as to be considered normal if unassociated with hypertension. It should not, however, be ignored. It may give early warning of developing pre-eclampsia and when associated with a hypertensive pregnancy may be a sign of deterioration or progression to eclampsia.

169

HYPERTENSION IN PREGNANCY

PRE-ECLAMPSIA

Pre-eclampsia is a disease of the second half of pregnancy characterised by hypertension, evidence of renal impairment (see below) and, commonly, excessive oedema.
Incidence: 5 to 7% of primigravid pregnancies. The disease here is 'primary' i.e. occurring in a patient whose blood pressure was previously normal and disappearing after pregnancy.

Pre-eclampsia may also be 'secondary' i.e. superimposed on pre-existing hypertension. The risk of superimposed pre-eclampsia in essential hypertension is approximately 30-35% and in renal disease greater than 60%.

Aetiology: The cause of the condition is unknown but there is a clear predisposition in certain groups:
1. Primigravid patients or in the first pregnancy with a given partner.
2. Increased risk with age.
3. Family history of pre-eclampsia or hypertension.
4. Pre-existing hypertension.
5. Multiple pregnancy.
6. Diabetic pregnacy.
7. Hydatidiform mole.
8. Severe Rhesus sensitisation.

Associated functional changes:

A great mass of data on the pathological and patho-physiological changes in this much studied disease has been accumulated. The significance of many of the observations remains uncertain. There are however some well recognised functional changes of immediate relevance to clinical management:

1. **Impaired renal function**
    Specific glomerular changes have been described as characteristic of 'true pre-eclampsia'. There is however evidence of both glomerular and tubular dysfunction.
    (a) Proteinuria (see above) means there has been increased escape of protein from the glomeruli. Levels should be quantified after exclusion of contamination and infection.
    (b) Uric acid retention: 80% of uric acid in the urine is secreted by the distal tubule. As this function is impaired there is a rise in plasma urate. Levels $>350\mu$mol/l are significant and may be an early indicator of the onset of pre-eclampsia.
    (c) Urea and Creatinine levels may rise. Levels > 6mmol/l and 100μmol/l respectively are significant.

HYPERTENSION IN PREGNANCY

PRE-ECLAMPSIA — Associated Functional Changes (continued)

2. **Disseminated Intravascular Coagulation** (DIC)
   This is evidenced by an increase in fibrin degradation products (from a normal of about $3\mu g/ml$ to 14) and a falling platelet count (from normal 300,000/mm^3 to 150,000). Platelet levels may fall much lower in severe cases and micro-angiopathic haemolysis secondary to small vessel blockage may be seen with fragmented red cells in the peripheral blood.

3. **Utero-placental perfusion**
   The investigation of this important area is particularly difficult but the studies done indicate that there is a significant decrease in utero placental perfusion in pre-eclampsia. The implications for fetal well-being are obvious and are an important consideration in the management of these patients. In practice, deterioration of placental function is often inferred from worsening renal impairment e.g. increasing proteinuria.

ECLAMPSIA

Pre-eclampsia is a disease of signs without symptoms. If it progresses towards eclampsia, however, the patient may complain of headache or visual disturbances due to rising blood pressure and abdominal pain, usually attributed to sub-capsular haemorrhage in the liver. The patient may be agitated, rest-less and hyper-reflexive and an epileptiform seizure follows.

An eclamptic convulsion

Incidence: A rare complication in the United Kingdom, < 1/1000 pregnancies.
Mortality — It remains a dangerous complication with a fetal mortality up to 30%.
Maternal mortality from cerebral haemorrhage, heart or renal failure is 2–3%.

171

HYPERTENSION IN PREGNANCY

ECLAMPSIA (continued)

Clinical Features

1. (Usually) signs of fulminating PE — very high BP, heavy proteinuria, acute oedema — with complaints of headache and visual upsets.
2. Twitching of face and hands.
3. Tonic phase with rigidity, apnoea, cyanosis.
4. Clonic phase with spasmodic movements, during which the patient may throw herself out of bed.
5. Period of unconsciousness.

Differential diagnosis

1. *Epilepsy.* Epilepsy has no association with hypertension.
2. *Subarachnoid haemorrhage* or *cerebral haemorrhage.* The coma deepens. Lumbar puncture may be necessary.
3. *Brain tumour.* This must be considered if the patient does not respond to anticonvulsive treatment or if coma deepens.
4. *Uraemia* from a cause other than pregnancy.

Complications

1. Hypertension causes *cerebral haemorrhage* or *thrombosis.*

   The blood pressure must be controlled by hypotensive drugs.

2. Repeated fits with periods of anoxia lead to *pulmonary oedema* and *cardiac failure.*

   The fits must be prevented by anti-convulsant drugs.

3. Liver necrosis may lead to *acute liver failure.*
4. Glomerular or tubular necrosis may lead to *anuria.*
5. Placental necrosis will lead to *fetal death.*

   When the patient develops eclampsia, the pregnancy must be terminated.

Post-mortem findings

There is widespread damage to the capillaries due to hypertension and to disseminated intravascular coagulation. The **Liver** shows subcapsular haemorrhage and tiny areas of necrosis which can be seen microscopically to be in the periportal region of the liver lobules. The **Brain** may show large haemorrhages in the pontine region or the internal capsule, or small areas of haemorrhage scattered throughout its substance. Haemorrhages are also found in the **Lungs, Adrenals** and all other organs, and microscopic inspection will reveal damage to the glomerular tufts and tubule cells of the **Kidney**, and to the vessels of the **Placenta**.

HYPERTENSION IN PREGNANCY

CLINICAL COMPLICATIONS OF HYPERTENSIVE PREGNANCY

1. Intra-uterine growth retardation — risk increased in proteinuric pre-eclampsia.
2. Fetal hypoxia and intra-uterine death.
3. Abruption of the placenta.
4. Eclampsia.
5. Cerebro-vascular accident.
6. Cardiac failure.
7. Renal failure.

To these may be added the risks to both mother and child of operative and/or premature delivery.

MANAGEMENT OF HYPERTENSIVE PREGNANCY

1. **Detection**
   There is no established, practical screening procedure other than good ante-natal care. Regular supervision, especially of recognised high risk groups, should be shared between the general practitioner and hospital specialist.

2. **Observations**

   These are the routine observations carried out on patients in whom hypertension has been confirmed. On them are based decisions about treatment. Nowadays many hypertensive patients are assessed on an outpatient basis in Day Care Units with only more severe cases being admitted. Similarly the severity of the condition would determine the frequency of these observations.
   - (a) Serial blood pressure recordings.
   - (b) Quantitation of proteinuria.
   - (c) Serial uric acid levels.
   - (d) Serial platelet counts.
   - (e) Assessment of fetal growth and well-being by kick charts, cardiotocography and ultrasound estimates of fetal weight and liquor volume (see Chapter 6).

3. **Treatment**
   - (a) Bed-rest in hospital — Hospital admission is indicated if the diastolic blood pressure remains at 100mmHg or more. The presence of proteinuria and evidence of fetal impairment are also indications for admission. Many patients with hypertension arising late in pregnancy require no other treatment before delivery.

HYPERTENSION IN PREGNANCY

MANAGEMENT — Treatment (continued)

(b) Hypotensive Agents — These may be used in three situations — chronic hypertension, pregnancy induced hypertension and in the treatment of a hypertensive crisis or imminent eclampsia (see below).

     Many obstetricians are cautious about such agents in spite of the risks of hypertension because of anxieties about the effects of the drugs on placental perfusion. Recent studies suggest there may be fetal benefits in treating both chronic and pregnancy induced hypertension, but the level of blood pressure at which such treatment should be employed is controversial. Most would favour a diastolic pressure remaining > 100mmHg.

1. Methyldopa is well established in the treatment of chronic hypertension. It does not reduce the incidence of superimposed pre-eclampsia but its safety in pregnancy is accepted.

2. Beta blockers have been found to achieve good blood pressure control and it has been suggested that they may slow the progression of the disease in pregnancy induced hypertension. There seems to be little to choose between agents such as Oxprenolol, Atenolol and Labetalol.

(c) Delivery is the ultimate treatment of hypertensive pregnancy and its timing depends on the observations of fetal and maternal well-being noted above. Prolongation of the pregnancy by means of bed-rest or drug therapy will reduce the risks of prematurity and improve the chances of vaginal delivery. Epidural block for both analgesia in labour and delivery by Caesarean section is excellent providing the platelet count is satisfactory.

IMMINENT ECLAMPSIA and ECLAMPSIA

If the premonitory signs described above under 'Eclampsia' are observed, the following emergency treatment should be instituted:

(a) If a fit has already occurred the first task is to **establish an airway** and **give oxygen** by face mask. An immediate intravenous injection of 20mg Diazepam will help to stabilise the situation.

(b) **Anti-convulsant therapy**

Maintenance therapy can be achieved by an infusion of Diazepam or Chlormethiazole. An alternative, which seems to be becoming more popular, is Phenytoin which can be given intravenously or intramuscularly. It has the advantage of not sedating the patient.

HYPERTENSION IN PREGNANCY

Imminent Eclampsia and Eclampsia — Treatment (continued)

(c) Hypotensive therapy

Hydralazine 10–20mg intravenously remains popular with obstetricians. It is short-acting and can be given by slow injection or infusion. Diazoxide can also be given intravenously and it seems that using lower doses (30–100 mg) than were favoured formerly is quite safe. Larger doses have been associated with neo-natal hyperglycaemia. Both Hydralazine and Diazoxide act by producing relaxation of smooth muscle in vessel walls and, in theory therefore, should not affect uterine blood flow.

(d) Delivery

If the baby has survived the eclamptic seizure delivery should be undertaken as soon as the situation has been brought under control. A Caesarean section will often be the method of choice today. There is, however, a tendency for eclamptic patients to start labour spontaneously and, if the cervix is favourable, amniotomy can be done and Oxytocin stimulation started. If Caesarean section is performed, a general anaesthetic has some obvious advantages but an epidural can be used provided there is no evidence of coagulation defect.

(e) Urinary Output

The bladder must be drained by catheter throughout, to avoid stimulation from a full bladder and to facilitate nursing. Urine volumes should be measured hourly and if there is oliguria or anuria a diuresis should be induced by an intravenous infusion of Mannitol. If renal failure persists after delivery it usually responds well to dialysis.

(f) Cardio-respiratory system

Signs of congestion and pulmonary oedema must constantly be looked for, and if there is any sign of cardiac failure, digitalisation will be required.

(g) Coagulation failure

There is invariably some degree of disseminated intravascular coagulation, and coagulation factors such as fibrinogen, platelets, FDP's, thrombin, should be monitored. Post-partum anaemia is common.

COAGULATION FAILURE IN PREGNANCY

Normal haemostasis depends on constriction of blood vessels, aggregation of platelets in response to damage to the vascular endothelium and the generation of fibrin to form clot. This system is balanced by the fibrinolytic mechanism which removes fibrin and restores vascular patency.

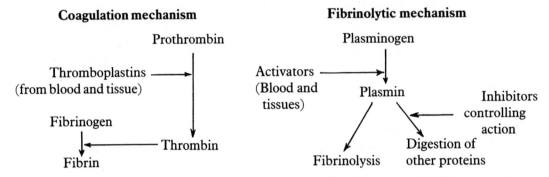

These two mechanisms are normally in a state of dynamic equilibrium. The coagulation mechanism is activated whenever vascular endothelium is breached. Fibrinolysis prevents vascular occlusion as soon as endothelial integrity is restored and removes the fibrin scaffold when no longer required in areas of repair.

Deficiency or absence of blood clotting can be brought about in two ways:-

1. Depletion of fibrinogen and other factors due to the formation of either a large blood clot or multiple small intravascular thrombi. Frequently both lesions are present due to escape of tissue thromboplastins into the blood stream.

2. Excessive production of plasminogen activators resulting in lysis of any clot formed.

These usually form two phases of the coagulation defect syndrome. Phase 1 depletion of fibrinogen is always present and, by the nature of the lesion causing it, is apt to initiate the phase of fibrinolysis.

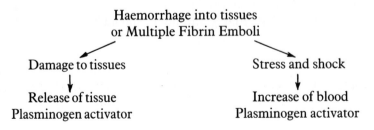

Phase 2 is particularly liable to occur in pregnancy since plasminogen activator is present in high concentration in the uterus and lungs.

COAGULATION FAILURE IN PREGNANCY

Once these two phases are in operation a further complication arises due to their interaction. Fibrin strand formation takes place in three steps.

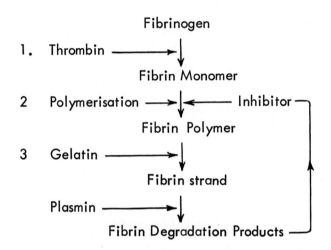

The products of fibrinolysis interfere with the second step and result in poor clot formation which is more susceptible to fibrinolysis. A vicious circle is therefore set up.

In addition to the coagulation defect the patient frequently exhibits symptoms of stress of a degree quite unrelated to the magnitude of the original causative condition. This is probably due to inadequate inhibition of the digestive action of plasmin.

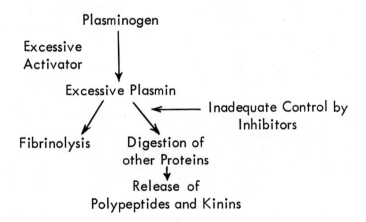

Kinins which are the result of digestion of α_2 globulins cause pain, increased permeability of capillaries, contraction of some smooth muscles and relaxation of others.

COAGULATION FAILURE IN PREGNANCY

The position may be summarised as follows:

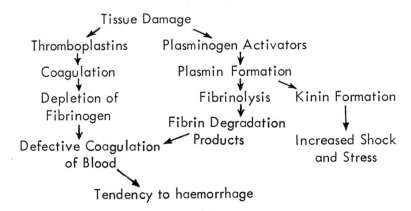

Tissue Damage

Thromboplastins   Plasminogen Activators

Coagulation   Plasmin Formation

Depletion of   Fibrinolysis   Kinin Formation
Fibrinogen
                         Fibrin Degradation
Defective Coagulation ← Products   Increased Shock
of Blood   and Stress

Tendency to haemorrhage

Aetiology

The coagulation failure syndrome is associated mainly with four conditions in pregnancy.

1. **Concealed Accidental Haemorrhage**

Clot — depletes fibrinogen, platelets and other clotting factors.

Damage to uterus and placenta — escape of thromboplastins and plasminogen activators into general circulation.

2. **Amniotic Fluid Embolism**   This catastrophic event is often fatal but fortunately rare. The diagnosis may only be made with certainty at post-mortem when emboli of vernix and bundles of squamous cells are identified in pulmonary vessels. It is a complication of artificial rupture of the membranes, Caesarean section and occasionally external version. There is sudden collapse associated with tachycardia, tachypnoea, cyanosis and hypotension. Multiple small emboli lodge in the lungs and venous pulmonary arterial pressures are increased. Multiple small intravascular fibrin clots are formed as well as amniotic emboli. Fibrinolysins are probably released from the damaged lung.

3. **Retention of a Dead Fetus**   A coagulation defect may occur in this condition but only if the dead fetus is retained for at least one month. Thromboplastins causing intravascular thrombi, and plasminogen activators are liberated from the degenerating placenta and fetus.

4. **Septic Abortion**   The mechanism is similar in this condition, various factors being liberated by the necrotic tissues. The condition is complicated by the presence of infection which may cause a kind of Schwartzmann reaction.

COAGULATION FAILURE IN PREGNANCY

Diagnosis and Treatment

Although a coagulation defect may be obvious the difficulty lies in diagnosing the phase. There are theoretically three phases.

1. *Coagulation.*   Thromboplastins may still be circulating in the blood even after the available fibronogen is consumed.
2. *Fibrinogen depletion.*   In this phase thromboplastins are no longer present but fibrinogen and other blood clotting factors are depleted.
3. *Fibrinolysis.*

The first phase is of extremely short duration and scarcely influences the approach to treatment. Difficulty lies mainly in differentiating phases 2 and 3 due to the fact that the patient's condition is usually critical and specific laboratory tests are too time-consuming.

Most cases of coagulation failure can be treated by combinations of whole blood and concentrates of red cells and platelets as indicated. The use of heparin to counteract widespread disseminated intravascular coagulation remains controversial and expert haematological guidance is essential.

CHAPTER 9

VAGINAL BLEEDING IN PREGNANCY

SUMMARY OF CAUSES

ECTOPIC PREGNANCY

6-8 weeks
Decidual Bleeding

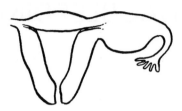

HYDATIDIFORM MOLE

ABORTION

Usually before
16 weeks

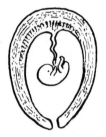

Usually before
16 weeks

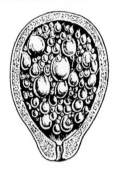

ANTE-PARTUM HAEMORRHAGE

After 28 weeks

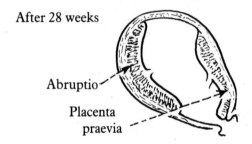

Abruptio

Placenta
praevia

Placental abnormalities (see Chapter 13)
e.g.
placental
circumvallata

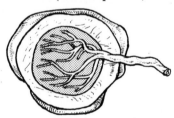

By definition, bleeding after 28 weeks; but these conditions may present in mid-trimester.

INTRA-PARTUM HAEMORRHAGE

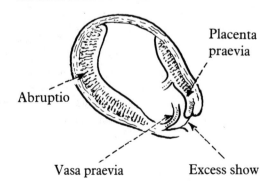

Placenta
praevia

Abruptio

Vasa praevia   Excess show

INCIDENTAL CAUSES

Cervical
carcinoma
(see
Chapter 10)

Cervical
ectopy

Cervical polyp

Varicosities
of cervix,
vagina or
vulva

Error
from urinary tract
or haemorrhoids

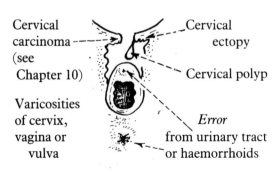

May present at any stage of pregnancy.

ECTOPIC PREGNANCY

Ectopic pregnancy is one in which the products of conception develop outside the uterine cavity. By far the commonest site is the fallopian tube.

The fallopian tube is about 10cm long. Its diameter varies from 1mm in the interstitial portion to about 5mm at the fimbriated end.

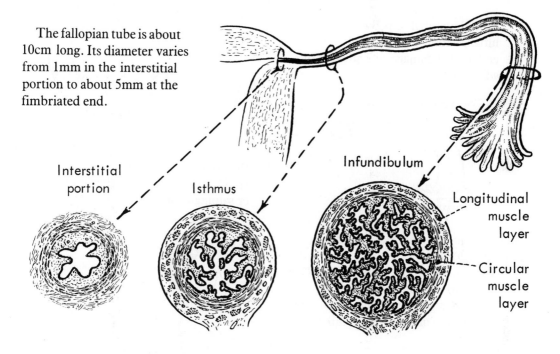

Interstitial portion

Isthmus

Infundibulum

Longitudinal muscle layer

Circular muscle layer

The musculature is of two layers, an inner circular and an outer longitudinal, and peristaltic movements are particularly strong during and after ovulation. The mucosa is arranged in plications or folds which become much more complete and plentiful as the infundibulum is approached.

The mucosa consists of a single layer of ciliated and secretory cells, resting on a thin basement membrane. There is little or no submucosa and no decidual reaction so muscle is easily invaded by trophoblast.

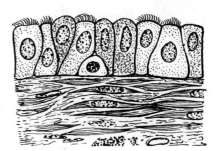

183

TUBAL PREGNANCY — AETIOLOGY

Ectopic implantation may be fortuitous or the result of a tubal abnormality which obstructs or delays the passage of the fertilised ovum.

1. Preceding tubal or pelvic inflammation with residual endothelial damage or distortion by adhesions.

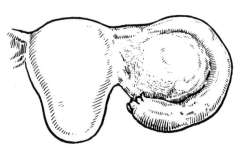

Tubal anastomosis

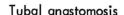
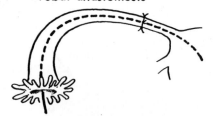

2. Previous tubal surgery e.g. attempted sterilisation, reversal of sterilisation or salpingostomy.

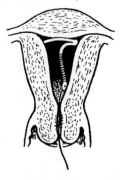

3. Intra-uterine contraceptive device (IUCD).
   Women who conceive with an IUCD in situ have an increased risk of ectopic pregnancy. This may be due to infection or an effect on tubal motility.

Diverticulum

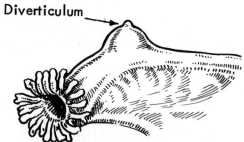

4. Congenital abnormality of the tube such as hypoplasia, elongation or diverticulum.

5. Migration of ovum across the pelvic cavity to the fallopian tube on the side opposite to the follicle from which ovulation occurred.

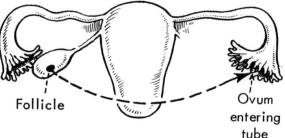

Follicle

Ovum entering tube

TUBAL PREGNANCY — IMPLANTATION

Because there is no decidual membrane in tubal mucosa, and no submucosa, the ovum rapidly burrows through the mucosa and embeds in the muscular wall of the tube, opening up maternal blood vessels and causing necrosis of muscle and connective tissue cells.

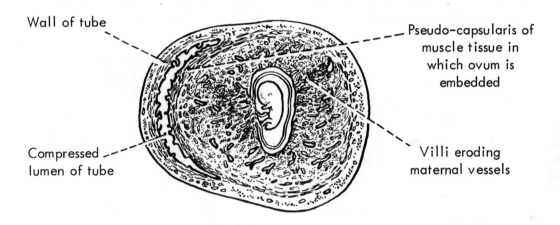

Wall of tube

Pseudo-capsularis of muscle tissue in which ovum is embedded

Compressed lumen of tube

Villi eroding maternal vessels

The ampulla is the commonest site of implantation, followed by the isthmus.

Interstitial implantation is rare but very dangerous because it ends in rupture of the uterine muscle with severe haemorrhage.

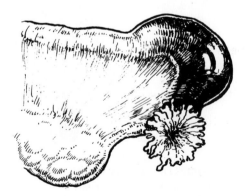

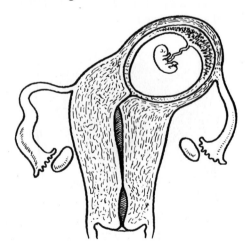

185

TUBAL PREGNANCY — OUTCOME

The muscle wall of the tube has not the capacity of uterine muscle for hypertrophy and distension and tubal pregnancy nearly always ends in rupture and the death of the ovum.

RUPTURE INTO LUMEN OF TUBE (TUBAL ABORTION)

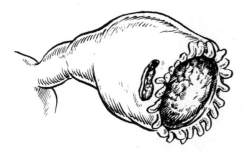

This is usual in ampullary pregnancy at about 8 weeks. The conceptus is extruded, complete or incomplete, towards the fimbriated end of the tube, probably by the pressure of accumulated blood. There is a trickle of bleeding into the peritoneal cavity, and this may collect as a clot in the pouch of Douglas. It is then called a pelvic haematocele.

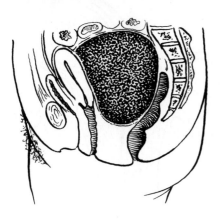

RUPTURE INTO THE PERITONEAL CAVITY

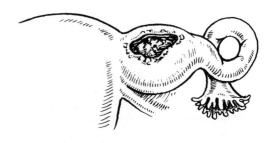

This may occur spontaneously, or from pressure (such as straining at stool, coitus or pelvic examination) and occurs mainly from the narrow isthmus before 8 weeks, or from the interstitial portion at 12 weeks. Haemorrhage is likely to be severe.

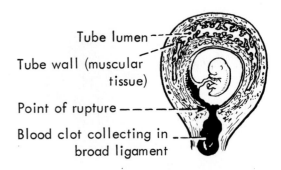

Tube lumen

Tube wall (muscular tissue)

Point of rupture

Blood clot collecting in broad ligament

Sometimes rupture is extraperitoneal between the leaves of the broad ligament — broad ligament haematoma. Haemorrhage in this site is more likely to be controlled.

TUBAL PREGNANCY — EFFECT ON UTERUS

The uterus enlarges in the first three months almost as if the implantation were normal, and may reach the size of a gravid uterus of the same maturity. This is a source of confusion in diagnosis.

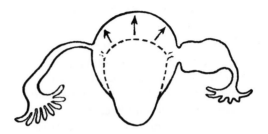

The uterine decidua grows abundantly, and when the ovum or embryo dies bleeding occurs as the decidua degenerates. Rarely it is expelled entire as a decidual cast and is replaced within a few weeks (perhaps before clinical diagnosis) by normal endometrium.

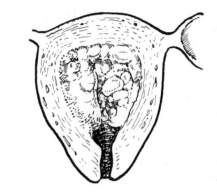

Enlargement of Non-Gravid Uterus

The picture shows a non-gravid uterus enlarged to the size of a 16 weeks' pregnancy. It was seen at laparotomy carried out in the 34th week of an abdominal pregnancy in which the placenta was attached to the pelvic floor and the broad ligament.

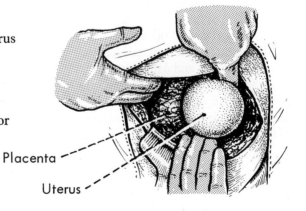

Placenta

Uterus

187

TUBAL PREGNANCY — SYMPTOMS AND SIGNS

Tubal pregnancy can present in many ways and misdiagnosis is common.

PAIN in the lower abdomen is always present and may be either stabbing or cramp-like — 'uterine colic'. It may be referred to the shoulder if blood tracks to the diaphragm and stimulates the phrenic nerve, and it may be so severe as to cause fainting. The pain is caused by distension of the gravid tube, by its efforts to contract and expel the ovum, and by irritation of the peritoneum by leakage of blood.

VAGINAL BLEEDING occurs usually after the death of the ovum and is an effect of oestrogen withdrawal. It is dark brown and scanty and its irregularity may lead the patient to confuse it with the menstrual flow and thus, inadvertently, give a misleading history. In about 25% of cases tubal pregnancy presents without any vaginal bleeding.

INTERNAL BLOOD LOSS will, if gradual, lead to anaemia. If haemorrhage is severe and rapid (as when a large vessel is eroded) the usual signs of collapse and shock will appear. Acute internal bleeding is the most dramatic and dangerous consequence of tubal pregnancy, but it is less common than the condition presenting by a slow trickle of blood into the pelvic cavity.

PELVIC EXAMINATION in the conscious patient will demonstrate extreme tenderness over the gravid tube or in the pouch of Douglas if an haematocele has collected. If the pregnancy is sufficiently advanced and rupture has not occurred, a cystic (and very tender) mass may be felt in the fornix; but often tenderness is the only sign elicited.

PERITONEAL IRRITATION may produce muscle guarding, frequency of micturition, and later a degree of fever, all leading towards a misdiagnosis of appendicitis.

SIGNS and SYMPTOMS of EARLY PREGNANCY may be present and help to distinguish the condition from other causes of lower abdominal pain. The menstrual history may be confusing, as noted opposite, and when implantation occurs in the isthmus, tubal rupture may occur before the patient has missed a period.

ABDOMINAL EXAMINATION will demonstrate tenderness in one or other fossa. If there has been much intraperitoneal bleeding there will be general tenderness and resistance to palpation over the whole abdomen.

TUBAL PREGNANCY — DIFFERENTIAL DIAGNOSIS

1. Salpingitis.
2. Abortion.
3. Appendicitis.
4. Torsion of pedicle of ovarian cyst.
5. Rupture of corpus luteum or follicular cyst.
6. Perforation of peptic ulcer.

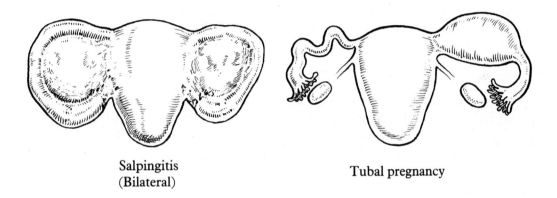

Salpingitis
(Bilateral)

Tubal pregnancy

1. SALPINGITIS

Swelling and pain are bilateral, fever is higher and a pregnancy test is usually negative. There may be a purulent discharge from the cervix.

2. ABORTION, threatened or incomplete.

Bleeding is the dominant clinical feature and usually precedes pain. The bleeding is red rather than brown and the pain is cramping or colicky like labour. The uterus is larger and softer and the cervix patulous or dilated. Curettage may help but naked eye appearances cannot be relied on.

3. APPENDICITIS

The area of tenderness is higher and localised at McBurney's point. There may be a swelling if an appendix abscess has formed but it is not so deep in the pelvis as a tubal swelling. Fever is greater and a positive pregnancy test and amenorrhoea unlikely.

189

TUBAL PREGNANCY — DIFFERENTIAL DIAGNOSIS

4. TORSION of PEDICLE of OVARIAN CYST

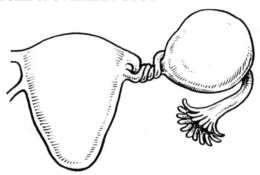

The mass so formed can usually be felt separate from the uterus, while a tubal pregnancy usually feels attached. Tenderness may be marked, and intraperitoneal bleeding may produce fever. Signs and symptoms of pregnancy are absent but there is a history of repeated sudden attacks of pain which pass off.

5. RUPTURE of CORPUS LUTEUM

It is virtually impossible to distinguish this by examination from a tubal pregnancy, but such a severe reaction is rare.

AIDS to DIAGNOSIS

1. Always take a **Careful history**. Inquire in detail about supposed LMP, its timing and appearance.

2. Always **Think** of tubal pregnancy; a woman with lower abdominal pain in whom there is a possibility of pregnancy should be regarded as having an ectopic until proved otherwise.

3. *Pregnancy test*. A negative test does not exclude an ectopic pregnancy but a positive test is helpful. Modern tests based on monoclonal antibodies or Beta **HCG** assay will indicate pregnancy at a very early stage. When combined with ultrasonic examination of the uterus they may indicate a need for further investigation.

4. *Ultrasound*. Its main value is to exclude an intra-uterine pregnancy. If this is done in the presence of a positive test, ectopic pregnancy is likely.

5. *Laparoscopy*. This has become the main means of diagnosis in suspected ectopic pregnancy.

TUBAL PREGNANCY — DIFFERENTIAL DIAGNOSIS

Laparoscopy (continued)

A light source is transmitted to the laparoscope through a flexible fibreglass cable, illuminating the cavity with a brilliant light which gives off no heat.

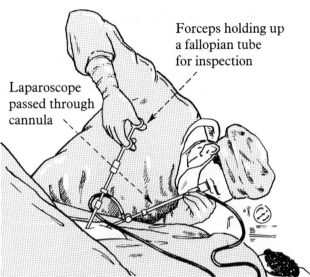

Forceps holding up a fallopian tube for inspection

Laparoscope passed through cannula

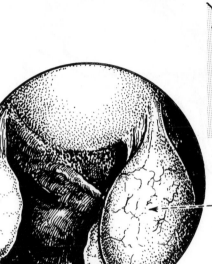

The laparoscope is particularly useful for identifying an unruptured tubal pregnancy which is still producing equivocal symptoms, and for excluding salpingitis and bleeding from small ovarian cysts.

In a few cases much blood and inflammatory adhesions will prevent a full inspection, and laparotomy must be done.

6. *Culdocentesis* (passing a needle through the posterior fornix into the pouch of Douglas). This may be helpful if laparoscopy is not available. Intraperitoneal blood does not readily clot and if such blood is obtained it is an indication for laparotomy. However, an unruptured tubal pregnancy will not be revealed by this procedure, nor will endometriosis; and if inflammatory adhesions fix the pelvic organs, the intestine may be perforated.

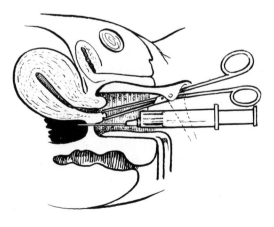

191

TUBAL PREGNANCY — TREATMENT

1. Once the diagnosis is made, the next step is laparotomy which should not be delayed.

2. If haemorrhage and shock are present, restore the blood volume by the transfusion of whole blood or a volume expander and proceed with operation. The patient's condition will improve as soon as the bleeding is controlled.

3. Salpingectomy is the treatment of choice. Blood and clot should be removed from the peritoneal cavity. Conservation and repair of the tube, even if it appears possible, is unwise because of the danger of recurrence. It should not be attempted unless there is a compelling reason such as a previous loss of the other tube in a patient who very much wants a child.

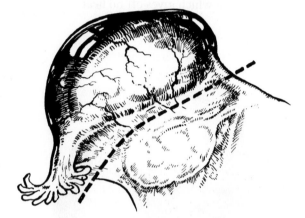

ABDOMINAL PREGNANCY

Abdominal pregnancy is very rare in the United Kingdom. The ovum is expelled from the tube and reimplants elsewhere in the pelvis; or implantation occurs primarily in the peritoneum.

Clinical features

1. There is a history of 'threatened abortion' with irregular bleeding.

2. Continual abdominal discomfort is felt, and fetal movements are painful.

3. Fetal abnormality is common and fetal mortality is high. Fetal death may be followed by suppuration with abscess pointing into bowel or bladder; or by calcification and lithopaedion formation.

The ovum may be expelled intra- or retro-peritoneally. The trophoblast develops its connection with the nearest blood supply (usually on the broad ligament and back of uterus); and in the retroperitoneal situation the proximity of great vessels will increase the risk of haemorrhage.

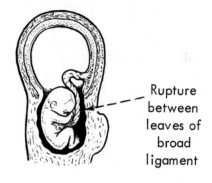

Rupture between leaves of broad ligament

Diagnosis is difficult

1. Palpation is unreliable even when fetal limbs are easily felt.

2. Ultrasound may show the fetus outwith the uterus and an abnormal fetal attitude due to lack of liquor.

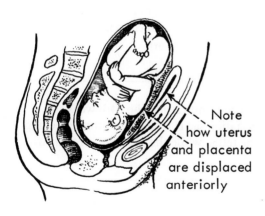

Note how uterus and placenta are displaced anteriorly

Treatment. Once diagnosed or strongly suspected, it is better to perform laparotomy in the interests of the mother. The fetus is removed, the cord tied and the abdomen closed. No attempt is made to detach the placenta unless it is clear that bleeding can be controlled. Recovery is apt to be slow while the placenta is being absorbed, and the pregnancy test will remain positive for about four weeks.

ABORTION

Abortion is the expulsion, dead, of the products of conception before 28 weeks' gestation.

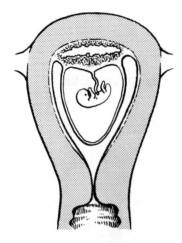

1.

Haemorrhage occurs in the decidua basalis leading to local necrosis and inflammation.

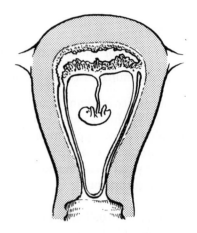

2.

The ovum, partly or wholly detached, acts as a foreign body and initiates uterine contractions. The cervix begins to dilate.

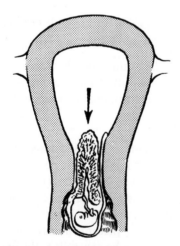

3.

Expulsion complete. The decidua is shed during the next few days in the lochial flow.

Up to 12 weeks, before the placenta is fully developed, abortion may be completed as shown.

From the 12th to the 24th week the gestation sac is likely to rupture expelling the fetus, while the placenta is retained.

From the 24th week onward the mechanism resembles normal labour although the placenta is more often retained.

ABORTION

Once an abortion is declared inevitable, because of the amount of blood loss or dilation of the cervix, it becomes either:

COMPLETE   or   **INCOMPLETE**

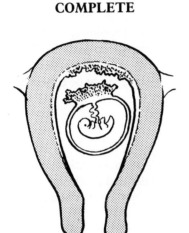
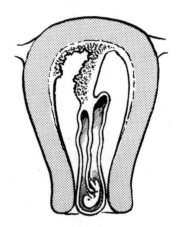

Uterine contractions are felt 'like a small labour', the cervix dilates and blood loss continues. The fetus and placenta (often with membranes intact) are expelled complete.

The uterus contracts and no further treatment is needed except perhaps for a haemorrhagic anaemia.

In spite of uterine contractions and cervical dilatation, only the fetus and some membranes are expelled. The placenta remains partly attached and bleeding continues.

This abortion must be completed by surgical methods.

Classification is based on a mixture of clinical and pathological concepts, and is sufficiently flexible to suit a condition in which diagnosis is often only presumptive. Sepsis can complicate any type of abortion and must often be due to criminal interference.

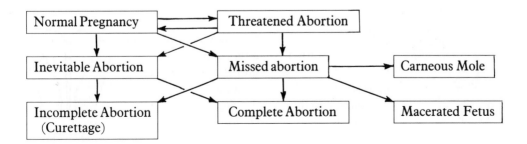

195

ABORTION

AETIOLOGY.   In most cases the cause is unknown.

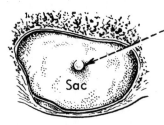

Abnormal development of the ovum

Of those embryos recovered from abortion about half are said to be abnormal either chromosomally or structurally. ABO blood group incompatibility between mother and fetus has been reported to be approaching 50%, more than twice as high as might be expected.

Maternal Conditions

High fever, congestive cardiac failure, severe Rh iso-immunisation, chronic renal disease are all associated conditions. 'Hormonal Imbalance' — not a well defined condition — usually refers to progesterone deficiency. This has not been convincingly shown to be a cause of abortion.

Uterine causes

Mechanical causes are rare but recognised:

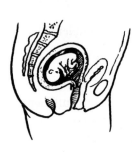

Incarceration of gravid uterus

The growing uterus cannot escape from the pelvis because of retroversion.

Cervical Incompetence

Lacerations or functional incompetence may make it impossible for the uterus to contain a gestation normally. Abortion occurs in mid-trimester (see page 203).

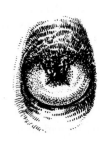

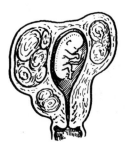

Fibroids

A uterus distorted by fibroids may be unable to accommodate the growing fetus.

Congenital abnormality of the uterus may interfere with the development of the growing fetus.

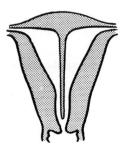

ABORTION

CLINICAL FEATURES

Haemorrhage is usually the first sign and may be very heavy if placental separation is incomplete.

Pain is usually intermittent, 'like a small labour'. It ceases when the abortion is complete.

Cervical dilatation means that abortion is inevitable.

Threatened Abortion. Abortion is said to threaten when any bleeding occurs before the 28th week. It may even be accompanied by pain, yet the abortion process may not have begun in utero and the pregnancy may continue. Some women have a tendency to bleed in the early months for no known reason. There may be shedding of decidua at the time of a missed period up to 12 weeks.

The patient is treated by bed-rest. An ultrasound scan should be carried out to confirm that the fetus is alive. Where this is so, the patient can be reassured and gradually mobilised.

Inevitable Abortion. Here bleeding may still be slight and the cervix still closed. Clinically the woman has a threatened abortion but bleeding is retroplacental and the ovum already dead. Painful uterine contractions will supervene and the cervix begins to dilate. Ultrasound confirms the pregnancy is not continuing and treatment is by evacuation of the uterus.

Incomplete Abortion. The patient will have had substantial bleeding and painful contractions. Tissue and blood clot may be found in the vagina. Bleeding may be controlled by an intramuscular injection of Ergometrine 0.5mg. This is usually combined with an analgesic such as Pethidine or Morphine. This will usually control the bleeding until surgical evacuation can be performed. Hypovolaemia may necessitate blood transfusion.

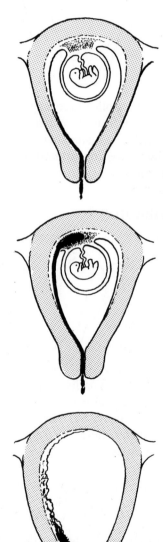

Blood clot

197

ABORTION — DIFFERENTIAL DIAGNOSIS

TUBAL PREGNANCY

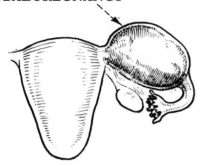

The swollen tube may not be felt separate from the enlarged uterus. There is usually a history of severe pain and slight bleeding but laparoscopy may be required.

FIBROIDS

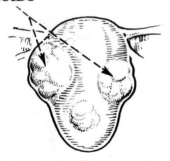

The irregularity of the mass should be felt unless the patient is very fat. Bleeding may be heavy but there will be no history of amenorrhoea. Abortion and fibroids may co-exist.

METROPATHIA HAEMORRHAGICA

Metropathia haemorrhagica may simulate abortion with a period of amenorrhoea followed by heavy bleeding. The distinction may only be made on histological appearances.

PYOSALPINX

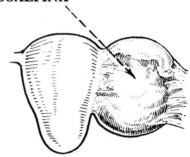

The uterus may be involved in adhesions and there is often irregular bleeding. There will be no evidence of pregnancy however, and there may be systemic signs of infection.

OVARIAN CYST

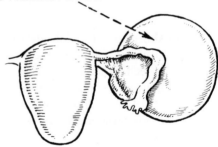

Luteal or follicular cysts may be associated with amenorrhoea and irregular bleeding. On examination the uterus should be felt separately.

Some uterine bleeding has no organic explanation and the patient accepts or supplies a diagnosis of abortion for want of anything better.

ABORTION — TREATMENT

SURGICAL TREATMENT of INCOMPLETE ABORTION

1. It must be done in theatre with the patient anaesthetised.

2. The patient may bleed:
   - (a) before admission to hospital
   - (b) while in hospital
   - (c) during the operation

   } Blood loss may be large and facilities for blood transfusion must be at hand.

3. The operator must, all the time, remember the ease with which a gravid uterus can be perforated by a metal instrument.

'Digital Curettage' is tried first.

Removal of placental tissue with ovum forceps.

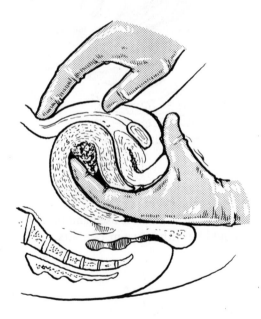

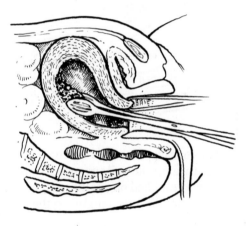

The surgeon presses on the fundus with the external hand and clears out as much of the cavity as he can reach with the internal finger.

The open blades are rotated to grasp tissue and then gently withdrawn. Before using any instrument inside the uterus an oxytocic, Syntocinon 10 units or . Ergometrine 0.25mg, should be given intravenously to cause contraction and thickening of the uterine wall.

ABORTION — TREATMENT

CURETTAGE. A blunt curette may be tried first but usually a sharp curette is required.

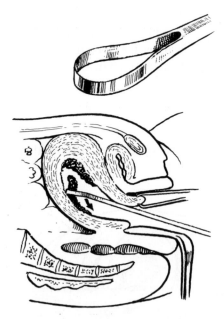

The concave side of the curette loop is pressed against the wall and pulled down. It is then reapplied on another part of the wall. Do not push the curette up the uterine wall.

PACKING the UTERUS. This is only necessary if bleeding continues from an empty uterus and oxytocin is not effective; or if the uterus still has products of conception but curettage is considered too dangerous.

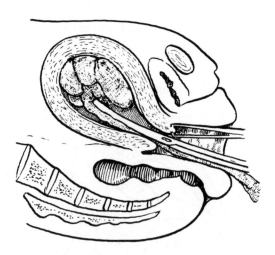

It is important to pack the whole cavity, not just the lower part.

Dry sterile gauze is used and the pack should be withdrawn in 12 hours.

MISSED ABORTION

The retention of an ovum, after its death, for a period of several weeks.

Death of the ovum occurs unnoticed; or is marked by some vaginal bleeding which ceases after treatment for threatened abortion. However enlargement of the breasts ceases and the uterus shrinks as liquor is absorbed. Pregnancy tests will be negative about a week after death and ultrasound confirms the diagnosis.

If retained for long enough, the gestation may end up as a

CARNEOUS MOLE   or   **MACERATED FETUS**

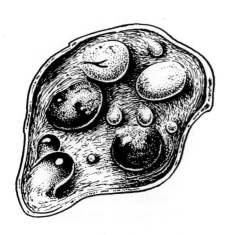 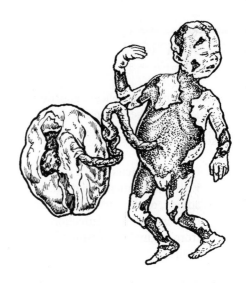

A carneous mole is a lobulated mass of laminated blood clot. The projections into the shrunken cavity are caused by repeated haemorrhages in the chorio-decidual space. In very early pregnancies (up to 12 weeks) complete absorption of the dead ovum may occur.

The skull bones collapse and override and the spine is flexed (changes known as 'Spalding's sign' when seen on X-ray). The internal organs degenerate and the abdomen is filled with bloodstained fluid. The skin peels very easily.

Pathological changes in the fetus such as mummification (fetus papyraceous) and calcification (lithopaedion) are exceedingly rare.

MISSED ABORTION

Treatment

If left alone most missed abortions will be spontaneously expelled, but during the waiting period there is a slight risk of coagulation defect and this should be looked for before embarking on evacuation of the uterus.

If the uterus is not larger than the size of an eight to ten week pregnancy it may be emptied by curettage. This operation requires experience and as bleeding is free until the uterus is emptied, transfusion facilities must be available.

If the uterus is too large for the curette, prostaglandin E_2 should be used by the extra-amniotic route.

SEPTIC ABORTION

Infection may complicate abortion once the cervix starts to dilate or instruments are introduced into the uterine cavity.

Causes

1. Delay in evacuation of the uterus. Either the patient delays seeking advice, or the surgical evacuation has been incomplete. Infection occurs from vaginal organisms after 48 hours.

2. Trauma, either perforation or cervical tear. Healing is delayed and infection is more likely to be a peritonitis or cellulitis. Criminal abortions are of course particularly liable to sepsis.

Infecting Organisms

These are usually the vaginal or bowel commensals.
1. Anaerobic streptococcus
2. Coliform bacillus
3. Clostridium welchii
4. Bacteroides necrophorus
Any of these organisms but particularly the last two may be the cause of septic shock (q.v.)

Clinical features

Slight bleeding continues with pyrexia and a raised pulse rate. Examination reveals pelvic tenderness and the patient displays anxiety.

Treatment

This should be active to minimise the risk of septic shock. Cervical and high vaginal smears and blood cultures are taken and a broad spectrum antibiotic such as a cephalosporin together with an agent effective against anaerobes prescribed. Curettage should be carried out as soon as possible; there is nothing to be gained by leaving infected material in utero. The septic uterus is particularly vulnerable to trauma.

HABITUAL ABORTION

Habitual abortion indicates the occurrence of at least 3 consecutive spontaneous abortions.

Aetiology A recurring factor must be suspected but this is seldom identified although search is made for any of the various conditions mentioned on page 196.

Treatment

Treatment is usually empirical and when success is obtained the psychological effects of close medical supervision cannot be discounted. Rest and the reassurance provided by ultrasound of a continuing pregnancy play a part.

Causes

1. CERVICAL INCOMPETENCE

Habitual abortion is often attributed to this cause especially if there has been a history of previous trauma such as a second trimester induced abortion, or some traumatic incident associated with childbirth. The condition is not a common one and tends to be over-diagnosed. The patient's history is the best guide to diagnosis and the following features differentiate cervical incompetence from other causes of abortion.

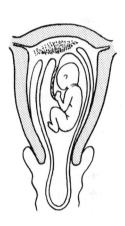

(a) Pregnancy ends in mid-trimester or early third trimester.
(b) The cervix may dilate silently allowing herniation of the gestation sac and rupture of the membranes.
(c) Bleeding is not a feature.

If the cervix is seen to be damaged it should be repaired, but often there is no visible or palpable lesion, and the treatment of **Cervical suture** (McDonald suture: Shirodkar suture: cervical cerclage) is applied empirically.

Technique of cervical suture

Under anaesthesia the cervix is grasped with a vulsellum and four bites of non-absorbable, inert suture are inserted at the level of the internal os. The suture is tightened to resist a No. 6 dilator and is removed at 37 weeks.

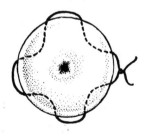

This treatment does not harm but is too often applied irrationally to patients who have suffered habitual abortion not obviously because of cervical incompetence. Difficulties arise when abortion becomes inevitable in spite of the suture which must then be removed to prevent damage to the cervix.

HABITUAL ABORTION

2. HORMONE DEFICIENCY

The corpus luteum, producing progesterone, is essential for the early maintenance of pregnancy but dependence on it ceases as early as 8–10 weeks. As a cause of abortion, therefore, progesterone deficiency remains controversial. There is certainly no theoretical justification for the administration of exogenous progestogens into the second trimester.

Evidence of progesterone deficiency can be sought by estimation of the serum progesterone level or, if radio-immunoassay is not available, by the following tests:

(a) Vaginal cytology

In pregnancy there is a proliferation of cells from the intermediate layers of the vaginal epithelium, the most abundant being the 'navicular' cell — an oval or boat-shaped cell with thickened borders, clear basophil cytoplasm and a vesicular nucleus.

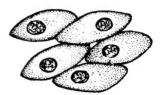

Navicular cells

When progesterone is deficient there is a change in the pattern and the number of cornified and pyknotic cells increases. These are cells of a more angular outline with small pyknotic nuclei, often eosinophil in reaction. When these cells surpass 20% of a cell count ('a high karyopyknotic index') a state of progesterone deficiency is diagnosed.

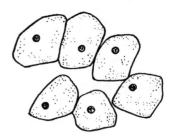

Pyknotic cells

(b) Ferning of cervical mucus

This is a microscopic inspection of dried cervical mucus in which crystals of sodium and potassium chloride are seen in the absence of the influence of progesterone.

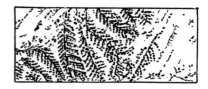

Both of these tests have been used in the normal menstrual cycle as tests of ovulation.

HYDATIDIFORM MOLE AND CHORIOCARCINOMA

Hydatidiform in the placenta is a form of trophoblastic neoplasia which may lead to a frankly malignant proliferation of trophoblast cells, known as choriocarcinoma.

Histology

To the naked eye the mole looks like a bunch of whitish grapes, often interspersed with blood clot. Microscopically, the villi show three changes:-

1. Trophoblastic proliferation of both the cytotrophoblast (Langhan's cells) and the syncytiotrophoblast.
2. Hydropic changes in the stroma, with 'cistern' formation.
3. Absence of fetal vessels.

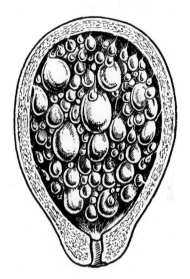

Naked eye appearance. Some villi may be up to 3cm in length.

Syncytium: sheets of cytoplasm containing dark oval nuclei

Avascular oedematous spaces

Cystic spaces (cisterns)

Cytotrophoblast: cuboidal cells with prominent nuclei

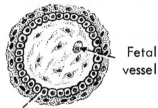

Normal villus

Fetal vessel

Chorionic epithelium

In a normal villus, the trophoblastic layers are single-celled with no proliferation, the stroma contains numerous cells, and there are fetal vessels.

205

HYDATIDIFORM MOLE AND CHORIOCARCINOMA

COMPLETE and PARTIAL MOLE

Hydatidiform moles are now classed as complete or partial. The distinction is made on histological and karyotype evidence and is of considerable clinical significance.

Complete Mole

This shows total hydatidiform change with no evidence of fetal circulation. Proliferation of the trophoblast cells is marked.

The karyotype is in most cases 46XX, derived entirely from the paternal contribution. Fertilisation is by haploid (23X) sperm which duplicates its chromosomes without cell division. Why there should be failure of the ovum contribution is not yet known. Complete moles are more likely to develop malignant change.

Partial Mole

This mole is associated with a fetus (even if the only evidence is traces of a microscopic fetal circulation), hydatidiform change is variable, and trophoblast proliferation, although present, is of moderate degree. The karyotype is abnormal and the commonest finding is triploid (69XXX or XXY), the result of fertilisation by more than one sperm. Partial moles are less likely to develop malignant change.

AETIOLOGY of HYDATIDIFORM MOLE

This is not known but factors include age, environment and probably genetic make-up. Mole is commoner in Asians than in Caucasians, and the European incidence is about 1:2000 compared with an extreme of 1:250 in the Philippines.

Maternal age

Hydatidiform mole occurs most commonly in women under 20 and over 45, the women in whom congenital abnormalities are most likely to be found. In Asian countries where there is a high birth rate, women tend to continue child-bearing until late in their reproductive life.

High parity and malnutrition

Although there is no evidence of any specific dietary deficiency as a cause, these factors are associated in every society with congenital abnormality. Asian countries have high birth rates and high perinatal and infant mortality rates. They also have to deal with the problems caused by malnutrition.

HYDATIDIFORM MOLE

CLINICAL FEATURES

This uncommon condition tends to be unsuspected, but should always be considered in cases of threatened abortion and hyperemesis gravidarum.

Symptoms

1. **Bleeding**
   This is almost the rule. A minor degree of intravascular coagulation appears to accompany molar pregnancy, platelets are reduced, and FDPs increased.

2. **Hyperemesis**
   This is probably due to the increase in HCG secretion, although this has never been established definitely as the cause of hyperemesis in normal pregnancy.

3. **Pallor and dyspnoea**
   Anaemia is often greater than expected, and there may be considerable intra-uterine bleeding.

4. **Anxiety and tremor**
   HCG, which is a glycoprotein similar to TSH, has weak thyroid stimulating properties.

Signs

1. **Uterine enlargement**
   Most patients present at about 14 weeks, and in a majority of cases the uterus is larger than expected. The presence of theca-lutein cysts in the ovary, which occurs in about 10% of cases, may add to this impression.

2. **Absent FH**
   It is very rarely a mole and fetus will coexist.

3. **Absent fetal parts**
   The uterus has a doughy feel.

4. **Signs of pre-eclampsia**
   Hypertension and proteinuria at 16 weeks are strongly suggestive of mole.

5. Unexplained degree of anaemia.

6. Passage of vesicles per vaginam (which make the diagnosis).

7. Signs of hyperthyroidism.

HYDROPIC ABORTION

This occurs in the first trimester. In the products of conception there is usually a mixture of normal chorionic villi and hydropic villi, but in the latter the chorionic epithelium is atrophic.

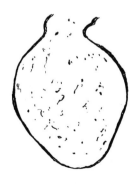

This may be confused with partial mole but the tropho blast is atrophic and the condition is non-neoplastic.

207

HYDATIDIFORM MOLE — DIAGNOSIS

ULTRASONOGRAPHY

Ultrasound has become the main method of diagnosing hydatidiform mole. It is extremely accurate provided that the mole is sufficiently developed, as the echoes produced from the mass of vesicles produce a characteristic 'snowstorm' appearance. The scan must be carried out by an experienced operator as the appearances of vesicle tissue can be mimicked by a septic abortion or a fibroma.

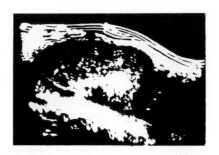

HUMAN CHORIONIC GONADOTROPHIN

Since most of the trophoblast cells secrete HCG, its assay is a measure of the amount of tumour tissue. Grossly elevated levels of HCG are found with hydatidiform moles. HCG is a glycoprotein of two polypeptide chains, alpha and beta. Beta is unique to HCG, and very accurate radio-immunoassays can now be made of beta HCG. For ordinary diagnostic and follow-up purposes however the standard HCG assay is satisfactory.

There are wide variations of the levels in normal pregnancy which reach a peak at about 14 weeks and thereafter fall.

To be diagnostic before 14 weeks, a serum level above 1000 IU/ml should be obtained. About one third of cases will be indeterminate and repeat assays will be required to make a diagnosis.

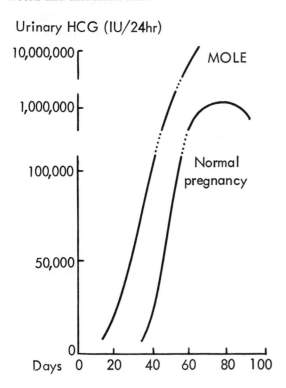

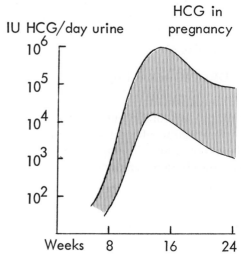

HYDATIDIFORM MOLE — TREATMENT

Once hydatidiform mole is diagnosed, the uterus should be evacuated.

Risks before evacuation

1. Haemorrhage.

2. Trophoblastic invasion and perforation of myometrium.

3. Dissemination of possibly malignant cells.

Risks during evacuation

1. Haemorrhage.

2. Perforation by instruments

3. Dissemination of possibly malignant cells.

There seems no doubt that active methods of evacuation such as hysterectomy, hysterotomy and the use of oxytocics are associated with a threefold increase in the need for subsequent chemotherapy to deal with varying degrees of malignancy. However the immediate safety of the patient may call for some of these measures, and the following plan of management is suggested.

1. After spontaneous abortion, the uterus should be completely emptied by suction.

2. If spontaneous abortion does not occur, an attempt should be made to empty the uterus by suction. This is usually quite simple up to about 14 weeks size.

If bleeding becomes severe, oxytocics must be given, and on rare occasions an emergency hysterectomy or hysterotomy may be unavoidable.

3. If the uterus is of such a size as to deter the obstetrician from attempting suction curettage, abortion should be induced using extra-amniotic prostaglandin together with Oxytocin if necessary. Subsequent surgical evacuation of the uterus may also be required. Hydatidiform mole is not a common condition, and very few obstetricians have profound practical experience in its surgical management. Rapid evacuation of a large uterus has been known to cause disseminated intravascular coagulation and fatal shock.

4. In the case of the older woman whose family is complete, hysterectomy may be justified, especially as dissemination of trophoblast cells can be almost completely prevented by early clamping of the uterine vessels.

HYDATIDIFORM MOLE — FOLLOW UP

Hydatidiform mole, although it can cause serious immediate complications, is particularly important because in about 10% of cases it will persist and undergo malignant change in varying degree. This outcome is much more common after complete rather than partial moles, but all patients must be followed up for prolonged periods by radioimmunoassays of serum or urinary HCG.

Indications for Chemotherapy

1. The high HCG levels associated with every mole persist for two months after evacuation.

2. Any detectable HCG in the serum after 6 months.

3. Persistent uterine bleeding, even if no trophoblastic material is obtained by curettage. This is an indication of myometrial invasion.

4. Evidence of trophoblastic metastasis usually to the brain or lungs.

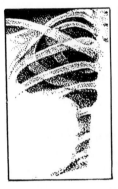 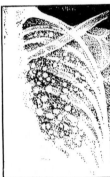

X-ray of the lung field may show one large shadow (cannon-ball metastasis) or numerous trophoblastic emboli (snowstorm).

Predisposing Factors in the need for Chemotherapy

1. Complete moles are far more likely to become malignant than are partial moles. Since the distinction is not always a simple one on histological inspection, it is important to obtain the karyotype of the molar tissue wherever possible. Complete moles are almost always of karyotype 46XX but a few have been reported as 46XY.

2. Abnormally proliferative trophoblast is likely to persist. (See over on histological appearance of malignancy.)

3. The use of any oxytocic agent or the application of surgery such as hysterotomy, is more likely than suction curettage to disseminate trophoblastic cells.

4. The use of oral contraceptives after evacuation. Exogenous sex steroids prolong the persistence of trophoblastic cells and delay the fall in HCG excretion, perhaps because of an immunosuppressive action.

INVASIVE MOLE AND CHORIOCARCINOMA

The classification of the various degrees of malignant change in hydatidiform mole is not universally agreed on. A simple system of nomenclature would be:-

1. Hydatidiform mole.
2. Intermediate degrees of neoplastic change
    (Invasive mole, Destructive mole, Villous choriocarcinoma).
3. Choriocarcinoma.

Both invasive mole and choriocarcinoma are rare conditions. The symptoms and signs are similar to those associated with hydatidiform mole but metastatic lesions occur; the more malignant the growth the earlier its appearance. Haemoptysis and cerebral haemorrhage are the normal results but local metastases to the vagina are also common.

INVASIVE MOLE
(Destructive mole, Villous choriocarcinoma)

CHORIOCARCINOMA
Chorionepithelioma, Avillous choriocarcinoma)

Proliferating cytotropho- blast cells

Wandering syncytial cells

Cytotrophoblast cells

Myometrium invaded by cytotrophoblast cells and syncytial cells

The trophoblast retains its villous structure but it invades the myometrium and may produce metastases.

Villous formation is absent. Trophoblast cells invade the myometrium and blood vessels resulting in gross haemorrhage and metastases.

It must be emphasised that the histological patterns vary widely. The more malignant growths show the greater cellular irregularity and mitotic activity. Choriocracinoma is usually found early in pregnancy arising in association with a mole but can follow abortion or even full time pregnancy.

Either of these conditions once diagnosed would be an indication for immediate chemotherapy.

INVASIVE MOLE AND CHORIOCARCINOMA — CHEMOTHERAPY

Chemotherapy is aimed at cure, which may be said to have occurred when no HCG can be detected in the serum. However even β-HCG cannot be demonstrated in concentrations lower than 3mlU/ml which represents the output of 5,000 trophoblast cells somewhere in the body, so HCG monitoring must be continued indefinitely.

Trophoblast disease chemotherapy is a specialised service confined in the United Kingdom to a single unit to which all cases may be referred. Deaths from trophoblast tumour are now rare in the UK.

METHOTREXATE

Methotrexate is the principal drug used, a derivative of folic acid, and one of the antimetabolite group which prevents cell replication.

Dosage is limited by side-effects on the bone marrow and alimentary tract, and there is a practical limit of tolerance when treatment must be stopped to allow recovery of normal tissue.

A moderate course would be 35mg i.m. every 48 hours for 4 doses. This is followed after 24 hours by 'rescue therapy' with folinic acid to diminish the toxicity of methotrexate.

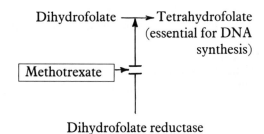

Dihydrofolate ——→ Tetrahydrofolate (essential for DNA synthesis)

Methotrexate

Dihydrofolate reductase

(Methotrexate has a much greater affinity for dihydrofolate reductase)

Treatment is monitored by assay of HCG and by blood cell counts. Methotrexate is excreted unchanged in the urine, and renal function must be adequate.

COMBINATION THERAPY

The use of multidrug chemotherapy is resorted to when methotrexate/folinic acid appears or becomes ineffective. The choice of drugs is individual for each patient, and their administration requires expert oncological supervision.

PROGNOSTIC FACTORS IN CHEMOTHERAPY FOR TROPHOBLAST NEOPLASM

ADVERSE

1. Histological evidence of choriocarcinoma.

2. Large tumour masses or widespread secondaries.

3. Delay in detection of persisting tumour cells.

4. Very high HCG levels.

5. Previous unsuccessful chemotherapy.

FAVOURABLE

1. Evidence of invasive mole only.

2. No evidence of recurrence or spread: small tumour mass.

3. Early diagnosis of persistence.

4. Relatively low and falling HCG levels. (HCG excretion is roughly quantitative of the amount of tumour.

IMMUNOLOGICAL FACTORS

Trophoblast tissue is in the nature of an allograft and one would expect an immunological reaction between the host and her tumour. In 90% of cases the tumour shows reactive signs consisting of lymphocytes, plasma cells and histiocytes, and the more marked this immunological reaction, the better the prognosis. The ABO system also influences prognosis which is worst in women of groups B and AB whose husbands are O or A.

PREGNANCY AFTER CHEMOTHERAPY

Methotrexate can be retained in the body for up to eight months, and the theoretical risk is of cytotoxic damage to oocytes resulting in an increased incidence of fetal abnormality. However this does not seem to be borne out in practice, although patients are advised to delay conception for a year so that possibly damaged ova may be shed. Barrier methods of contraception should be used rather than oral contraception, or the IUD which may cause misleading irregular haemorrhage.

ANTE-PARTUM HAEMORRHAGE

Ante-partum haemorrhage is bleeding from the genital tract after the 28th week of pregnancy and before the birth of the baby. This is a practical definition as it includes the incidental causes of bleeding illustrated in summary at the beginning of this chapter. These are dealt with elsewhere. An alternative definition, no longer favoured, is bleeding from the placental site. This encompasses the two conditions of Placenta Praevia (inevitable haemorrhage) and Abruptio Placentae (accidental haemorrhage). A substantial number of cases of ante-partum haemorrhage remain unexplained even when the placenta is examined after delivery for signs of premature separation.

PLACENTA PRAEVIA (INEVITABLE HAEMORRHAGE)

A low implantation of the placenta in the uterus, causing it to lie alongside or in front of the presenting part.

The cause is unknown. The incidence is greater in multigravidae and there is an association with fetal abnormalities. Twin pregnancy with its large placental bed is prone to low implantation of at least a part of the placenta. Placenta praevia is divided into four types or degrees, of which the first two are the commonest.

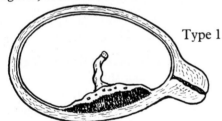
Type 1

The lower margin of the placenta dips into the lower segment. ('Low implantation'.)

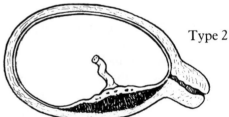
Type 2

The placenta reaches the internal os when closed but does not cover it.('Marginal'.)

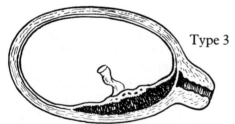
Type 3

The placenta covers the internal os when closed, but not when fully dilated.('Partial' or 'Incomplete'.)

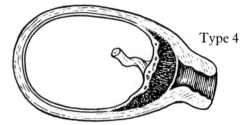
Type 4

The placenta covers the os even when the cervix is fully dilated. ('Central'or 'Complete'.)

Allocation to a particular type is usually made by palpation prior to delivery, or by observation at Caesarean section; so there is a subjective bias. In addition the degree of dilatation of the cervix at the time of assessment may alter a classification; what was type 1 at 2cm dilatation may become type 2 at 4 or 5cm.

ANTE-PARTUM HAEMORRHAGE

PLACENTA PRAEVIA   (continued)

Signs and symptoms

The formation of the lower segment by stretching leads to separation of the placenta and escape of blood from the maternal sinuses. This commonly occurs around the 32nd week but may begin as early as the late mid-trimester of pregnancy. The loss may be slight or considerable and tends to be recurrent. The bleeding is *painless* because blood is not normally retained within the uterine cavity.

Diagnosis

The presence of the placenta in the lower segment pushes the presenting part upwards and may encourage malpresentation or an oblique or transverse lie. The abdomen is soft and non-tender and the patient's general condition should reflect the amount of visible blood loss. Confirmation of the diagnosis is obtained by localisation of the placenta by ultrasound. This is very accurate but in minor degrees of placenta praevia (especially on the posterior wall) it may be impossible to be sure if the placenta encroaches on the lower segment. Soft tissue radiography and isotope localisation of the placenta are not now normally used.

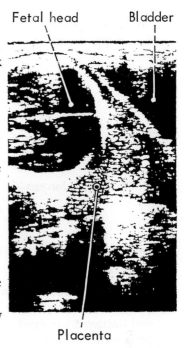

Fetal head   Bladder

Placenta

Management

If the pregnancy is immature (less than 37 weeks) the aim is to treat conservatively. The patient must remain in hospital and cross-matched blood should be available. Conservative management will be abandoned if the bleeding becomes severe or persistent. Placenta praevia is a treacherous condition and bleeding is unpredictable.

Examination in Theatre and Delivery

If the pregnancy continues to 37–38 weeks, the degree of placenta praevia can be confirmed by vaginal examination in theatre. This is carried out under anaesthesia and the theatre is set and staffed for Caesarean section. The vaginal fornices are carefully palpated for evidence of the placenta and if not encountered a finger is then passed through the cervix to explore the lower segment. If the surgeon is convinced of the diagnosis and the degree of placenta praevia he may omit this examination for fear of provoking haemorrhage. The treatment of placenta praevia today is invariably Caesarean section except in type 1 when the membranes may be ruptured and, if no bleeding occurs, spontaneous delivery may be awaited.

As a rule the lower segment operation is done even with an anterior placenta when the operator passes his hand around or below the placenta to extract the baby. If the examination has provoked torrential haemorrhage classical section may have a slight advantage in speed. Because of the poor retractile quality of the lower segment there is sometimes difficulty in obtaining control of bleeding after delivery of the baby and placenta. Hysterectomy may be ultimately necessary.

215

ANTE-PARTUM HAEMORRHAGE

PLACENTA PRAEVIA (continued)

If dangerous haemorrhage occurs and facilities for Caesarean section are not available, attempts might be made to control the bleeding by pressure of the presenting part on the placenta.

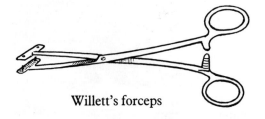

Willett's forceps

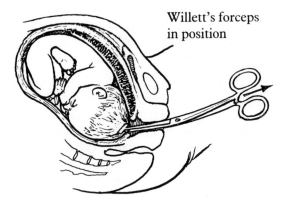

Willett's forceps in position

Where the head is presenting, Willett's forceps may be applied to the fetal scalp and traction maintained. With a breech presentation it may be possible to bring down a leg if at least two fingers can be passed through the cervix.

These are desperate measures which will almost certainly result in fetal death. They are only applicable when the mother herself is at risk from uncontrollable haemorrhage.

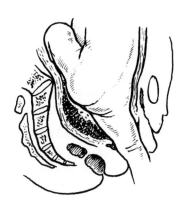

ANTE-PARTUM HAEMORRHAGE

ABRUPTIO PLACENTAE (ACCIDENTAL HAEMORRHAGE)

This means the separation of a normally situated placenta. It usually leads to bleeding per vaginam ('revealed') but often blood remains in the uterus as a retro-placental clot and sometimes there is no external bleeding ('concealed'). Where there is both external bleeding and evidence of retro-placental clot the haemorrhage is described as 'mixed'.

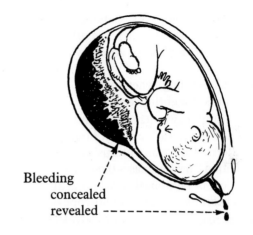

Aetiology

The aetiology of abruptio is unknown but several factors have been postulated as linked causes:

Bleeding
concealed
revealed - - - - - - - - - - - - - ➤

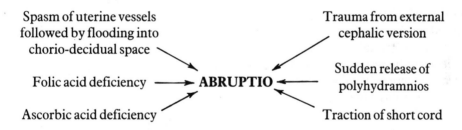

Spasm of uterine vessels followed by flooding into chorio-decidual space

Trauma from external cephalic version

Folic acid deficiency ⟶ **ABRUPTIO** ⟵ Sudden release of polyhydramnios

Ascorbic acid deficiency

Traction of short cord

Certain patients seem susceptible to abruptio but again the reason is unknown.

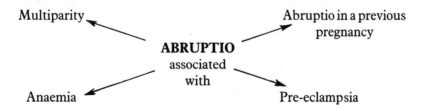

Multiparity

Abruptio in a previous pregnancy

ABRUPTIO
associated
with

Anaemia

Pre-eclampsia

The incidence of abruptio has fallen greatly with the reduction in the number of multiparous patients and better general health of the pregnant population.

ANTE-PARTUM HAEMORRHAGE

ABRUPTIO PLACENTAE (continued)

Signs and Symptoms

1. The patient complains of abdominal pain which may be severe and constant. Pain is greatest when there is a substantial 'concealed' bleed and may be minimal or absent where bleeding is entirely 'revealed'.
2. Vaginal bleeding, where present, usually makes the diagnosis straightforward.
3. The uterus may be tense and tender due to the retention of clot and the extravasation of blood into the uterine wall. The term 'Couvelaire uterus' is used to describe this condition. In severe cases blood may spread into the broad ligament or peritoneal cavity. It is difficult to detect the fetal heart by ordinary stethoscope or to feel uterine contractions.
4. There may be evidence of hypovolaemia depending on the extent of haemorrhage.
5. In severe cases the fetal heart may be absent.

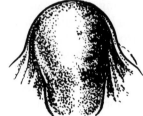

Couvelaire uterus

Differential diagnosis

Mild and early cases of abruptio are difficult to distinguish from normal labour with 'excessive show'. The diagnosis of an established mixed haemorrhage is not usually difficult but concealed abruptio may need to be distinguished from:

    (a)   Acute polyhydramnios
    (b)   Degeneration of fibroid
    (c)   Peritonism from perforation of a peptic ulcer, appendicitis or other cause.

Complictions of Abruptio

1. **Coagulation failure**

    In severe cases of mixed and concealed abruption coagulation failure may supervene due to the consumption of clotting factors and/or the development of fibrinolysis (see Chapter 7).

Clot ≡ depletes fibrinogen

Damage to uterus and placenta ≡ escape of thromboplastins and plasminogen activators into general circulation.

    All patients with ante-partum haemorrhage should have a clotting screen carried out on admission to hospital. An undetected or uncorrected coagulation defect may lead to catastrophic bleeding and shock. It is essential to correct the defect before delivery occurs. Transfusion with whole blood, fresh if possible, is the best treatment. Fresh-frozen plasma and concentrates of platelets may also be indicated and expert haematological guidance is desirable.

ANTE-PARTUM HAEMORRHAGE

ABRUPTIO PLACENTAE

Complications (continued)

2. **Renal failure**

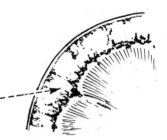

Severe hypovolaemic shock may cause ultimate renal failure with first haemoglobinuria, then oliguria or anuria. This may be due to either tubular damage or cortical necrosis. Urinary output should be monitored carefully in all cases of severe abruption.

The complications and dangers of this condition may be summarised as follows:

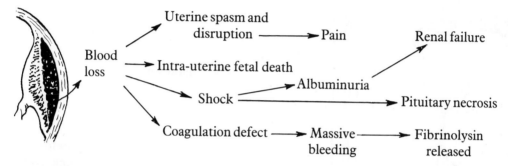

It is recognised that the risk of either coagulation failure or renal failure occurring will be reduced by rapid and liberal transfusion to restore the circulating blood volume together with speedy emptying of the uterus. Similarly the baby's chances of survival will be increased by improved perfusion of the placental site.

Management

1. **Minor or uncertain cases**

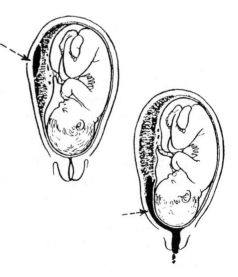

Minor retro-placental bleeding sometimes occurs producing a tender area in the uterus. There is a complaint of pain but little systemic upset. Similarly slight external bleeding will cause little disturbance. In both of these situations treatment is by bed-rest, sedation if required and observation. The haemoglobin should be estimated and a clotting screen carried out. Placenta praevia is excluded by ultrasound scan. Symptoms usually settle quickly and the patient is mobilised and the pregnancy may safely be allowed to continue. Fetal growth should be closely observed and at delivery the placenta should be examined for evidence of old blood clot or the presence of a crater.

219

ANTE-PARTUM HAEMORRHAGE

ABRUPTIO PLACENTAE

Management (continued)

2. **Established Abruptio**

    (a) Rapid assessment of maternal and fetal state.
    (b) Blood taken for haemoglobin, cross-match and clotting screen.
    (c) Sedation and analgesia to treat shock and pain.
    (d) Blood transfusion to correct hypovolaemia. The rate and volume of transfusion are best monitored by a central venous pressure (CVP).
    (e) Expedite delivery.

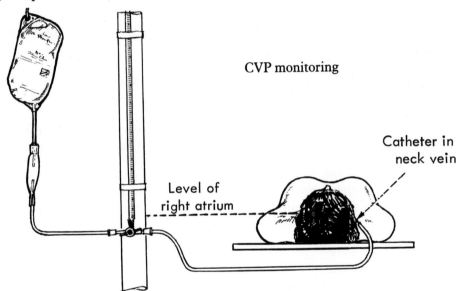

CVP monitoring

Catheter in neck vein

Level of right atrium

3. **Delivery**

    If the baby is dead an attempt should be made to achieve vaginal delivery. Vaginal examination and amniotomy are performed and labour is usually rapid. It is quite common to find on vaginal examination that the cervix is already considerably dilated. The presence of uterine contractions may not have been detected due to the hardness of the uterus caused by the abruption. If the fetal heart is detected on admission by ultrasound, Caesarean section is increasingly favoured to deliver the baby. As already noted the baby's condition will be improved by rapid restoration of the circulating blood volume. There may be poor retraction of the uterus following the delivery of the placenta and thus an atonic post-partum haemorrhage may add to the dangers the mother already faces. Intravenous oxytocics should therefore be given and Ergometrine, with its tonic action on the uterus, is the drug of choice. Following delivery careful supervision of urinary output is essential and the presence of anaemia should be sought.

A CLINICAL APPROACH TO ANTE-PARTUM HAEMORRHAGE

Many cases of relatively minor ante-partum haemorrhage do not fit clearly into the descriptions of placenta praevia and abruptio placentae already given. The diagnosis is not obvious and both mother and baby appear well. Conservative or 'expectant' management is appropriate and the following approach is suggested:

1. Hospital admission and bed-rest.
2. General assessment of the mother and baby including haemoglobin estimation and coagulation screen.
3. An early speculum examination to exclude local causes or confirm that the bleeding is from the uterine cavity (i.e. the placental site). A digital examination should NEVER be done.
4. Localise the placenta by ultrasound.
5. Mobilise when fresh bleeding has stopped.
6. Give anti-D immunoglobulin to Rhesus negative mothers without antibodies.
7. The patient may go home when the bleeding has stopped and placenta praevia has been excluded.
8. Continue ante-natal supervision to exclude growth retardation.
9. Examination in theatre at 38 weeks, finally to exclude placental praevia, may be advisable.
10. Careful examination of the placenta and membranes after delivery to try to identify the cause of the bleeding.

MULTIPLE PREGNANCY AND OTHER ANTENATAL COMPLICATIONS

MULTIPLE PREGNANCY

Multiple pregnancy is the term used when more than one fetus is present in the uterus. Twins are found in about 1 in 80 pregnancies in Caucasians, but are commoner in Negroes and least frequent in Mongol races. The difference is due to variation in binovular twinning, the instance of monovular twins being the same in all races.

Hellin's Rule (a mathematical approximation) gives triplets as 1 in 80^2 (6,400) pregnancies and quadruplets as 1 in 80^3 (512,000) pregnancies.

Sonar scan in early pregnancy sometimes shows twins where ultimately only one fetus is delivered.

There is a higher incidence of multiple pregnancy among women taking ovulation-producing drugs.

Twins may be monovular (monozygotic or monochorionic) — from one ovum, or binovolar (dizygotic or dichorionic) — from two ova.

Binovular twins are 3 or 4 times as common as monovular twins.

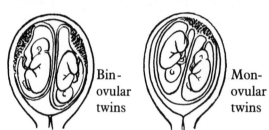

Bin-ovular twins

Mon-ovular twins

The incidence of binovular but not monovular twins is influenced by age, parity and heredity. Twinning is commoner in older mothers and with increasing parity. A family history (probably only maternal) increases the risk.

The importance of multiple pregnancy is its contribution to perinatal loss, which is several times higher than in comparable single pregnancies. This is due mainly to prematurity and fetal abnormality. Most complications of pregnancy are more frequent and increased strain on the mother is obvious.

DIAGNOSIS

1. **Early pregnancy:** In Centres where routine scanning is practised, most twins are diagnosed by ultrasound.

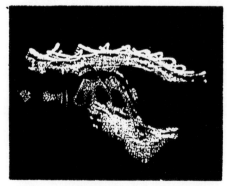

Twin gestation sacs at 8 weeks

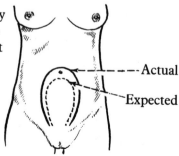

Multiple pregnancy is suspected clinically by finding that the uterus is progressively bigger than the dates suggest.

- - - Actual

Expected

224

Diagnosis (continued)

Other possible causes of apparently abnormal uterine enlargement in early pregnancy are:

(a) **Mistaken Dates** — bleeding after conception being considered as a period.

(b) **Polyhydramnios** — rare in early pregnancy

(c) **Fibroids**
These tend to
flatten and soften
in pregnancy but
may be irregular

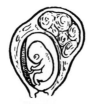

(d) **Abdominal Cyst**
It is usually
possible to
differentiate two
masses.

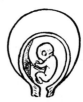

(e) **Hydatidiform Mole**
Usually
accompanied by
staining. Urinary
HCG excretion
will be much
elevated.

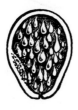

(f) **Retention of Urine**
'Catheter will
cure'. It may be
associated with
retroversion and
incarceration of
the uterus.

Ultrasound will differentiate all these conditions.

2. **Late pregnancy:** The uterus is more globular and larger than normal for the dates. Polyhydramnios may be present. It is commoner in monovular than in binovular twins. The conceptus is not as easy to define as a single fetus but three poles (head or breech) must be identified to be sure of the diagnosis.

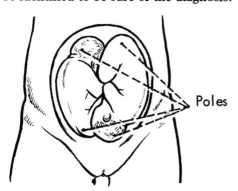

Poles

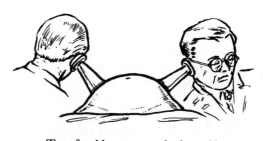

Two fetal hearts may be heard but they must be heard at the same time and differ in rate by 10 beats.

Clinical suspicion of twins must always be confirmed. This will usually be by ultrasound but occasionally, in late pregnancy, an X-ray may be required, especially if there is the possibility of more than 2 babies.

MULTIPLE PREGNANCY

COMPLICATIONS

The major complications are illustrated below but it must not be forgotten that the so-called minor complications of pregnancy such as heartburn, varicose veins, haemorrhoids and other pressure effects may all add to the mother's burden.

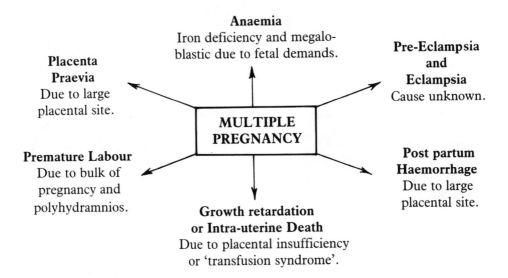

Anaemia
Iron deficiency and megaloblastic due to fetal demands.

**Placenta
Praevia**
Due to large
placental site.

**Pre-Eclampsia
and
Eclampsia**
Cause unknown.

**MULTIPLE
PREGNANCY**

Premature Labour
Due to bulk of
pregnancy and
polyhydramnios.

**Post partum
Haemorrhage**
Due to large
placental site.

**Growth retardation
or Intra-uterine Death**
Due to placental insufficiency
or 'transfusion syndrome'.

MANAGEMENT

1. **Pregnancy:** Antenatal care is conducted in the usual fashion looking for the above complications. A good quality diet is advised and iron and folic acid supplements should be given. Routine hospital admission used to be advised in an attempt to prevent premature labour. This is less common now but admission should be readily available to a tired and over-burdened mother.

   The development of ultrasound and cardiotocography now allows assessment of the growth and well-being of the individual fetus in a way not previously possible. A growth-retarded fetus may thus be identified. Serial cardiotocography should be carried out in the last weeeks of pregnancy.

Twin CTG's
simultaneously
performed

TWIN 1

TWIN 2

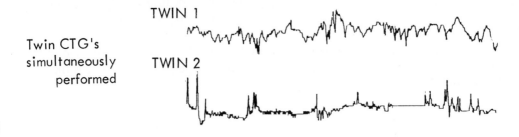

MULTIPLE PREGNANCY

MANAGEMENT (continued)

2. **Labour and Delivery:** Twins may present in various ways but in at least three quarters of cases the first presents by the vertex.

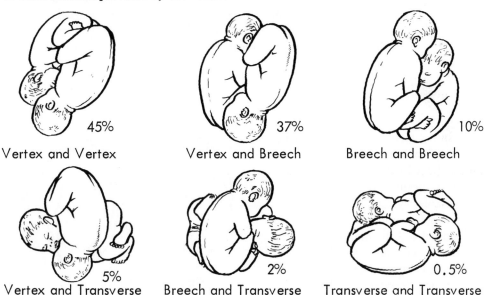

Vertex and Vertex 45%

Vertex and Breech 37%

Breech and Breech 10%

Vertex and Transverse 5%

Breech and Transverse 2%

Transverse and Transverse 0.5%

The lie of the second baby is unimportant until the first is born.

Labour is usually straightforward. There is an increased risk of cord prolapse with the smaller presenting part or malpresentation, and vaginal examination should be carried out when the membranes rupture.

Both fetal hearts should be monitored, the first by a scalp electrode and the second externally. Epidural analgesia is ideal, if available, as it permits any necessary intervention, especially with the second twin, during delivery. This should take place in an operating theatre with appropriate facilities and staff available. In addition to the obstetrician and midwives an anaesthetist and paediatrician should be present.

After the delivery of the first baby the cord is double clamped in case there are monovular twins and a risk of the second bleeding from the cord of the first.

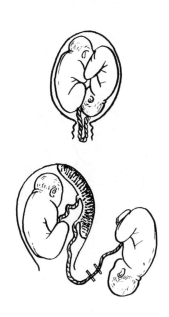

MULTIPLE PREGNANCY

DELIVERY (continued)

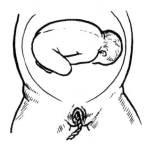

When the first baby is delivered the lie of the second is checked and if necessary corrected by external version to a vertex or a breech; if that is not possible then internal podalic version and breech extraction is performed (see Chapter 12).

Delay in the birth of the second twin gives risk of fetal loss as the placental site shrinks with the birth of the first and the reduction in uterine size also alters the uterine vascular system. To avoid this the second sac is ruptured once the lie is longitudinal and the mother is asked to bear down. This often stimulates contractions. Oxytocin may also be used if delay occurs. Spontaneous delivery or assisted breech delivery may then follow.

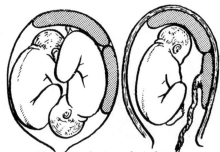

Placental site shrinking

Delay can be dealt with by forceps or vacuum extraction if the head presents. Intravenous Oxytocin should be given with the birth of the second twin to promote uterine retraction.

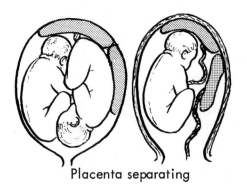

Placenta separating

Rarely the first placenta is born before the second baby. Bleeding is not usually severe. The uterus is actively contracting and the reduction in size of the placental site and the pressure of the fetus on it helps to control the blood loss.

The second birth should be completed without delay, and the placenta delivered as quickly as possible – manually if need be – and an oxytocic drug given.

MULTIPLE PREGNANCY

OTHER COMPLICATIONS

Locked twins

Locked twins is a very rare condition in which parts of one interlock with the other causing an impasse. It most commonly occurs with the first as breech and the second as a vertex. The head of the second slips down with the shoulders of the first and prevents the engagement of the head of the first in the pelvis.

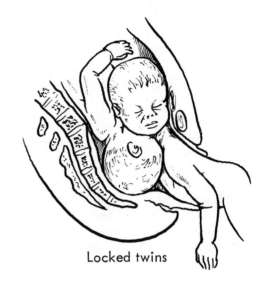

Locked twins

Early recognition is essential as the condition has a high fetal mortality. The treatment is to push the lower head out of the pelvis to free the head of the first fetus and allow delivery. If displacement is not possible the first baby will die and a destructive procedure is required to allow delivery of the trunk and then the second twin.

Conjoined twins are due to imperfect separation of monovular twins and delivery is not possible vaginally except in rare instances or with marked prematurity.

Triplets and quadruplets have similar problems and difficulties. Premature labour is much commoner because of the increased bulk and perinatal mortality higher. As in other obstetric abnormalities delivery by Caesarean section is invariably the method of choice.

MULTIPLE PREGNANCY

PLACENTAE and MEMBRANES

The placentae may be separate or appear as one so that the diagnosis of monovular or binovular twins is uncertain. The membranes between the sacs are examined.

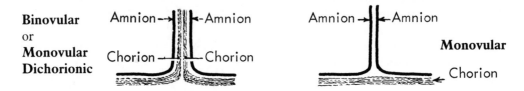

Binovular
or
Monovular
Dichorionic

Amnion → ← Amnion

Chorion → ← Chorion

Amnion → ← Amnion

Monovular

← Chorion

Binovular twins have two amnions sandwiching one or two chorions (the two chorions sometimes fuse), but sometimes monovular twins may be dichorionic if division of the embryonic disc has occurred before the formation of the amnion. Monovular monochorionic twins may have one or two amniotic sacs. Genotyping may be necessary to determine whether like-sex dichorionic twins are binovular or monovular.

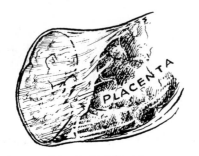

Fetus papyraceous

Sometimes a twin does not develop but becomes amorphous or shrivelled and flattened. This is called fetus papyraceous or compressus. It may be readily apparent or may be found wrapped in the membranes of the placenta.

The '**transfusion syndrome**' is sometimes found with monovular twins. This is dependent on a placental arterio-venous shunt. The arterial system of one leads closely to the venous system of the other and the arterial twin pumps some of its blood into the other circulation starving itself and making the other bulky, plethoric and polycythaemic.

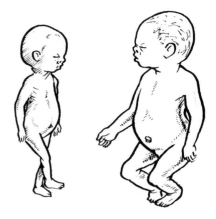

PREMATURE LABOUR

Pre-term labour is defined as the onset of labour before 37 completed weeks of pregnancy.

INCIDENCE: 5–10% of births but a major cause of peri-natal loss.

CAUSES: Certain conditions are associated with an increased risk of premature labour:

(a) Social factors:	Low socio-economic groups.
	Low maternal age.
	Low maternal weight.
	Smoking.
(b) Overdistension of the uterus:	Multiple pregnancy.
	Polyhydramnios.
(c) Uterine anomaly:	Congenital.
	Cervical incompetence.
(d) Fetal anomaly	
(e) Infection:	Maternal pyrexial illness.
	Amnionitis (premature rupture of the membranes).
(f) Antepartum haemorrhage	
(g) Trauma:	Injury.
	Surgery during pregnancy.

Many cases are unexplained and the mechanisms involved in stimulating uterine action are not clear.

PREVENTION   Improvements in the nutrition and general health of the population and a reduction in smoking should be beneficial.

Cervical suture is employed where there is evidence of incompetence of the cervix (see Chapter 9).

The prophylactic use of oral beta-sympathomimetic drugs in high risk situations such as twin pregnancy has been described. Doubts about their safety and effectiveness have not yet been resolved.

PREMATURE LABOUR

TREATMENT

A decision whether to attempt to stop pre-term labour will depend on the period of gestation, the estimated birth weight and the neo-natal paediatric facilities available. Improvements in paediatric care have reduced the need for efforts to postpone delivery.

Beta-Sympathomimetic Drugs: Salbutamol and Ritodrine stimulate the inhibitory sympathetic control of uterine muscle. They have several side-effects including maternal tachycardia, hyperglycaemia and reduction in the serum potassium level. A pulse rate of between 130–140 is acceptable, but overdosage may cause serious cardiac arrythmias. There have been persistent reports of postpartum pulmonary oedema following the use of betamimetics in association with corticosteroids (given to induce lung maturation) due perhaps to a combination of vasodilatation and sodium and water retention, and the two drugs should probably not be combined. Cardiac disease and diabetes are contraindications to the use of betamimetics.

Dosage: A pump is used, starting at 50 micrograms/minute IV, and gradually increasing until contractions are stopped or the maternal pulse is above 140. This dosage is usually required for at least 12 hours and once the uterus is controlled, oral therapy may be substituted.

Calcium Antagonists: Nifedipine (Adelat) is used in the treatment of ischaemic heart disease, and appears to act by inhibiting the flow of calcium ions in muscle fibres. This group of drugs also inhibit uterine muscle, but have not so far been found to offer any advantage over the beta-sympathomimetic drugs.

Prostaglandin Inhibitors: Drugs such as Indomethiacin inhibit the production of prostaglandin synthetase and undoubtedly reduce uterine activity. However they have been found in large doses to cause premature closure of the fetal ductus arteriosus and should not be used.

Corticosteroids: Prior to 32 weeks the use of a corticosteriod (Betamethasone) given by IV infusion has been employed to promote fetal lung maturation. It may be combined with a beta-sympathomimetic drug to try to postpone delivery for a few days. Side effects have been reported (see above) and a decision to employ Betamethasone should be taken in consultation with a paediatric colleague.

In practice, the use of drugs to inhibit uterine activity has on the whole been disappointing. Assessment of effectiveness is difficult because of the uncertainty surrounding symptoms of labour. If the drug is given early enough to be followed by a cessation of activity, it is always possible that the patient was in 'false labour'; and when the cervix is 3 cm dilated and the existence of labour is not in doubt, it is likely to be irreversible anyway.

PREMATURE RUPTURE OF MEMBRANES

This means rupture of the membranes, before labour, prior to 37 completed weeks.

CAUSES
Often not clear but the following conditions should be considered:

Cervical incompetence,	Fetal abnormality,
Polyhydramnios,	Infection.

DANGERS
Intra-uterine infection (which may cause fetal death), Premature labour.

MANAGEMENT

1. Admit to hospital.
2. 4-hourly temperature chart.
3. Detailed ultrasound scan for fetal abnormality.
4. Examine liquor for evidence of lung maturity (phosphatidyl glycerol). The specimen is obtained via sterile speculum and digital examination should be avoided.
5. Delivery is advised if lung maturity confirmed or clinical evidence of infection appears.
6. Otherwise treat conservatively. A pregnancy may sometimes continue for several weeks without infection developing.

Antibiotics are sometimes prescribed prophylactically, but resistant organisms will appear if their use has to be continued for some time. After birth, however, the baby will be treated.

POSTMATURITY

This term applies to unduly prolonged pregnancy — commonly considered to be 294 days from the first day of the last menstrual period.

Postmaturity remains a common indication for induction of labour, mainly because of fears about fetal anoxia. The placenta shows signs of 'ageing' structurally and functionally after term and the perinatal mortality rate begins to rise in pregnancies running beyond 42 weeks.

The risk of prolonged pregnancy will vary with other factors e.g. increased maternal age and hypertension.

A selective approach to intervention is, therefore, desirable and this is aided by modern methods of assessment:

1. Routine early ultrasound gives an accurate assessment of maturity.
2. A 'post dates' assessment of the fetus can be carried out at, say term + 10 days.
   (a) Ultrasound will estimate fetal weight, fetal attitude (increased flexion with diminished liquor) and liquor volume (largest pool measured).
   (b) Cardiotocography (repeated as considered appropriate) will give direct information about fetal well-being.

233

PROLAPSE AND PRESENTATION OF THE CORD

Prolapse occurs after rupture of the membranes when the presenting part is ill-fitting or abnormal. It is associated with multiparity and prematurity, disproportion and malpresentation, fetal abnormality and polyhydramnios.

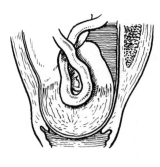

Prolapsed cord at the vulva

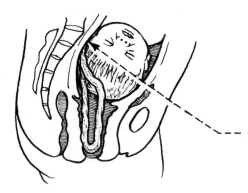

Once the cord is out of the uterus, and especially when out of the vagina, the fetal blood supply is obstructed, either because of the drop in temperature, or spasm of the vessels, or compression between the pelvic brim and the presenting part. If delivery is not effected within about 40 minutes, fetal death is likely.

The presence of prolapse may not be recognised until cord appears at the vulva; or cord may be palpated on vaginal examination done to assess progress of the labour or because of the sudden onset of acute fetal distress. It is essential to make a vaginal examination as soon as the membranes rupture in all patients who display an ill-fitting or non-engaged presenting part.

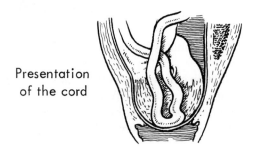

Presentation of the cord

Occult presentation of the cord

Presentation of the cord means that the cord is palpable at the cervix through intact membranes. Occult presentation means that the cord is lying alongside the presenting part but will not be palpable on vaginal examination. It is a particularly dangerous condition and may be a cause of unexpected fetal distress.

PROLAPSE OF THE CORD

TREATMENT

1. Determine the presence or absence of cord pulsation and fetal heart sounds. If the fetus is dead the labour may be left to proceed normally (if no other complication is present).
2. If the fetus is still alive, Caesarean section must be carried out as soon as possible unless vaginal delivery by forceps or breech extraction is likely to be straightforward.
3. While arrangements are being made for operation, the cord should be pushed back into the vagina and kept up with a gauze pack or by hand. An attempt is made to prevent compression of the cord between the presenting part and the pelvis by getting the mother to adopt a suitable position. The foot of the bed should be raised.

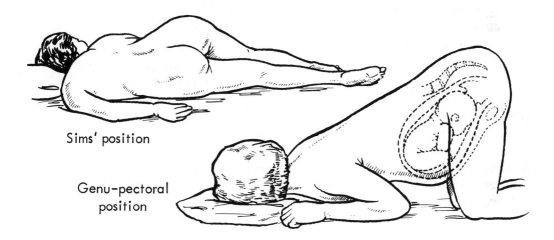

Sims' position

Genu-pectoral
position

4. Handling of the cord should be minimised as far as possible.
5. Prolapse of the cord, although often fatal for the child, carries no risk for the mother unless proper precautions are neglected for the sake of saving time. However great the need for haste, the mother must be properly prepared, and cross-matched blood made available.
6. Presentation of the cord when discovered by vaginal examination is an indication for section; but as the membranes are intact there is no immediate danger for the fetus, and more time is available.

POLYHYDRAMNIOS

Amniotic fluid has normally a volume of 500–1500 ml and if it is excessive it is called polyhydramnios. Two litres will be detectable clinically.

SIGNS

1. The uterus is bigger than expected.
2. Identification of the fetus and fetal parts is difficult.
3. The fetal heart is difficult to hear.
4. Ballottement of the fetus is easy.
5. A fluid thrill is detected.
6. Abdominal girth at umbilicus is more than 100 cm before term. The abdominal girth varies a little – an ebb and flow.

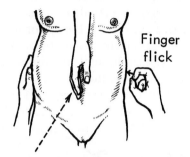

Finger flick

Hand on abdomen to cut transmission of impulse round abdominal wall

CAUSES

Excess liquor amnii is associated with fetal abnormality — especially anencephaly, spina bifida, oesophageal atresia, hydrops fetalis and monovular twins.

Haemangioma of the placenta is found on rare occasions with polyhydramnios.

Maternal conditions associated with polyhydramnios are diabetes and the more severe forms of heart disease and pre-eclampsia.

The development of polyhydramnios is usually gradual and in the last trimester. The symptoms are due to the bulk and weight of the uterus.
1. Discomfort and dyspnoea.
2. Indigestion.
3. Oedema, increase of varicose veins and haemorrhoids.
4. There may be abdominal pain.

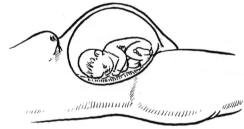

Polyhydramnios.

POLYHYDRAMNIOS

Polyhydramnios may be acute – developing quickly, usually 24–30 weeks. Acute abdominal pain and a feeling of bursting are often the presenting symptoms. Frequently there is vomiting. The abdominal skin is glazed, sometimes oedematous and often with fresh striae. The uterus is tense and tender and may be mistaken for concealed accidental haemorrhage, but there is no shock.

Polyhydramnios, whether acute or chronic, may lead to abortion or premature labour.

MANAGEMENT

A detailed ultrasound scan of the fetus should be carried out in an attempt to find a cause for the condition. If the fetus appears normal then the aim is to conserve the pregnancy. Rest and sedation may help and occasionally amniocentesis with drainage becomes necessary in an attempt to relieve distressing symptoms.

Amniocentesis

The placental site is localised by ultrasound and a needle or plastic catheter introduced into uterine cavity.

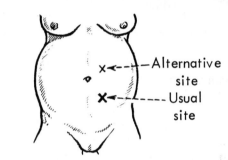

Amniocentesis (paracentesis) sites

1. The bladder is emptied.
2. A local anaesthetic is introduced into the skin of the abdomen over the lower left quadrant. If there are twins, the upper sac is more commonly affected and the chosen area is then just above the umbilicus.
3. The needle is pushed through into the uterus (if blood is obtained another site is chosen) and slow removal of 10dl of liquor will probably relieve the patient.

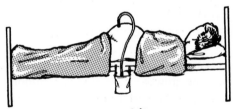

Drainage of liquor

Unfortunately the removal of liquor in this way sometimes stimulates uterine activity and the abdomen also tends to fill up again quickly.

If the fetus is found to be abnormal labour may be induced. An attempt should be made to drain the liquor slowly as the very rapid escape of a large volume of fluid may cause separation of the placenta and the problems of Abruption.

237

POLYHYDRAMNIOS

DIFFERENTIAL DIAGNOSIS

1. Multiple pregnancy — no fluid thrill.

2. Ovarian cyst — The cyst tends to press the pregnancy and cervix down into the pelvis.
    The polyhydramnios tends to lift the pregnancy out of the pelvis and the cervix is high.

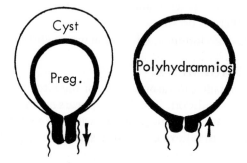

3. Hydatidiform mole — noted in early pregnancy but usually accompanied by bleeding.

4. A full bladder — this is usually caused by the uterus being incarcerated in the pelvis.

   Ultrasound will differentiate all these conditions if there is still doubt after clinical examination.

OLIGOHYDRAMNIOS

   This is a rare condition where the liquor may be reduced to a few ml. of milky fluid. Intra-uterine growth retardation is commonly associated with a degree of oligohydramnios and in cases of renal agenesis there is virtually no liquor.
   Absence of liquor makes the fetal skin dry and leathery and may produce pressure effects, e.g. talipes or torticollis, because of the lack of the amniotic fluid cushion and space.

UNSTABLE LIE

This term is used when the longitudinal axis of the fetus is repeatedly changing in relation to the uterus. Variable lie is an alternative title. Transverse, oblique or longitudinal lies may be found but no lie persists. The patient is usually multiparous.

CAUSES
1. Lax abdominal and uterine muscles.
2. Polyhydramnios.
3. Distortion of lower uterine pole: e.g. placenta praevia or pelvic tumour.
4. Abnormal fetus.

Congenital malformation of the uterus tends to give a stable malpresentation.

Unstable lie is not a problem till the last four or five weeks of pregnancy. The foreseen danger is that labour will commence or that the membranes will rupture while there is a malpresentation leading to obstructed labour and/or cord prolapse. For this reason it is common practice to suggest hospital admission at about 38 weeks to patients with unstable lie. As the pregnancy proceeds the likelihood of the onset of labour or rupture of the membranes increases.

The liquor amnii is at a maximum about 35 weeks (approximately one litre) and less at term (5dl or so). With fetal growth it appears even less relatively and this may stabilise the lie and presentation.

METHODS OF CONTROL
1. Time – as the liquor decreases and the fetus increases, the instability lessens and may lead to normal labour.
2. External version to longitudinal lie is usually easy. It may be repeated frequently in the hope that the liquor and fetal changes will give stability.
3. Polyhydramnios and an apparently normal fetus would encourage paracentesis as a method of stabilisation.
4. An abnormal fetus incompatible with life such as an anencephaly would justify termination of pregnancy, but not the risk of a Caesarean section.
5. Uterine stimulation by Oxytocin near term may be used if the lie is favourable, and if uterine activity develops then the membranes are ruptured.
6. The membranes may be ruptured to stabilise the presentation and Oxytocin then used to stimulate labour. This may be unsuccessful and a transverse or oblique lie recurs in which case Caesarean section is required.
7. Abnormal conditions such as tumours and suspected placenta praevia would be treated on their merits.
8. All cases which have had an unstable lie should be examined carefully in early labour to check that all is still satisfactory. If the membranes are intact and the lie other than longitudinal, external version may be possible.
9. Elective section may be used as being safest for a fetus which is plainly at risk.

SPECIAL CASES

1. THE ELDERLY PRIMIGRAVIDA

This uncomplimentary and rather emotive term is commonly applied to a woman who becomes pregnant for the first time at the age of over 35 years.

It is of course an arbitrary figure and the patients of this age who are young in mind and body, and have conceived without difficulty will usually do very well. Pregnancy in some women in this group, however, has occurred after a long period of infertility and there is an awareness in the minds of her attendants that the prospect of her conceiving again may be relatively low. The overall peri-natal mortality in this group is raised as is the incidence of operative delivery.

The following antenatal complications are increased in frequency and may merit special investigation.

(a) Abortion.   (d) Intra-uterine growth retardation.

(b) Down's syndrome.   (e) Premature labour.

(c) Hypertensive disorders.   (f) Gynaecological disorders e.g. fibroids.

2. DYSTOCIA DYSTROPHIA SYNDROME

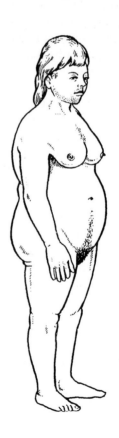

This term is used to describe women of a particular physical type who often present as elderly primigravidae, have had difficulty in conceiving and have a poor reproductive performance.

The woman is short and of stocky build.

There is a tendency to obesity, a male distribution of hair and an android pelvis.

Her hands are broad and square looking, and the fingers are short and of equal length.

The pelvic soft tissues tend to be rigid and lacking in elasticity.

Pre-eclampsia is relatively common.

There is a tendency for the pregnancy to become post-mature and occipito-posterior positions are common.

Labour is often prolonged and inco-ordinate and operative delivery is common.

3. THE GRAND MULTIPARA

This term is rarely used in these days of limitation of family size, but it is worth remembering that rising parity is associated with a rising peri-natal mortality rate. The increase in fetal loss in fourth and subsequent pregnancies is striking (see graph).

The mother of high parity is subject to the problems of increasing age and its effects, the harassment of a young family and the exhaustion this can cause, especially if there is little respite between pregnancies. The result may be self-neglect and poor attendance for antenatal care. Inevitably these factors are most harmful in lower socio-economic groups.

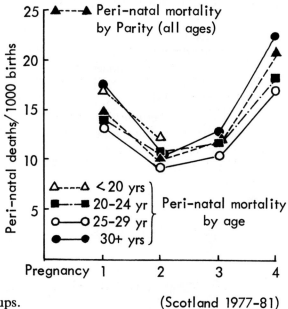

(Scotland 1977–81)

The incidence of the following complications is increased:

Anaemia.
Unstable lie due to muscular laxity.
Abruptio placentae.
Uterine rupture.
Post partum haemorrhage.

UTERINE DISPLACEMENTS AND ANOMALIES

RETROVERTED GRAVID UTERUS

This condition is probably a result of conception occurring in an already retroverted uterus. The commonest outcome is spontaneous correction between the 9th and 12th weeks, but sometimes the uterus becomes incarcerated in the pelvis as it grows, especially in the presence of some obstruction to correction such as adhesions or pelvic contraction.

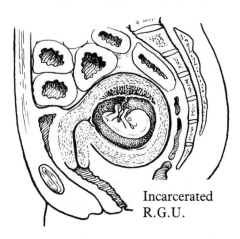

Incarcerated
R.G.U.

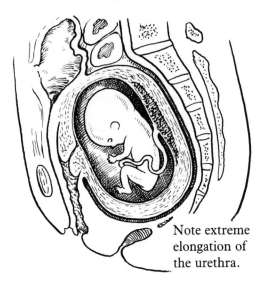

Note extreme
elongation of
the urethra.

The patient complains of pelvic pain and backache and defaecation is painful. The urethra is compressed and elongated causing frequencey, retention overflow and infection, and sometimes acute retention and rupture of the bladder. In addition the vesical blood supply is obstructed and gangrene of the bladder has been reported.

If uncorrected the pregnancy usually aborts but it can continue by a process of sacculation – hypertrophy and distension of the anterior wall of the uterus, which allows growth into the abdomen. If such a pregnancy reaches maturity delivery must be by section.

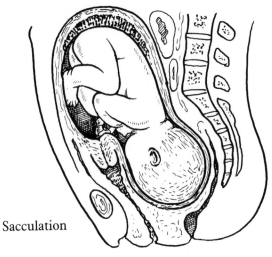

Sacculation

UTERINE DISPLACEMENTS AND ANOMALIES

RETROVERTED GRAVID UTERUS (continued)

Diagnosis

Urinary frequency and incontinence in early pregnancy always call for pelvic examination.
In retroversion the cervix is high behind the symphysis and difficult to reach, the bladder is
pushed up, and the soft uterus is felt in the pouch of Douglas.

Differenital Diagnosis

Urinary retention and pouch of Douglas swelling may also be due to:–
Haematocele from tubal pregnancy. Tenderness is extreme.
Fibroids are as a rule harder and more irregular.
An ovarian cyst may push the uterus up and forwards.
An ultrasound scan will help to differentiate these lesions.

Treatment

1. If a symptomless retroverted gravid uterus is detected, pelvic examination should be
    carried out every week until the uterus has emerged from the pelvis by the 12th or 13th
    week.
2. If urinary or other symptoms are present, the patient should be admitted and rested in bed
    for 48 hours with an indwelling catheter. A large watch-spring pessary may be inserted at
    the same time and the patient should lie more or less prone. If this simple treatment fails
    an attempt at correction by manipulation should be made with the patient under
    anaesthesia.

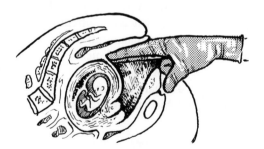 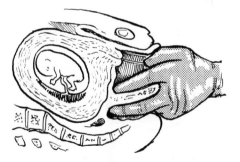

1. The cervix is pulled down with
    forceps with the patient in the knee
    elbow position. The fundus is pushed
    up through the posterior fornix.

2. Another method is to use finger
    pressure alone, via rectum and
    vagina.

243

UTERINE DISPLACEMENTS AND ANOMALIES

FORWARD DISPLACEMENT OF THE UTERUS ('PENDULOUS ABDOMEN')

If the pelvis is contracted and prevents descent, or if the abdominal muscles are weak (a consequence of repeated pregnancies) the uterus will project forward. A compensatory lordosis develops and the woman suffers great discomfort from backache and the stretching of the abdominal muscles. The condition causes delay in engagement of the presenting part apart from any disproportion, and may contribute to uterine rupture. A supporting corset may help during the pregnancy.

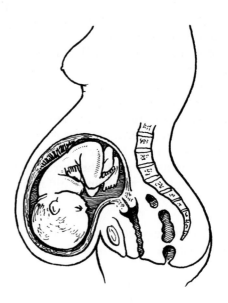

LATERAL DISPLACEMENT OF THE UTERUS

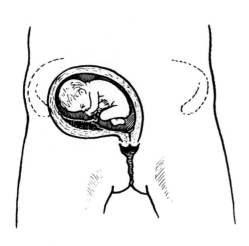

This may be discovered between the 6th and 10th weeks when the softening of the isthmus is at its maximum (see Hegar's sign). It is of no clinical significance except that it may be mistaken for a tubal pregnancy or pregnancy in a bicornuate uterus.

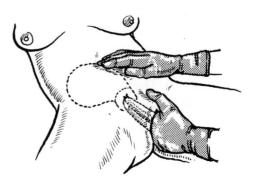

UTERINE DISPLACEMENTS AND ANOMALIES

PROLAPSE OF THE UTERUS

This may co-exist with pregnancy and will be aggravated in the early months by the softening and stretching of the tissues. The cervix projects well beyond the vulva and becomes oedematous and ulcerated. A ring pessary will maintain the uterus in the correct position until it is too big to descend through the pelvis (usually about the 20th week).

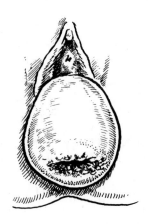

TORSION OF THE UTERUS

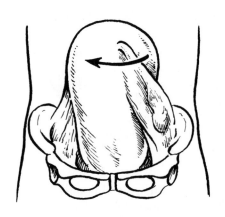

Some dextro-rotation is normal in pregnancy, probably because the pelvic colon takes up some of the space available in the left pelvis. Occasionally this rotation reaches 90° and if seen at Caesarean section care must be taken not to incise the left broad ligament and arteries. Torsion so severe as to interfere with the blood supply is unknown except as a complication of pregnancy in one horn of a double uterus when it is usually mistaken for concealed accidental haemorrhage.

UTERINE DISPLACEMENTS AND ANOMALIES

CONGENITAL ABNORMALITIES

These are the result of imperfect fusion of the two Müllerian ducts. The uterus, cervix and vagina, separately or together, can be single, double or intermediate; so classification is difficult and nomenclature confused. The anomalies described here are representative.

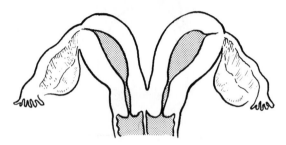

Double uterus, cervix and vagina
(Didelphys – 'double womb')

Uterus Didelphys

When both horns are well developed the pregnancy proceeds normally. Diagnosis is difficult but a double vagina and cervix may be observed, although easily missed at routine pelvic examination.

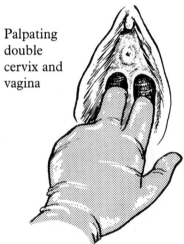

Palpating double cervix and vagina

Torsion of one horn can occur more easily than in the normal uterus and may occur during version, causing fetal death and symptoms of accidental haemorrhage. The non-gravid horn develops its own decidua and hypertrophies, and has been known to occupy the pelvis and obstruct labour.

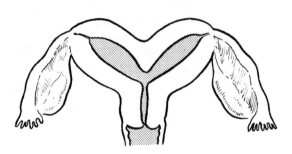

Uterus bircornis, unicollis, single vagina

Uterus Bicornis Unicollis

It is impossible to diagnose this condition except at laparotomy or perhaps during removal of a retained placenta which is more common with these abnormalities. This uterus encourages breech presentation – the head occupies one horn, the feet the other.

UTERINE DISPLACEMENTS AND ANOMALIES

CONGENITAL ABNORMALITIES (continued)

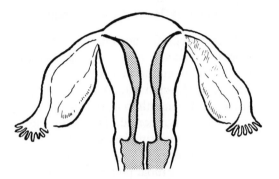

Uterus Septus

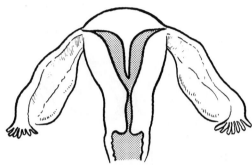

Uterus Subseptus

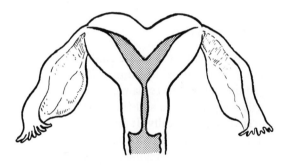

Uterus Arcuatus
('Cordiform Uterus')

This group can only be diagnosed when the uterus is opened at Caesarean section, although the arcuate uterus is often suspected on abdominal palpation through a thin abdominal wall. As a group they predispose to abortion, and to some complications of later pregnancy such as abnormal or unstable lie, and retained placenta.

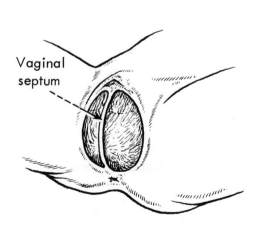

Vaginal septum

Vaginal Septa

These can occur on their own in otherwise normal genital tracts and are often incomplete. Sometimes the second stage may be delayed because of a septum preventing the advance of the head. The best treatment is to await this situation, and then when the septum is stretched, inject a little local anaesthetic, ligate, and divide with scissors.

UTERINE DISPLACEMENTS AND ANOMALIES

CONGENITAL ABNORMALITIES (continued)

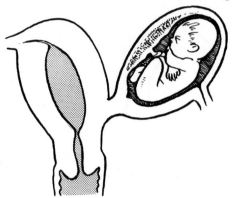

Pregnancy in Rudimentary Horn (Cornual Pregnancy)

Even though the horn has no access from the vagina, a 'wandering' sperm may fertilise an ovum on that side. Rupture with severe haemorrhage usually occurs at about the 4th month, but continuation to term has been reported. The non-pregnant horn hypertrophies, and the condition is usually (and fortunately) diagnosed as a tubal pregnancy, as the symptoms are similar. The treatment is excision of the gravid horn.

Angular Pregnancy

The ovum implants in the angle of the uterus near the tubal opening. The condition causes severe pain as the pregnancy progresses and the uterus enlarges asymmetrically. It may continue to term but there is a tendency to abortion, and tubal pregnancy may be diagnosed because of the patient's continual complaint of pain and the irregular swelling.

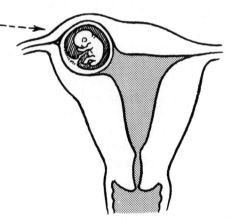

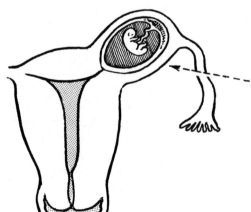

Interstitial Pregnancy

This is an ectopic implantation in the interstitial portion of the tube and is discussed under Ectopic Pregnancy. it is included here because of the similarity which it presents clinically and on palpation to angular and cornual pregnancies.

TUMOURS COMPLICATING PREGNANCY

The important ones are carcinoma of the cervix, fibroids and ovarian cysts.

FIBROIDS

Pregnancy in the presence of fibroids is rather rare. They contribute to infertility and are usually found in older women.

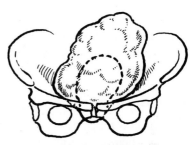

Multiple fibroids
at 12 weeks

Diagnosis: Fibroids are harder than any other pelvic mass likely to be met with and more likely to be multiple, but diagnosis is often presumptive. Twins, tubal pregnancy, ovarian cysts, salpingitis, cornual or angular pregnancies must all be considered. But fibroids are usually symptomless and can be left alone.

Degeneration: Fibroids are subject to 'red degeneration' (infarction) during pregnancy, when they become tender and painful and cause symptoms of fever. Sedation only is required until the condition subsides in a few days; but sometimes laparotomy may have to be done to exclude appendicitis. Degeneration may also complicate the puerperium.

Pressure Symptoms: If the fibroids are very big or are impacted in the pelvis, dysuria, dyschezia, abdominal distension, varicose veins and even dyspnoea may be complained of. Treatment should always be conservative unless an obstruction develops. Myomectomy in pregnancy is a very haemorrhagic operation, and likely to be followed by abortion.

Management of Labour: If the fibroid appears to be obstructing descent and engagement, Caesarean section should be carried out, but if not the labour should proceed normally. If there is doubt about obstruction the labour should be continued for a period to see if dilatation of the cervix causes the fibroid to be moved aside.

If delivery is by section, myomectomy should not be done at the same time. Fibroids regress considerably in the months following pregnancy and the uterine incision may be placed anywhere, through the fundus if necessary, to avoid interfering with the fibroids which will bleed excessively.

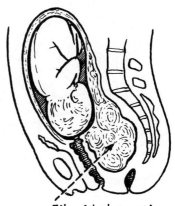

Fibroid obstructing
labour

TUMOURS COMPLICATING PREGNANCY

OVARIAN CYSTS

These tumours are generally removed at once because of their tendency to mechanical complications and the possibility of malignancy.

The commonest type is the simple cyst (70%) or the dermoid (25%). About 5% are malignant.

Diagnosis

Palpation is much easier in early pregnancy before the uterus occupies most of the pelvis. An ovarian cyst is more mobile than a hydro- or pyosalpinx, and less tender than a tubal pregnancy.

Diagnosis of cystic masses outside the gravid uterus has been simplified by the development of ultrasonography.

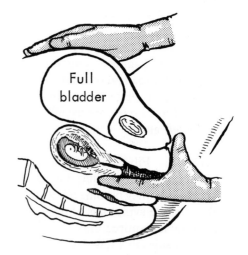

Eliciting Hegar's sign

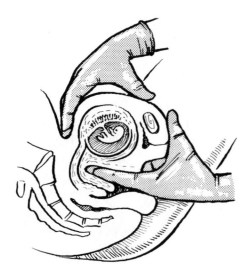

Palpating a full bladder

1. A full bladder especially when dislodged from the pelvis by the gravid uterus, is often mistaken for a cyst.
2. A normal gravid uterus from the 2nd to the 4th month has a very soft isthmic region (see Hegar's sign, page 73) and it is easy to mistake the cervix for the uterus and the corpus for a cyst.
3. The cyst may be a large corpus luteum. It is a good working rule to observe rather than operate on any single cyst up to the size of say a tangerine orange. Even then a corpus luteum is occasionally removed.

TUMOURS COMPLICATING PREGNANCY

OVARIAN CYSTS (continued)

Complications in the Cyst

1. Torsion is the commonest and may lead to rupture. The symptoms are acute, with sudden onset of abdominal pain, vomiting and pyrexia. These subside, to occur again a few days later. Pelvic examination will reveal a tender cystic mass and the distinction from tubal pregnancy may be impossible.

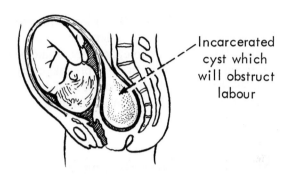

Incarcerated cyst which will obstruct labour

2. Pressure symptoms may arise if the cyst becomes incarcerated in the pelvis or is of very large size. These will include dysuria, pain, abdominal distension, varicose veins, dyschezia.

3. Suppuration. This is most likely in the puerperium as a result of trauma sustained during delivery.

Complications in the Pregnancy

1. There is an increased tendency to spontaneous abortion if the cyst is large.
2. A cyst in the pelvis will obstruct labour, causing malpresentation or non-engagement of the head.

- -

Treatment

The principle is to remove the cyst as soon as its presence is detected and its nature diagnosed. Laparotomy in early pregnancy is not usually a problem as little handling of the uterus is required to gain access to the cyst. If a cyst is discovered at or near term and is well clear of the pelvis, labour can be induced and the cyst removed a few days later. If the cyst is likely to obstruct labour Caesarean section and removal of the cyst should be performed.

The most difficult decisions arise in mid-pregnancy when laparotomy to remove the cyst might involve considerable uterine handling. The obstetrician must decide whether removal of the cyst can safely be postponed until the fetus is viable.

TUMOURS COMPLICATING PREGNANCY

CARCINOMA OF THE CERVIX

Treatment

Proper treatment of the condition requires the termination of the pregnancy. The implications of delaying treatment for the sake of the fetus should be fully discussed with the mother. If the baby is viable, delivery should be by Caesarean section following which normal treatment can be given. In early pregnancy hysterotomy may be carried out or external irradiation applied which will cause fetal death and abortion. Treatment in this case would be completed by the subsequent insertion of Caesium.

The positive cervical smear in pregnancy

The management of the positive cervical smear in pregnancy has been greatly simplified by the use of colposcopy. A colposcopic examination may provide adequate reassurance or allow a punch biopsy to be taken safely to make a definitive diagnosis.

CHAPTER 11

NORMAL LABOUR

LABOUR

Labour is the process of birth. In response to uterine contractions the cervix dilates, the birth canal is formed and the baby descends through the pelvis.

UTERINE ACTION

The fibres of the myometrium **Contract** and **Relax** like all muscle.

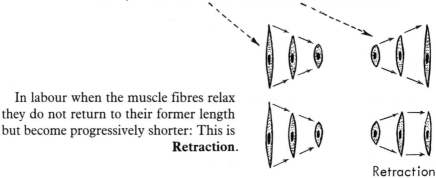

In labour when the muscle fibres relax they do not return to their former length but become progressively shorter: This is **Retraction**.

Retraction

The uterine capacity is thus progressively reduced and the thickness of the uterine wall increased.

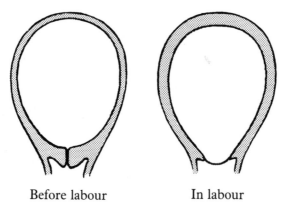

Before labour   In labour

As labour progresses the contractions increase in frequency, strength and duration. The muscle of the lower segment of the uterus (see Chapter 2) is thin and relatively passive, and the cervix consists mainly of fibrous connective tissue.

LABOUR

UTERINE ACTION (continued)

The effect of the progressive retraction of the upper segment muscle is to stretch and thin the lower segment and cause effacement and dilatation of the cervix. The junction of the upper and lower segments is called the physiological retraction ring.

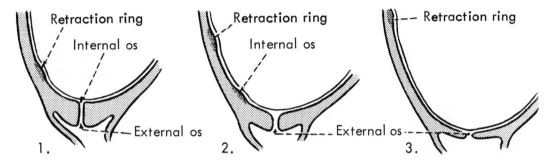

Effacement is most striking in the primigravida. In the parous patient dilatation and effacement usually occur together.

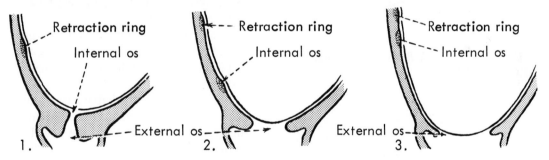

The effacement and dilatation of the cervix loosens the membranes from the region of the internal os with slight bleeding and sets free the mucus plug or operculum. This constitutes the 'Show' and allows the formation of the forewaters.

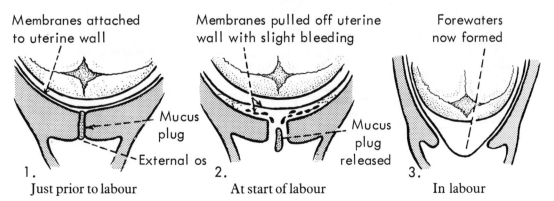

255

CHANGES IN BIRTH CANAL

AT BEGINNING OF LABOUR

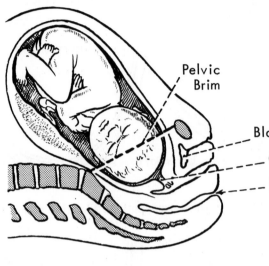

Pelvic Brim

Bladder

Cervix beginning to open

Normal anus

Labour is divided into **Three Stages:**
First Stage... start to full dilatation of the cervix.
Second Stage...full dilatation to birth of baby.
Third Stage... birth of baby to delivery of placenta (afterbirth).

The fetus is descending during first and second stages of labour.

The birth canal is formed by dilatation of cervix and vagina and by stretching and displacement of muscles of pelvic floor and perineum.

The bladder is pulled above the pubis because of the attachments to the uterus; the urethra is stretched and the bowel is compressed.

BIRTH CANAL AT BEGINNING OF SECOND STAGE

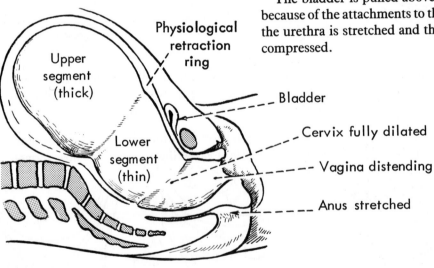

Upper segment (thick)

Physiological retraction ring

Lower segment (thin)

Bladder

Cervix fully dilated

Vagina distending

Anus stretched

CHANGES IN BIRTH CANAL

At the **End** of the **Second Stage** the birth canal has been fully formed. The outlet of the canal is at right angles to the inlet. This angulation is called the Curve of Carus

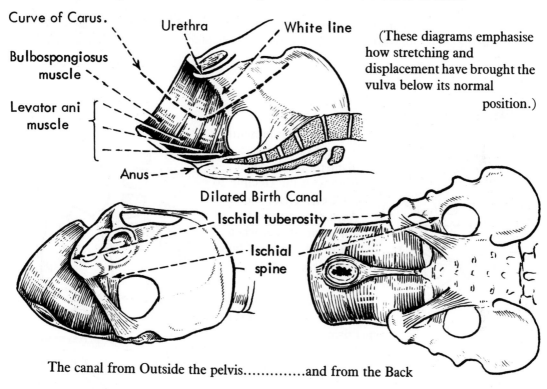

Curve of Carus.

Bulbospongiosus muscle

Levator ani muscle

Urethra

White line

Anus

(These diagrams emphasise how stretching and displacement have brought the vulva below its normal position.)

Dilated Birth Canal

Ischial tuberosity

Ischial spine

The canal from Outside the pelvis..............and from the Back

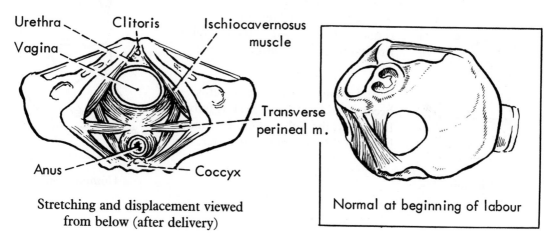

Urethra

Vagina

Clitoris

Ischiocavernosus muscle

Transverse perineal m.

Anus

Coccyx

Stretching and displacement viewed from below (after delivery)

Normal at beginning of labour

257

THE MECHANISM OF LABOUR

The mechanism of labour is the series of passive movements of the baby, particularly its presenting part, as it descends through the birth canal.

Illustrated is the mechanism of labour where the vertex presents in the left occipito-lateral (LOL) position (see Chapter 5).

NORMAL MECHANISM

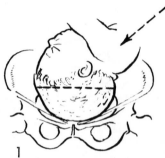

The **Head** is presenting in the **Transverse** diameter of the pelvic brim with the **Occiput** to the **Left**. There is often **Asynclitism** prior to engagement, i.e. when one or other parietal bone is the leading part.

1

The diagram shows the posterior parietal bone leading – this is posterior asynclitism. (If the anterior parietal bone is leading there is anterior asynclitism.)

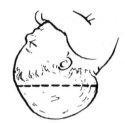

2

Asynclitism

At the **Beginning** of **Labour** the fetus is in an attitude of **Flexion** but the neck is not yet fully flexed so the **Occipito-Frontal** is the **Presenting** diameter.

As **Labour progresses** the fetus becomes compact. The neck is fully flexed and the **Suboccipito-Bregmatic** becomes the **Presenting** diameter.

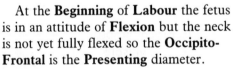

3

Flexion

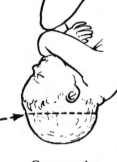

4

Compaction

258

NORMAL MECHANISM

Descent and **Engagement** occur.

Engagement is descent of presenting diameters through pelvic brim.

The leading part – the vertex – is now near the level of the ischial spines.

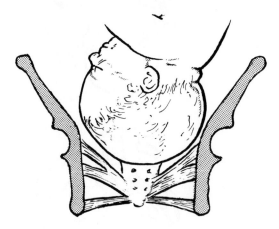

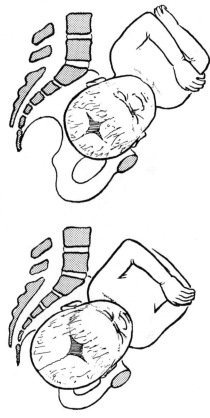

Descent continues and occiput rotates in cavity of pelvis anteriorly to the right oblique diameter bringing occiput to the left obturator foramen anteriorly.

Now in left occipito-anterior (L.O.A.) position.

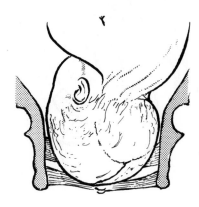

The L.O.A. position is partly attributed to the presence of the sigmoid colon in the left posterior quadrant of the pelvis.

Note how the neck is twisting.

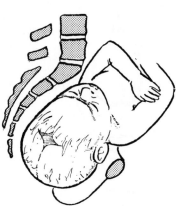

259

NORMAL MECHANISM

Descent continues and occiput reaches pelvic floor. Occiput now rotates to the front. This is **Internal rotation.** The head is now occipito-anterior (O.A.). Note twisting of the head and shoulders. The shoulders are in the left oblique of the brim.

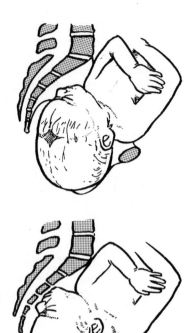

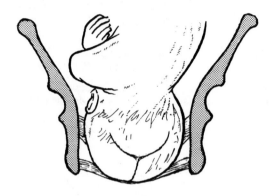

It is a maxim that the fetal part which first comes in contact with the pelvic floor rotates anteriorly (Internal rotation).

Rotation is through 45° from oblique and is called Anterior or Short rotation.

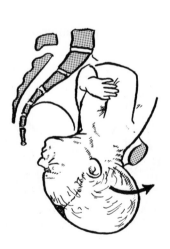

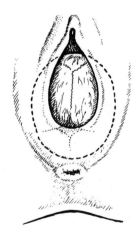

Occiput is now below the symphysis. A further descent of the fetus pushes head forwards with a movement of extension and the occiput is delivered.

Increasing extension round the pubis delivers the Bregma, Brow and Face.

NORMAL MECHANISM

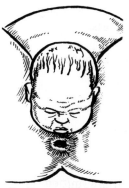

Delivery of Head

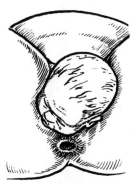

Restitution

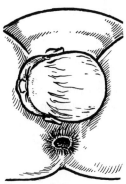

External Rotation

Descent and **Delivery** of the head has brought the shoulders into the pelvic cavity.

The head on delivery is oblique to the line of the shoulders. The bisacromial diameter is in left oblique diameter of the cavity.

The bisacromial diameter is the distance between the acromion processes and is 11cm.

The head now rotates to the natural position relative to the shoulders. This movement is known as **Restitution**.

Descent continues and the shoulders rotate to bring the bisacromial diameter into the antero-posterior diameter of the pelvic outlet.

This descent and rotation causes the head to rotate so that the occiput lies next to the left maternal thigh. This is **External rotation**.

The anterior shoulder now slips under the pubis and with lateral flexion of the fetal body the posterior shoulder is born. The rest of the body follows easily.

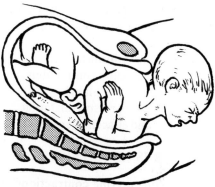

Delivery of Head

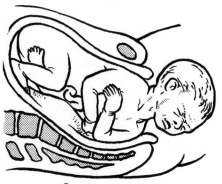

Restitution

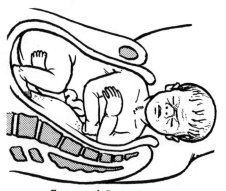

External Rotation

261

DIAGNOSIS OF LABOUR

The point of onset of labour is often uncertain as dilatation and effacement of the cervix may be present before labour, particularly in parous women. 'Show' is not always present and observation over a period of time may be needed to establish the diagnosis.

True labour
Regular contractions.
'Show'.
Progressive dilatation
and effacement of cervix.

False or **Spurious Labour**
Irregular contractions
No 'Show'
No progressive dilatation or
effacement of cervix

LABOUR IS RECOGNISED BY:

1. **Palpable uterine contractions** which are regular in frequency and intermittent in character. The interval between contractions is 10 minutes or less and each contraction may last half a minute or longer.

    The uterus becomes firm and rises, altering the abdominal contour. This is due to the rising forwards of the uterus so that it approximates to the direction of the birth canal. This movement is easier if the patient is upright. Ambulation may therefore give mechanical advantage.

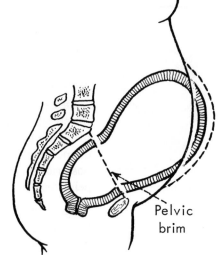

Pelvic brim

Altered abdominal contour with contraction

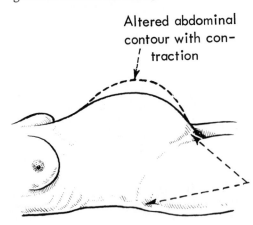

The discomfort is felt in upper sacral region and lower abdomen.

DIAGNOSIS OF LABOUR

Recognition of Labour (continued)

2. **'Show'** — a little blood and mucus discharged from the vagina. This is from separation of the membranes at the lower pole causing bleeding which mixes with the operculum of the cervix.

3. **Dilatation of the Cervix**. This is accompanied by the formation of forewaters or bag of waters.

Cervical dilatation is guaged by vaginal or rectal examination and is expressed in the diameter across the cervix or by proportions of dilatation.

  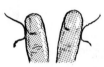 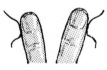

1 Finger	2 Fingers	3 Fingers	4 Fingers
2cm	3.5cm	5.5cm	7.5cm
	⅓ DILATED	½ DILATED	¾ DILATED

(These are Clinical Estimations)

PROGRESS IN LABOUR

PROGRESS IN LABOUR IS GAUGED BY:

1. Increasing strength, frequency and duration of **uterine contractions** — assessed by palpation, external abdominal transducer or intrauterine catheter (see page 271).

2. **Dilatation of the cervix**. This may be estimated by vaginal or rectal examination.

Vaginal examinations must be done with antiseptic precautions

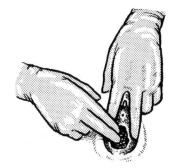

After cleansing the vulva the labia are parted with the gloved hand.

The fingers of the right hand are introduced gently into the vagina.

Points to be noted:
1. Degree of dilatation and effacement of the cervix.
2. Presence or absence of forewaters.
3. State of the liquor if any (clear? meconium stained?).
4. Position of the presenting part. This is determined by palpating the suture lines and fontanelles in relation to the pelvic diameters.
5. Level of the presenting part. This is judged by its relationship to the brim or ischial spines.

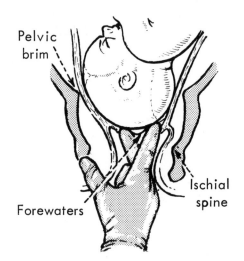

The diagram shows a well-flexed head in the LOL position which is almost engaged (the suboccipito-bregmatic diameter is just above the brim), the cervix is about 3 fingers dilated and the forewaters are present.

PROGRESS IN LABOUR

2. **Dilatation of Cervix** (continued)

Rectal examination

This carries no risk of infection but gives less information than vaginal examination and is not so accurate. It is excellent for gauging the level of the presenting part.

The upper vagina and rectum lie close to each other. Only one finger can be introduced.

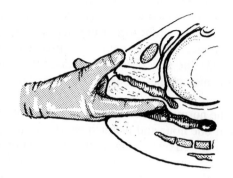

3. **Descent of presenting part —** this can be recognised by
   (a) abdominal palpation and
   (b) changing fetal heart positions.

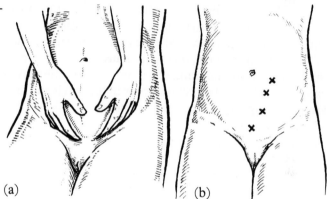

(a)   (b)

On vaginal examination descent is judged by Zero Station Notation.

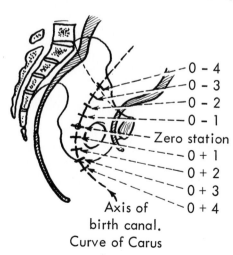

```
                    0 - 4
                    0 - 3
                    0 - 2
                    0 - 1
                    Zero station
                    0 + 1
                    0 + 2
                    0 + 3
   Axis of          0 + 4
   birth canal.
   Curve of Carus
```

Zero is the level of the ischial spines, that is the mid pelvis, and estimations are in centimetres above and below zero.

The leading part at zero = just engaged

Compare with fifths above the brim – page 275.

PROGRESS IN LABOUR

The **First Stage** of labour in a primigravida lasts up to 12 hours and sometimes longer and in a parous woman is usually 4–8 hours.

The effects of the increasing strength of contractions on the mother will be obvious in her appearance. During them she is preoccupied and slips into the breathing pattern she has learned. She may become distressed with the contractions. Commonly spontaneous rupture of the membranes occurs as the first stage proceeds.

The normal **Second Stage** of labour in a primigravida lasts about one hour and is much shorter in the parous woman. It is recognised by a change in the character of the contractions. They become more powerful and expulsive with a desire to bear down, and the secondary forces now come into action. The diaphragm is fixed, the patient holds her breath and the abdominal muscles contract. Sometimes the mother feels nauseated and may vomit. She may have the feeling that the bowel is about to move, due to pressure on the rectum, and this may have an inhibiting effect on her until the reason is explained. The head descends deeply in the pelvis and may be visible or palpable through the perineum.

MANAGEMENT OF LABOUR

GENERAL CONSIDERATIONS

The aim should be to provide the mother with a relaxed, friendly atmosphere within which her well-being and that of the baby can be closely supervised. The presence of her husband, partner or mother should be encouraged. The mother's preferences in respect of the conduct of her labour and delivery should be met as far as possible. Where a particular preference is considered ill-advised this should be explained and usually the matter is easily resolved.

The Labour Suite should provide a sitting room furnished with comfortable chairs of various heights and types. Radio and television may provide entertainment and distraction. There should be a separate delivery room with a bed to which the mother can retire if she wishes. Modern delivery beds can be adapted to look like normal beds for the first stage of labour, while providing features to allow operative procedures to be carried out as required.

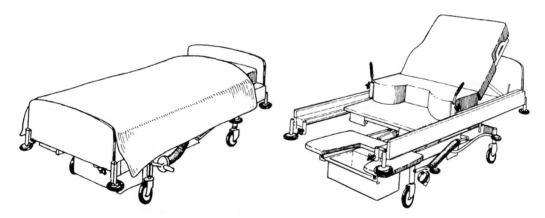

If the mother is in bed during the first stage she should (a) sit propped up using e.g. bean bags or (b) lie tilted by a wedge to avoid the supine position and thus possible hypotension.

(a)   (b)

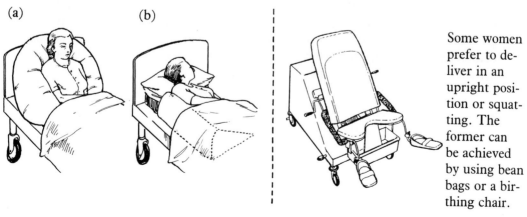

Some women prefer to deliver in an upright position or squatting. The former can be achieved by using bean bags or a birthing chair.

MANAGEMENT OF LABOUR

CARE OF THE MOTHER

1. **General** — The mother should not be left alone. Fears can be allayed and confidence engendered by a supportive midwife. Minimal perineal shaving may be done in case an episiotomy is required. If the rectum is full a suppository is given to reduce the risk of faecal soiling in late labour. A bath or shower can be refreshing.

2. **Diet** is withheld because delayed gastric emptying leads to the danger of inhalation of stomach contents should a general anaesthetic be required. The routine administration of antacids has now been stopped in many hospitals but H_2-antagonists such as Cimetidine may be given intramuscularly if surgical intervention seems likely.

3. **Pulse rate,** blood pressure and urinary output are measured regularly and if ketosis or dehydration develops this is treated by intravenous fluids.

4. **Progress** in labour is assessed as already described (see page 264).

5. **Analgesia** is given as required. The method chosen depends on the mother's preference, her reaction to her contractions and the likely length of her labour.

   (a) *Inhalation* — Entonox is a 50/50 mixture of oxygen and nitrous oxide. It may be used near the end of the first stage or during the second stage of labour.

   The device is designed for self-administration by inhalation through a mask or mouthpiece attached to a cylinder.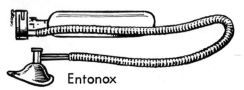

   Entonox

   (b) *Narcotic drugs* — Pethidine 100–200mg, Morphine 10–20mg and Pentazocine (Fortral) are the mainstay for women in established labour. The first two may be combined with Promazine (Sparine) to reduce the incidence of nausea. All three drugs depress fetal respiration and Naloxone (Narcan Neonatal) should be used intravenously or intramuscularly if the baby is affected.

   (c) *Continuous epidural anaesthesia* — Local anaesthetic (0.25% or 0.5% Bupivicaine) is instilled at 3–4 hour intervals through a catheter inserted into the epidural space. This gives the patient complete freedom from pain of labour. Most obstetricians consider epidural anaesthesia justified if the patient asks for it and it is the method of choice in some cases e.g. hypertension, premature labour.

MANAGEMENT OF LABOUR

CARE OF THE MOTHER (continued)

(c) *Continuous epidural anaesthesia* (continued)

Its use has transformed the management of difficult or prolonged labour and it has been of great benefit to many women. The absence of maternal distress must not mislead the obstetrician into ignoring signs of obstructed labour and the effect of prolonged contractions on the mother and fetus. Its disadvantage is that after its administration the patient must lie on her side to avoid the possibility of hypotension. It may also lead to prolongation of the second stage of labour by abolishing involuntary expulsive efforts and thus lead to a higher incidence of operative vaginal delivery. This is by no means inevitable where weaker concentrations of Bupivicaine are used and midwives are used to managing such labours. Operative delivery, including Caesarean section, can be done under epidural block.

Epidural anaesthesia should be administered by an experienced anaesthetist, and supervised by him throughout labour even if the 'top-ups' are given by the midwives.

The epidural space is about 4mm wide and lies between the dura and the periosteum of the vertebral canal. It is limited above at the foramen magnum where dura and periosteum fuse, and below by the ligament covering the sacral hiatus.

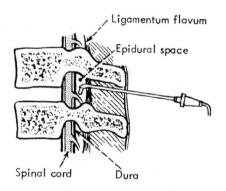

Local anaesthetic can be injected into this space which is traversed by the spinal nerves, and produce the same effect as a spinal block without the risk of headache, meningism or nerve root trauma.

Complications

1. Mild hypotension (about 20%).
2. Sepsis.
3. Needle inserted into cerebrospinal space. (This is a failure of the technique.)
4. Bladder atony and increased need for catheterisation (about 40%).
5. Total spinal block. This occurs if the local anaesthetic is injected into the cerebrospinal space. Respiration is paralysed and there is hypotension. This is an acute anaesthetic emergency.

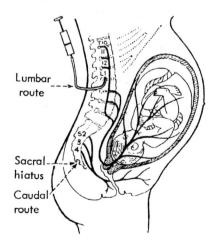

269

MANAGEMENT OF LABOUR

CARE OF THE MOTHER (continued)

6. **Second stage**   The mother is allowed to make involuntary expulsive efforts provided full dilatation of the cervix has been confirmed. Premature pushing can make the cervix oedematous and delay progress.

   Organised pushing should not be started until the baby's head is visible. This is hard work and the mother will tire quickly.

CARE OF THE BABY

Assessment of the baby's condition in labour depends essentially on observations of the fetal heart rate. The presence of **Meconium** in the liquor should always be noted but is, at best, only a warning that there may be a problem. It is postulated that fetal anoxia leads to an increased output by the vagus, stimulating the fetal gut and resulting in the passage of meconium.

(a) **Fetal heart recordings** — The traditional method of recording the fetal heart intermittently, between contractions, by the Pinard stethoscope suffers from the grave drawback that changes in the heart rate are first seen in association with uterine contractions, and must be related to them in time.

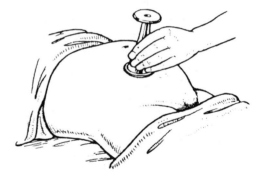

Continuous fetal heart recording, as presently established however, has the disadvantage of tying the mother to her delivery bed. While its use is mandatory in high-risk labours, it can be used intermittently in normal mothers by detaching the electrode from the monitor to permit mobility and recording continuously when the mother wishes to be in bed or in a chair.

The development of telemetric monitoring will render some of these conflicts obsolete.

MANAGEMENT OF LABOUR

Continuous Fetal Heart Rate Monitoring

The fetal monitor provides a continuous printed record of the fetal heart rate, and uterine contractions, and also gives an immediate indication of the FH through a ratemeter, a flashing light, and an audible signal.

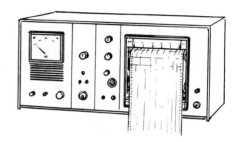

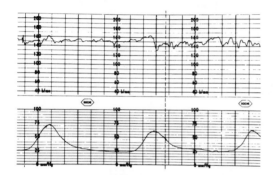

The FHR may be recorded through an ultrasonic transmitter-receiver (a transducer) or through the fetal ECG obtained by an electrode implanted in the fetal scalp. Uterine contractions are indicated by an external tocograph, a very delicate pressure gauge, or more accurately by an intrauterine catheter.

Ultrasonic Recording

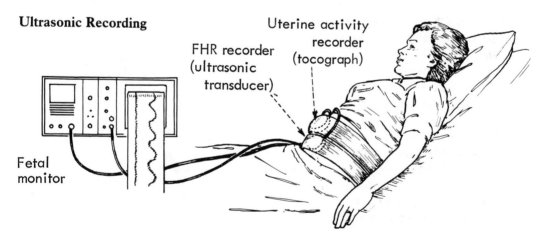

Very high frequency sound waves (2 million per second) are transmitted from the central crystal, and enough of the waves reflected from the fetal heart surface are picked up by the six receivers.

As the heart surface is moving, the returning waves have a different frequency (Doppler effect) and the rate at which these different frequencies are received is recorded by the monitor.

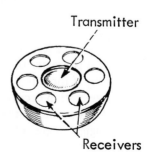

271

MANAGEMENT OF LABOUR

Fetal ECG Recording

The monitor records the rate at which the R wave of the fetal ECG is obtained from the scalp electrode. This gives a better tracing than ultrasonic recording but is a little more complicated — the membranes must be ruptured and the presenting part accessible — while the midwife can set up ultrasound apparatus at any stage in the labour.

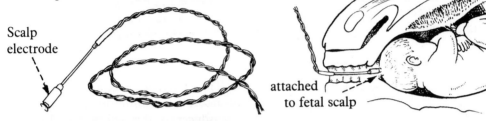

Scalp electrode

attached to fetal scalp

Interpretation of Intrapartum FHR Tracings

1. The average baseline rate should be between 120 to 160 beats per minute. Sustained tachycardia may be a warning of fetal distress and prolonged or severe bradycardia is ominous.

2. *Baseline variability.* The normal FHR fluctuates by ± 10 beats/min every 5 seconds or so — evidence of fetal ability to react normally to the stress of labour. Loss of this variability, especially in association with tachycardia, indicates severe hypoxia. (This is sometimes referred to as 'beat-to-beat variation'.)

3. *Response of FHR to uterine contractions.* The uterine contraction acts as a stress to the fetus, producing a transient reduction in oxygenated blood supply. The normal FHR should be maintained with the contraction or show only a slight deceleration of less than 40 beats/min. If it is greater than this and especially if there is a 'lag phase' or late deceleration occurring after the period of uterine contraction, a pathological degree of hypoxia may be present.

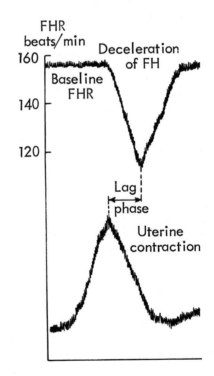

MANAGEMENT OF LABOUR

Response of FHR to uterine contractions (continued)

Decelerations may be classified as:

(a) *Early*, where the lowest rate of the FH coincides with the peak of contractions. These may be normal in late labour but should not be ignored if persistent or severe.

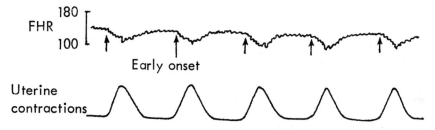

(b) *Late*, where the lowest rate of the FH follows the peak of contraction. These are indicative of hypoxia.

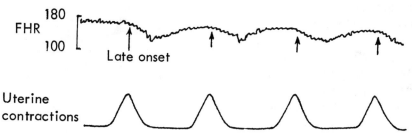

(c) *Variable*, where the pattern and timing of deceleration varies with contractions. These are thought to be due to cord compression. They are quite common and may be related to the mother's position. They should not however be ignored if persistent or associated with other adverse features.

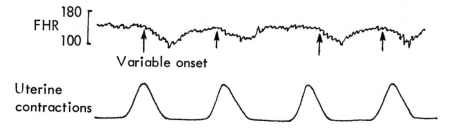

MANAGEMENT OF LABOUR

CARE OF THE BABY (continued)

(b) Fetal blood sampling

During the arduous work of normal labour the mother gradually develops a metabolic acidosis (a depletion of her buffer reserves), but the pH is maintained at 7.38 ± 0.03. In dysfunctional labour the acidosis may be of such degree as to bring about an actual lowering of the pH.

Normal fetal pH is much more acid at 7.30 ± 0.05, but in the presence of hypoxia it compensates by the anaerobic catabolism of its glycogen stores, leading to an accumulation of lactic acid and a fall in pH.

To obtain a sample of fetal blood for pH estimation, a special tube (amnioscope) is passed through the cervix which must be sufficiently dilated. By using a special guarded knife a blob of blood is obtained from the scalp which can be sucked up and analysed in a pH meter.

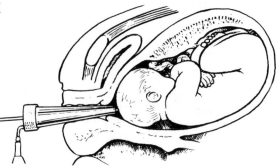

There is a small risk of scalp haemorrhage which may be difficult to control, and the sampling has to be repeated every two or three hours which may distress the patient.

Indications for fetal scalp blood sampling (FBS)

It will be seen that this technique takes time and trouble, and causes inconvenience to the patient and her attendants. However until electrodes for the continuous monitoring of fetal pH and O_2 become generally available, FBS is the only available test for confirming or excluding fetal hypoxia which may be suggested by FHR monitoring or the presence of meconium.

pH levels between 7.20 and 7.25 are suspicious and require repeat estimation if the labour is allowed to proceed. Levels below 7.20 are indicative of significant fetal acidosis and delivery is indicated.

PARTOGRAMS IN THE MANAGEMENT OF LABOUR

The partogram, a graphic display of progress in labour, has become widely used in many different situations.

Friedman conceived a graph of cervical dilatation and time (a cervicogram) and applied it to the clinical management of labour.

This principle has been modified and adapted by many workers and it is now a partogram, showing the progress and management of labour.

Most partograms show the dilatation of the cervix and the descent of the head in fifths as described by Crichton (abdominally) or by zero notation (vaginally).

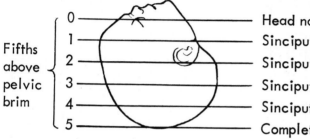

Fifths above pelvic brim

- 0 — Head not palpable.
- 1 — Sinciput felt: occiput not felt.
- 2 — Sinciput felt: occiput just felt.
- 3 — Sinciput easily felt: occiput felt.
- 4 — Sinciput high: occiput easily felt.
- 5 — Completely above brim.

Philpott took 1cm per hour dilatation as being a reasonable gradient. He drew an 'Alert' line starting at 1cm and four hours later an 'Action' line. Others have varied the charts to differentiate between primigravid and parous cases.

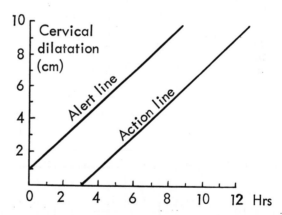

Having been introduced initially to illustrate dilatation of the cervix and to give warning of failure of normal progress, partograms are now used to illustrate all the routine observations on mother and baby together with uterine action and drug therapy.

PARTOGRAM (Diagrammatic)

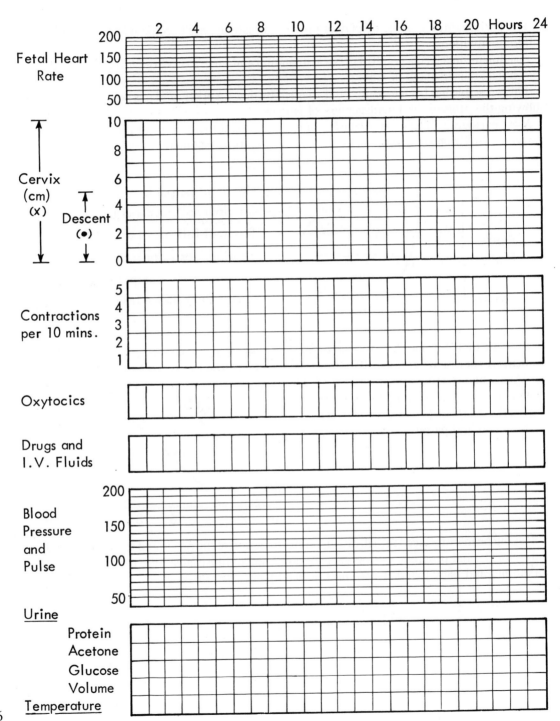

MANAGEMENT – DELIVERY

As in the rest of her labour the mother will commonly be accompanied by her partner, even at operative delivery.

To help create a more informal and 'homely' atmosphere, many hospitals have abandoned the use of sterile gowns and masks for attendants, only sterile gloves being worn.

Most women are delivered in the dorsal position but the left lateral or an upright position may be preferred. If delivery is conducted in the dorsal position, the mother should be tilted by the use of a wedge to avoid supine hypotension.

For mother
> Sterile drapes for legs and thighs.
> Sterile sheet and pad to go below
>   buttocks and on bed.
> Sterile towel to cover abdomen.

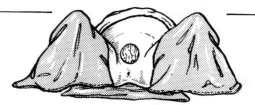

For episiotomy and **repair** of **perineal wounds**
> Local anaesthetic
>   syringe and needles.
> Scissors — for cutting
>   perineum (episiotomy).
> Sutures and needles
>   for repair.

For baby care (see Care of Newborn and Asphyxia.)
> Sterile towel — for reception.
> Mucus suction catheter.
> Oxygen.
> Laryngoscope.
> Warm cot.
> Syringes, needles and
>   ampoules of
>   Naloxone (Narcan)

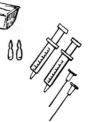

For swabbing and **wiping clean**
> Bowls with lotions.
> Swabs and cotton wool.
> Gamgee pads.

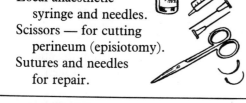

Cotton wool for wiping baby's eyes

For care of cord
> Pressure forceps to
>   clamp cord,
>   or cord clamp or
>   cord ligatures.
> Scissors to cut cord.

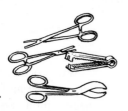

For controlling bleeding
> Oxytocic drugs.
> Syringe and needles.
> Pressure forceps for
>   bleeding points
>   in perineum.
> Bowl to collect and
>   measure third stage
>   blood loss and to
>   receive placenta.

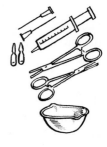

MANAGEMENT – DELIVERY

With the further descent and rotation of the head the perineum distends, the anus dilates and the vagina opens with contractions. There is regression between contractions but each contraction gives further progress and delivery is imminent.

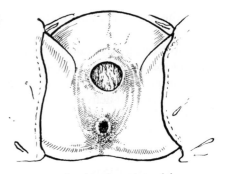

Delivery is a sterile and antiseptic procedure

Delivery of the baby may be conducted in the left lateral or in the dorsal position.

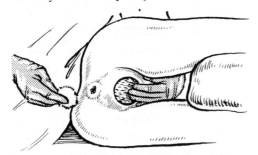

In the left lateral position the right leg is supported.

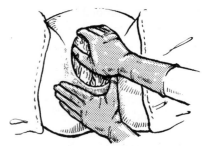

In the dorsal position the anal region is not so well seen.

A sterile pad soaked in antiseptic lotion is placed over the anus. The sinciput may be felt behind the anus at the tip of the sacrum.

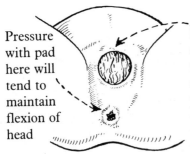

Pressure with pad here will tend to maintain flexion of head

Pressure downwards on head will promote flexion and allow occiput to slip under pubis. The distending diameter is usually the occipito-frontal.

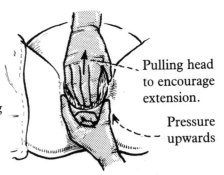

Pulling head to encourage extension.

Pressure upwards

Crowning of the head is when there is no recession between contractions and is due to the biparietal diameter having passed through the bony pelvis.

When occiput is free extension is encouraged and head is delivered. The neck region is now explored and if the cord is felt it is pulled to give some slack. The baby's eyes are wiped.

MANAGEMENT – DELIVERY

Restitution now occurs and then external rotation as the shoulders descend in pelvis.

The head is now grasped — fingers of the left hand beneath chin and jaw and the right fingers below the occiput.

The head is now taken towards the anus to dislodge the anterior shoulder from behind the pubis.

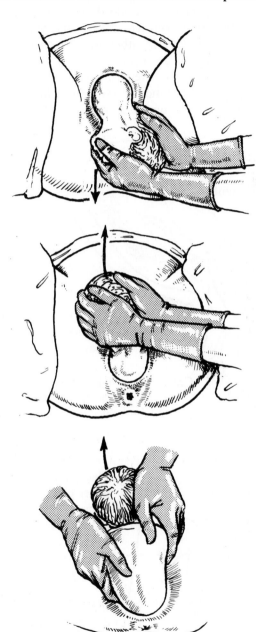

After the birth of the anterior shoulder the head is now lifted up over the pubis. This allows the posterior shoulder to slip over the perineum and be delivered. Traction should not be necessary, just guidance.

The perineum is often torn by the birth of the shoulders especially if the delivery is hurried and not allowed to occur with uterine contraction.

The shoulders are now gripped and the trunk delivered by lifting up over pubis. This can sometimes be aided by taking the shoulders posteriorly first and then upwards. The trunk and legs are thus delivered.

The baby's mouth and nose are drained by posture and suction. The baby soon cries and is now laid between the mother's legs or on her abdomen and the cord is divided between clamps or ligatures.

MANAGEMENT – THIRD STAGE

The first and second stages of labour are now complete and the THIRD stage has started.

The management of the Third Stage begins during the delivery of the baby. It is almost universal practice, in normal cases, to give Syntometrine (Syntocinon 5 units and Ergometrine 0.5mg) intra-muscularly either with the crowning of the head or with the delivery of the anterior shoulder. The Syntocinon acts in $2\frac{1}{2}$–3 minutes and the aim is to reduce the risk of the third stage and immediate post-partum haemorrhage. If the injection is given with the crowning of the head and the rest of the delivery proceeds in an unhurried manner, the drug will be taking effect on the uterus as the delivery of the baby is completed.

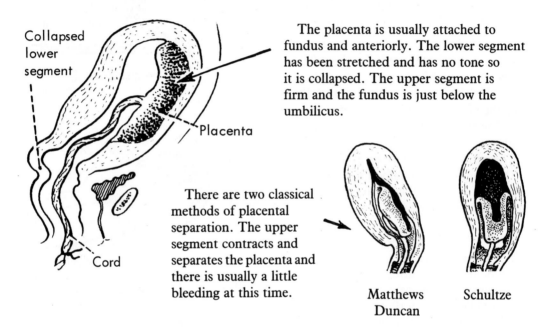

The placenta is usually attached to fundus and anteriorly. The lower segment has been stretched and has no tone so it is collapsed. The upper segment is firm and the fundus is just below the umbilicus.

There are two classical methods of placental separation. The upper segment contracts and separates the placenta and there is usually a little bleeding at this time.

Matthews Duncan

Schultze

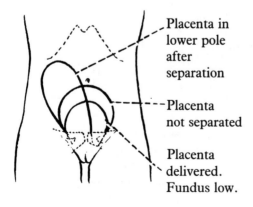

Placenta in lower pole after separation

Placenta not separated

Placenta delivered. Fundus low.

The placenta now descends into the lower segment and gives it form. The fundus thus rises above the umbilicus, is hard and, no longer containing the placenta, is narrower and often displaced laterally.

The placenta is then expelled or removed, and as the lower segment is again empty it collapses and the fundus is now narrow, hard and found halfway between the pubis and umbilicus.

MANAGEMENT – THIRD STAGE

The management of the third stage is now explained in the light of this physiological description. It is best conducted in the dorsal position.

1. The height, width and consistency of the fundus may be felt by gentle palpation. Rubbing the fundus may cause irregular uterine activity which partly separates the placenta and causes bleeding.

2. It is useful to put a ligature or clamp on the cord at the vulva. Descent of the placenta will cause the ligature to move away from the vulva. A bowl is placed against the perineum to collect any blood.

3. The signs of the placental separation are:

    > Narrow, hard, ballotable fundus.
    > Slight bleeding.
    > Lengthening of the cord.

4. The separated placenta may be removed by traction on the cord while the other hand maintains pressure upwards on the fundus (Brandt-Andrews' method). - - - - - - ➤

    Cord traction has become established as the commonest way of delivering the placenta. Alternatively the mother may be asked to expel it by bearing down once separation has occurred. The risks of cord traction are uterine inversion (see Chapter 13) or avulsion of the cord.

5. When the placenta appears at the vulva it is caught by both hands and the membranes are twisted gently to allow them to peel off completely. A bowl placed against the perineum allows blood loss to be assessed. Normal loss is about 250ml.

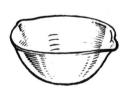

Murdoch's bowl

6. The uterine fundus is now rubbed up to assure firm contraction.

7. The vagina, labia and perineum are inspected for tears or other injuries. The vulva is swabbed down and a sterile pad placed over it to collect the lochial discharge.

8. The placenta is now examined. It is suspended by the cord to show the extent of the membranes and any deficiencies. It is then placed maternal side uppermost to see if it is complete. An incomplete placenta is an indication for immediate exploration of the uterus.

CHAPTER 12

ABNORMAL LABOUR

INDUCTION OF LABOUR

Termination of a pregnancy by inducing labour may be indicated because of a suspected or confirmed risk to the mother or baby, or both.

Such indications are:

Hypertensive disorders.
Prolonged pregnancy.
Compromised fetus e.g. growth retardation.
Maternal diabetes.
Rhesus sensitisation.

Hypertensive disease and prolonged pregnancy have long been the largest groups. Induction in such cases has often been carried out on epidemiological data as opposed to established risk in an individual case. Modern methods of fetal assessment aim to establish the risk in an individual and thus avoid needless intervention.

Other indications for induction are:

Fetal abnormality or death — the main reason for intervention is to alleviate distress in the mother.

Social — induction may be requested by a mother for a variety of social or domestic reasons. The obstetrician may reasonably agree to such requests if the findings are favourable for delivery and if there are no features which would make intervention unusually hazardous.

The effectiveness of modern methods of induction may tempt the obstetrician to be over-enthusiastic in their use. Any intervention should carry the implication of delivery by whatever means necessary and must therefore be justifiable.

METHODS OF INDUCTION

As labour approaches, the cervix normally shows changes known as 'ripening' so that it becomes 'inducible' and is then called a 'favourable' cervix. The condition of the cervix is the most important factor in successful induction and, where ripening has not occurred, there is a greater chance of a long labour, fetal hypoxia and operative delivery.

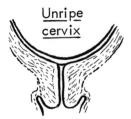

Unripe cervix

An unripe cervix is hard, long, closed and not effaced.

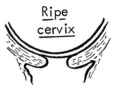

Ripe cervix

A ripe cervix is soft, effaced or becoming effaced and admits the finger.

INDUCTION OF LABOUR

METHODS OF INDUCTION (continued)

Cervical Score					
	0	1	2	3	
Dilatation (cm)		<2	2-4	>4	
Length (cm)		>2	1-2	<1	
Consistency	Firm	Average	Soft		
Position	Post.	Mid Anterior			
Level	0-3	0-2	0-1:0	0+	
				Total	

The Bishop score

This is an accepted method of recording the degree of ripeness before labour (cf. the Apgar Score applied to the newborn baby). It takes account of the length, dilatation and consistency of the cervix and the level of the fetal head. A score of 9 or higher is favourable.

(a) RIPENING THE CERVIX

The collagen fibres of which the cervix is composed can be much softened in consistency by the local application of prostaglandin. A vaginal tablet of Dinoprostone 3mg (Prostin E2) may be inserted into the posterior fornix to soften and efface the cervix. This will permit amniotomy and may even result in the initiation of labour. In special circumstances, e.g. fetal death in utero, a Dinoprostone solution may be infused extra-amniotically through a Foley catheter.

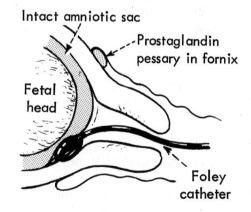

Intact amniotic sac

Prostaglandin pessary in fornix

Fetal head

Foley catheter

INDUCTION OF LABOUR

(b) **AMNIOTOMY** (Artificial Rupture of Membranes)

This is done to initiate labour (surgical induction) or, during labour, to try to accelerate the course, or to allow a fetal scalp electrode to be applied or to permit estimation of the fetal pH. Amniotomy appears to release a local secretion of endogenous prostaglandins.

Two methods are commonly described:-

1. FOREWATER AMNIOTOMY

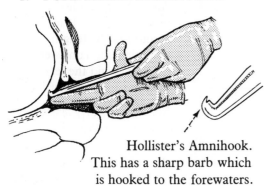

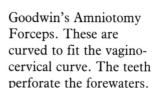

Hollister's Amnihook.
This has a sharp barb which
is hooked to the forewaters.

Goodwin's Amniotomy
Forceps. These are
curved to fit the vagino-
cervical curve. The teeth
perforate the forewaters.

The operation may be done blindly by passing the instrument along the fingers or by direct vision using a speculum.

2. HINDWATER AMNIOTOMY

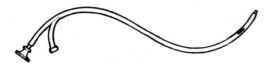

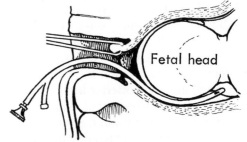

Fetal head

The instrument used is a Drew-Smythe cannula. It is passed above the fetal head by palpation or visually to puncture the amnion in the region of the neck.

Hindwater rupture is seldom used now. It is not so effective as forewater rupture. There is risk of injury to uterus or placenta. Occasionally copious bleeding leads to fetal death. (Kleihauer's test should be done if there is bleeding). Amniotic embolism can occur and cause maternal death.

The procedure is carried out by an aseptic technique and sometimes sedation may by required to permit adequate examination. The colour and quantity of the liquor removed should be noted. The absence of the umbilical cord should be checked at the start and finish of the operation.

INDUCTION OF LABOUR

Complications of Amniotomy

Failure to induce effective contractions

Labour may not become established after amniotomy alone and it is usual to stimulate the uterus further by intravenous oxytocin after an interval of 3 hours or so if contractions are inadequate.

Placental separation (Abruptio)

This may be caused by the sudden reduction in the volume of liquor where there has been polyhydramnios.

Bleeding

This is not uncommon when the hindwaters are ruptured. The cannula may start fetal or maternal bleeding which can be so severe that section is indicated. The best method of identifying the source of blood is by Kleihauer's test, a laboratory procedure, by which a blood slide is so stained a to show the fetal cells standing out in a field of 'ghost' maternal cells (See Chapter 8).

Prolapse of the cord

This will only happen with an ill-fitting presenting part, and it used to be considered, probably wrongly, that this complication was less likely if the hindwaters rather than the forewaters were ruptured. Cord prolapse, occult or frank, should give warning signs on the FHR monitor.

Infection

The uterus is inevitably infected from the vagina within 24 hours of amniotomy, and both mother and child are at risk. Infection may perhaps be delayed by observing careful antiseptic techniques, and by exhibiting antibiotics whenever delay is anticipated.

Pulmonary embolism of amniotic fluid

This rare condition presents as severe shock of rapid onset, with intense dyspnoea and often bleeding. It is associated with amniotomy and strong uterine contractions, and must be distinguished from eclampsia, abruptio, ruptured uterus, and acid aspiration.

Treatment must include positive pressure ventilation, and correction of the inevitable coagulation defect. Post mortem examination of the maternal lungs will show fetal cells and lanugo, and mucin, but how the mucin gets there is not known.

There is a rare condition called *vagitus uterinus* which is sometimes met after amniotomy. Vagitus means the crying of a baby, and faint kitten-like cries can be heard from inside the uterus, presumably due to fetal respiration. It is regarded as an unfavourable sign.

(c) I.V. OXYTOCIN

Synthetic oxytocin by continuous intravenous infusion is commonly used after amniotomy to stimulate uterine contraction. It is also used occasionally with intact membranes e.g. to help stabilise the fetus with a variable lie prior to amniotomy. Like amniotomy I.V. oxytocin is also used to augment or accelerate labour.

INDUCTION OF LABOUR

I.V.OXYTOCIN (continued)

Synthetic oxytocin does not have a pressor factor, unlike natural oxytocin, but it is a powerful drug and sometimes unpredictable, as uterine sensitivity can show a wide variation. It must be administered with great care by the doctor or midwife who should be present all the time.

EFFECT ON UTERINE ACTIVITY
This varies with time and the progress of labour. Since too little oxytocin is useless and too much may cause fetal hypoxia or uterine rupture, it is necessary to adjust the dosage to the individual patient's response.

Activity of uterus (may be calculated in various ways, such as multiplying the strength of the contraction by its duration).

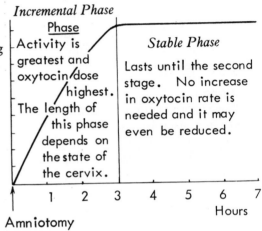

Incremental Phase

Phase
Activity is greatest and oxytocin dose highest. The length of this phase depends on the state of the cervix.

Stable Phase

Lasts until the second stage. No increase in oxytocin rate is needed and it may even be reduced.

1 2 3 4 5 6 7
Hours

Amniotomy

Units of Syntocinon in 500 ml Hartmann's solution	Drops per minute				
	10	20	40	60	80
	Dose of Syntocinon in mU/min				
2	2.66	5	11		21
8		21	43		85
16			85	128	171
32			171	256	341

The best method of administration is by an infusion pump and drop counter. A solution of 2 units of syntocinon in 5dl Hartmann's solution is used beginning at 10 drops per minute (2.66m.units/minute). This is increased every 15 minutes until satisfactory contractions are established.

INDUCTION OF LABOUR

Complications of Oxytocin

Poor uterine action

This may occur where amniotomy has been carried out in spite of an unfavourable cervix. Ripening of the cervix with Prostaglandin should be used first in these circumstances. Sometimes, in spite of apparently satisfactory uterine action, little dilatation of the cervix occurs and labour has to be terminated by Caesarean section. This is due to inco-ordinate uterine action (see page 291).

Abnormal fetal heart rate patterns

Prolonged or excessive oxytocin administration can cause fetal hypoxia by over-stimulation of the uterus. Continuous fetal heart rate monitoring is required for all patients undergoing oxytocin stimulation.

Hyperstimulation

Overdosage can cause excessive, painful contractions and even a prolonged spasm (tetanic contraction). If hyperstimulation becomes evident the infusion should be stopped to allow the uterus to relax. To assess the proper dosage of oxytocin an intra-uterine cannula may be required although this technique is too invasive for routine use.

Rupture of the uterus

The possibility of rupture must be borne in mind when using oxytocin. It is unlikely in a primigravida but has been reported. It is more to be expected in the parous woman or in the patient who has had a previous section or hysterotomy. The use of an intra-uterine cannula is advisable in such patients and epidural anaesthesia, which might mask early signs of rupture, should be used with caution.

Water intoxication

This may result from the prolonged administration of high doses of oxytocin in large volumes of electrolyte-free fluid. This should not be an issue in labour using normal dosage of oxytocin in an agent such as Hartmann's solution.

ACCELERATION OF LABOUR

The progress of spontaneous labour can be speeded up by amniotomy and oxytocin infusion. By using these techniques most women can be delivered within 12 hours. Prolonged labour is thus avoided together with its possible accompaniment of maternal exhaustion, fetal distress and intra-uterine infection. Such interventions should not, however, be automatic and their indiscriminate application has aroused hostility in some mothers. If acceleration is considered desirable the reason for this should be explained and discussed with the mother.

ABNORMAL UTERINE ACTION

The physiology of the uterus is by no means as clearly understood as that of the heart, but its patterns of action in labour have in the past been extensively studied by means of pressure gauges both intra- and extra-uterine. From such work has emerged a theory of UTERINE POLARITY which has not yet been altogether superseded, although it is being challenged as more experience is gained with accelerated labour.

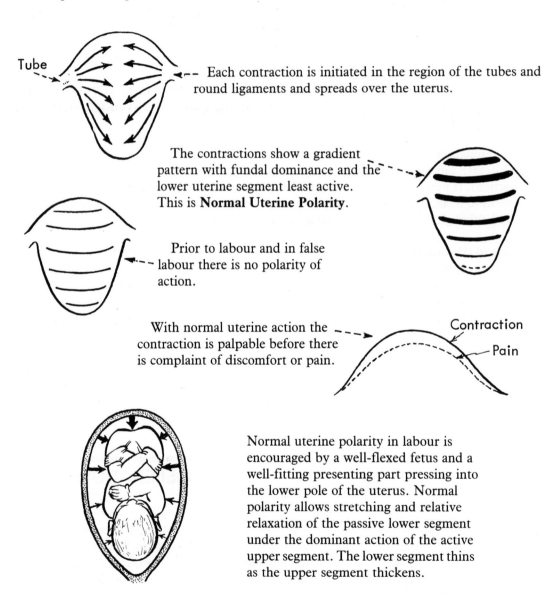

Tube

Each contraction is initiated in the region of the tubes and round ligaments and spreads over the uterus.

The contractions show a gradient pattern with fundal dominance and the lower uterine segment least active. This is **Normal Uterine Polarity**.

Prior to labour and in false labour there is no polarity of action.

With normal uterine action the contraction is palpable before there is complaint of discomfort or pain.

Contraction

Pain

Normal uterine polarity in labour is encouraged by a well-flexed fetus and a well-fitting presenting part pressing into the lower pole of the uterus. Normal polarity allows stretching and relative relaxation of the passive lower segment under the dominant action of the active upper segment. The lower segment thins as the upper segment thickens.

ABNORMAL UTERINE ACTION

NORMAL POLARITY

Within the concept of normal polarity or well coordinated uterine action, 2 abnormal patterns can be recognised:

1. **Weak contractions** (Hypotonic inertia)

   Uterine action is weak and infrequent and progress in labour is slow. The course of this labour is altered simply by acceleration by amniotomy combined with intra-venous oxytocin if required.

2. **Excessively strong contractions**

   These can cause precipitate labour and delivery. This may produce fetal distress due to persistent pressure on the placental site or rapid moulding of the fetal head. Should there be mechanical obstruction to progress in this situation (e.g. a malpresentation) there is a risk of uterine rupture.

ABNORMAL POLARITY has been postulated in 3 situations:

1. **Incoordinate uterine action**

   Contractions appear of satisfactory strength and are painful but unproductive. The normal relationship of upper to lower segment is disordered. This is a phenomenon of primigravid labours and may be associated with occipito-posterior positions or minor degrees of disproportion. The role of oxytocin in this situation is controversial. Some protagonists of accelerated labour do not accept this as a real condition.

2. There may be **localised tonic contraction** or **constriction ring** which grips round a narrow part of the fetus, usually between the head and shoulders. This may be recognised at Caesarean section.

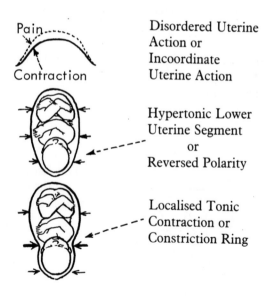

Disordered Uterine Action or Incoordinate Uterine Action

Hypertonic Lower Uterine Segment or Reversed Polarity

Localised Tonic Contraction or Constriction Ring

3. **Cervical rigidity**

   This may be acquired or congenital. Trauma or surgery to the cervix may induce scarring or there may be an absence of normal elasticity. Failure to recognise this in labour can lead to uterine rupture.

CONTRACTED PELVIS

Pelvic types are described fully on **pages 64,65.**
A contracted pelvis is one in which an important diameter is 1cm less than that of the normal gynaecoid pelvis.

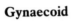

Gynaecoid

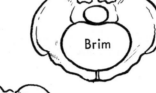

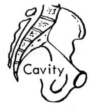

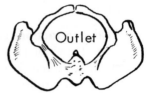

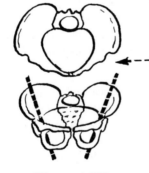

The **Anthropoid** pelvis can be considered normal for clinical purposes as its measurements are equivalent to a gynaecoid pelvis turned through 90°, although there is a tendency for the head to engage and descend in the antero-posterior axis.

The anthropoid pelvis is frequently found in association with a high assimilation of the sacrum — the fifth lumber vertebra is incorporated in the sacrum making a sixth segment. The effect is to alter the angle of the pelvic brim so that it is about 75° rather than the normal 55°. This makes engagement more difficult and delayed. The long sacrum makes the pelvis deeper so that the head has further to travel in the confines of the pelvic cavity.

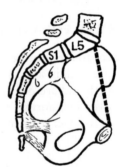

High
assimilation

The **Android** pelvis is a pelvis with decreasing capacity the deeper the head descends. The greatest difficulty is at the outlet. It is sometimes called the funnel pelvis.

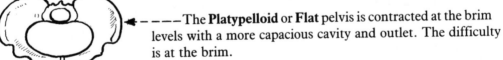

The **Platypelloid** or **Flat** pelvis is contracted at the brim levels with a more capacious cavity and outlet. The difficulty is at the brim.

A pelvis of pure type is not always found and many pelves have mixed characteristics. For example, an android brim has a normal diagonal conjugate diameter and if the rest of the pelvis has gynaecoid characteristics, the reduced brim capacity may not be noticed.

CONTRACTED PELVIS

CAUSES

Major pelvic deformity is rare in the UK and most pelvic abnormalities encountered are minor ones of pelvic shape or size related to the mother's height and build.

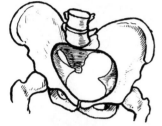 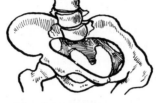 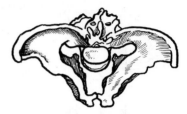

Naegele's pelvis   Nutritional deformity   Bony disease

A. Genetic (a) Without deformity — generally contracted (justo-minor) pelvis
           (b) With deformity (e.g. achondroplasia, Naegele's pelvis – absence of one sacral
                                                 ala)

B. Bony disease e.g. tuberculosis, osteomyelitis.
C. Trauma e.g. old fracture of pelvis.
D. Nutritional e.g. rickets, osteomalacia. An extreme type of this deformity is illustrated.

ANTE-NATAL ASSESSMENT

Pelvic size is related to maternal height and if the mother is less than 155cm pelvic contraction should be suspected.

It was formerly routine practice to carry out pelvic assessment at 36 weeks. This is commonly omitted nowadays. It is argued that rarely will a pelvis be so contracted as to preclude a trial of labour (see page 295). Undoubtedly a better assessment of pelvic size and possible disproportion can be carried out in labour, perhaps helped by analgesia or an epidural block.

Where performed, however, the following information is sought:

1. The diagonal conjugate can be measured if the sacral promontory is reached, in which case the pelvis is smaller than normal.

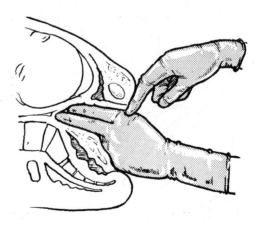

CONTRACTED PELVIS

ANTE-NATAL ASSESSMENT (continued)

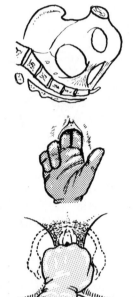

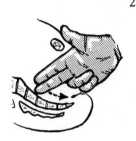

2. The sacral curvature and length are palpated and also the sacro-coccygeal junction and its mobility. The sacro-spinous ligaments on each side are located by feeling the ischial spine. Each ligament should accommodate two fingers easily. The thickness and prominence of the ischial spines are noted and especially any tendency to encroach on the cavity.

3. The sub-pubic angle is estimated by putting two fingers under the symphysis and spreading them. The angle should not be less than 90°.

4. The inter-tuberous diameter should be as wide as the normal fist.

Radiological assessment of the pelvis (other than an erect lateral film) is rarely performed on the antenatal period.

Disproportion arises when the presenting part is too big for the pelvis. The assessment of disproportion is a clinical judgement and is a comparison between the fetal head and the pelvic brim. The head may be too big or the pelvis too small. Malposition or malpresentation of a normal head can cause disproportion.

The fetal head is the best pelvimeter and if the head engages in the antenatal period there is unlikely to be a problem. If the head is not engaged an attempt may be made to make it engage by asking the patient to sit up and lean forwards.

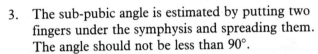

1. Head behind pubis – there should be no problem of disproportion.

2. Head flush with pubis – may or may not mould and engage.

3. Head over-riding pubis and will not enter brim-cephalo-pelvic disproportion probable.

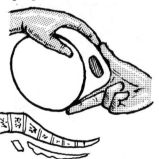

The assessment of disproportion may also be made by trying to push the head to the pelvic brim with one hand and the fingers of the other gauge descent while the thumb feels for overlap (Munro Kerr's method).

TRIAL OF LABOUR

This term is used when the outcome of the labour is uncertain. Even with ultrasound estimates of the fetal weight and biparietal diameter and knowledge of the mother's pelvic characteristics clinically and/or radiologically, it is not always possible to predict the outcome, hence the term 'Trial of Labour'. Its use reminds the mother's attendants of the uncertainty of the situation, demands extra vigilance on their part and requires ready access to Caesarean section if the trial is judged to have failed.

A trial of labour is undertaken in head presentations only and should never be used in breech presentation. The phrase was originally used to describe the testing of brim disproportion. This is too narrow to be clinically useful but the term should be confined to tests of mechanical disproportion and not be used for other procedures such as 'scar testing' after Caesarean section.

The uncertain factors in labour which will influence the outcome of the trial are:

1. Quality of the uterine activity.
2. Ability of the baby's head to mould safely.
3. The wellbeing of mother and baby.

Ideally the trial will begin with spontaneous labour and intact membranes. Induction would be employed only if medically indicated and stimulation of uterine activity with oxytocin should be used cautiously. Good uterine activity is essential, however, and more trials fail because of poor contractions than because cephalo-pelvic disproportion is clearly established. Progress in labour and fetal wellbeing are closely monitored and a low threshold for intervention by Caesarean section should be observed.

MALPOSITION AND MALPRESENTATION

Malposition means incorrect positioning of the vertex. This includes occipito-posterior (OP) positions and deflection of the head short of brow presentation.

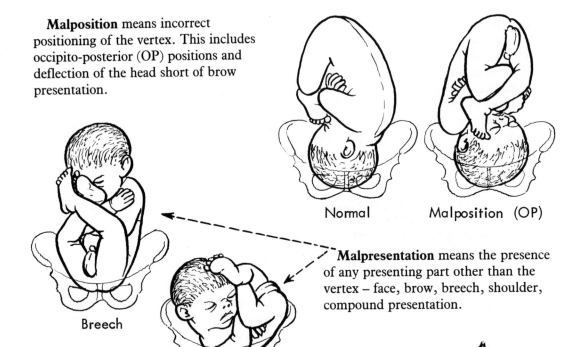

Normal   Malposition (OP)

Breech

Shoulder

Malpresentation means the presence of any presenting part other than the vertex – face, brow, breech, shoulder, compound presentation.

Well-fitting   Ill-fitting

DANGERS

1. Ill-fitting Presenting Part.
    The forewaters are not protected from the forces of uterine contractions, and are forced through an incompletely dilated cervix ('sausage-shaped forewaters').

2. Membranes rupture early and the cord may prolapse past the presenting part.

3. Contractions may be irregular and poorly sustained. If moulding occurs, and the presenting part becomes a better fit, the labour will perhaps progress more normally; otherwise dilatation of the cervix is likely to cease temporarily after the forewaters have ruptured.

4. In parous woman labour may proceed quickly in spite of an ill-fitting presenting part.
    With a malpresentation such as brow or shoulder there is a danger of obstructed labour and uterine rupture if unrecognised.

DIAGNOSIS OF MALPRESENTATION

1. ABDOMINAL EXAMINATION

(a) A lie other than longitudinal will lead to shoulder presentation.

(b) If lie is longitudinal the presentation is either head or breech.

(c) If the head presents the leading part is either vertex, face or brow. The last two may be suspected by recognising unusual width of the head.

2. VAGINAL EXAMINATION

The mouth and anus may be mistaken.

Mouth

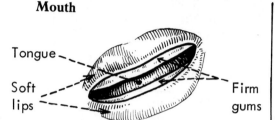

The mouth may be mistaken for the anus because of oedema masking laxity of the orifice.

Anus

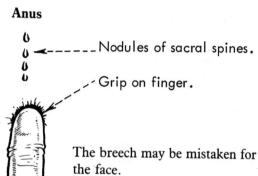

The breech may be mistaken for the face.

If in doubt do not use force as other tissues such as eyes or genitalia may be damaged.

Sacrum

The sacrum is recognised by the shape, nodular ridge of the spines and possibly the foramina and the posterior portion of iliac crest. The spine nodules are continuous with the vertebrae above.

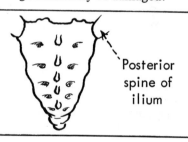

Supra-orbital ridges

Supra-orbital ridges are recognised by double curve, root of nose, orbits and frontal suture. All may be partly obscured by caput.

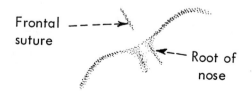

Nose

The nose is recognised by the 'saddle', and its firm elasticity.

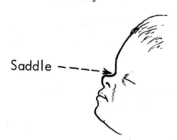

297

DIAGNOSIS OF MALPRESENTATION

VAGINAL EXAMINATION (continued)

The Foot and Hand may be mistaken.

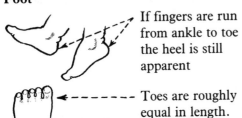

Foot

If fingers are run from ankle to toe the heel is still apparent

Toes are roughly equal in length.

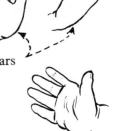

Hand

If fingers are run from wrist to palm then the 'heel' disappears

Fingers are not equal and the thumb is separate.

Right or left is identifiable by the position of the great toe or thumb.

Shoulder

The shoulder is identified by the humerus, scapula, acromion process, coracoid process, clavicle and ribs. All of these cannot be palpated at once.

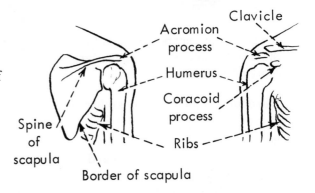

The Knee and Elbow may be mistaken.

Knee

The knee has a hollow as the knee cap is not yet formed.

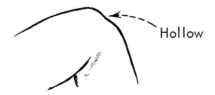

Elbow

The elbow has the point of the olecranon process.

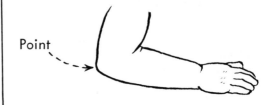

OCCIPITO-POSTERIOR POSITION

Occipito-posterior position is a malposition of the head and occurs in 13% of vertex presentations. The presenting part is the vertex and the denominator is the occiput.

Postulated Causes

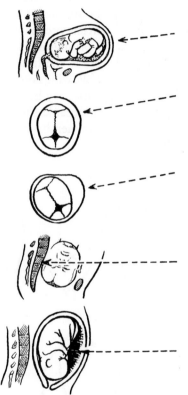

Pendulous Abdomen – This is found in multiparae.

Anthropoid pelvic brim – This favours direct O.P. or direct O.A.

Android pelvic brim – The transverse diameter of the brim being near the sacrum encourages the biparietal diameter to accommodate posteriorly.

A flat sacrum with a poorly flexed head leads to further deflexion and O.P.

The placenta on the anterior uterine wall tends to encourage the fetus to flex round it.

R.O.L. position of the head and the normal right obliquity and dextro-rotation of the uterus favours deflexion of the head and R.O.P. descent. There is some assistance from the pelvic colon in the left posterior pelvic quadrant.

Chance is clearly an important cause.

299

OCCIPITO-POSTERIOR POSITION

DIAGNOSIS

Palpation

A.
    The fetal back is found to one side or may be difficult to identify.

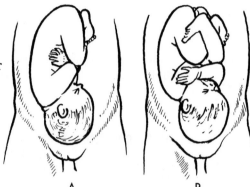

A.   B.

B.
    The fetal head is postero-lateral and will be free above the brim in late pregnancy, even in a primigravida. The limbs are to the front and give hollowing above the head. This may be particularly noticeable after rupture of the membranes.

Auscultation

    The fetal heart is heard best well out in the flank but descends to just above the pubis as the head rotates and descends.

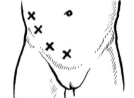

Vaginal examination

    The membranes tend to rupture early, often before labour is established. If the membranes are intact they may protrude through the cervix giving finger-like forewaters, or may fill the upper vagina and obscure the presenting part. The presenting part is the vertex, but there is deflexion (incomplete flexion) so the anterior

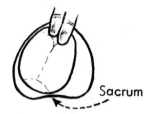

Sacrum

fontanelle is readily felt in the anterior part of the pelvis near the ileo-pectineal eminence. The sagittal suture aims towards the sacro-iliac joint. The posterior fontanelle is not readily felt till the head is in lower pelvic cavity.

OCCIPITO-POSTERIOR POSITION

MECHANISM

Two types of occipito-posterior (O.P.) are described.

A. Flexed O.P. with suboccipito-frontal and biparietal diameter engaging 10cm x 9.5cm.

B. Deflexed O.P. with occipito-frontal and biparietal diameters engaging 11.5cm x 9.5cm.

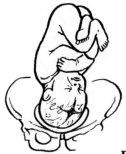

Engagement occurs in the transverse or the right oblique diameter of the brim. Descent occurs in the right oblique diameter of pelvis giving the right occipito-posterior position (R.O.P.). Descent continues to pelvic floor.

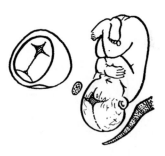

Further progress depends on flexion of head

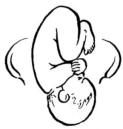

A. If flexion of the head increases in descent then the occiput strikes pelvic floor first and rotates anteriorly through the right occipito-lateral (R.O.L.). position – and then to the R.O.A. position and to the direct O.A. position.

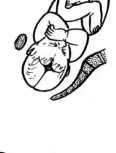

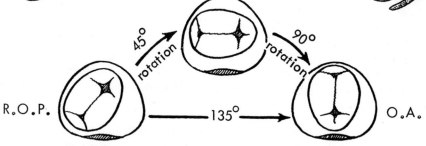

R.O.P.   45° rotation   90° rotation   135°   O.A.

The occiput has thus rotated through the angle of 135° to bring the occiput to the symphysis pubis. This is know as **Long** rotation. The mechanism is thereafter the same as for the occipito-anterior position.

301

OCCIPITO-POSTERIOR POSITION

MECHANISM

B. If flexion of head remains incomplete in descent then rotation of the occiput anteriorly on the pelvic floor may not occur; but rotation of the occiput posteriorly may occur bringing the occiput into the hollow of the sacrum. This is known as SHORT rotation (45°) and gives the persistent occipito-posterior (P.O.P.) position or direct O.P. position.

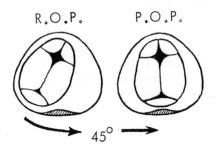

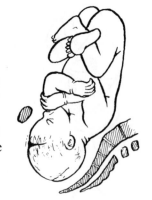

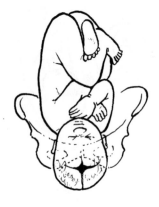

The mechanism now is difficult for flexion of the head is restricted by the fetal chest though the brow is pressed to the pubis and some flexion occurs. The soft tissues are stretched more than in O.A. and the fetus is delivered face to pubis.

If this does not occur then an impasse is reached and labour becomes obstructed.

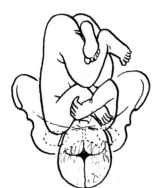

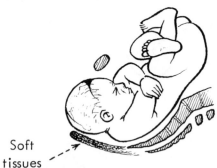

Soft
tissues

Sometimes the long rotation of the O.P. is arrested and the head is left in the occipito-lateral position in the cavity of the pelvis. This is one form of transverse arrest of the head.

OCCIPITO-POSTERIOR POSITION

LABOUR

Occipito-posterior positions may lead to disorganised labour especially in the primigravida. Contractions may be painful and accompanied by troublesome backache, but uterine action is incoordinate and progress slow. Good analgesia is necessary and an epidural block is ideal. Accurate assessment of the quality of uterine action by an intra-uterine catheter may be helpful and Syntocinon can be employed. Retention of urine is common in such labours and catheterisation may be required. The mother may feel an urge to bear down before the second stage is reached, probably due to pressure on the sacrum and rectum. Premature expulsive efforts can delay progress by causing oedema of the cervix and an epidural is again helpful in this situation.

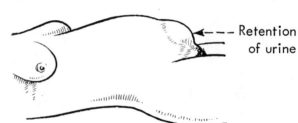

Retention of urine

DELIVERY

Two thirds of the cases will deliver spontaneously as O.A.
12% will deliver spontaneously face to pubis. The perineum is distended by the occipito-frontal diameter, and an extensive episiotomy will be required.

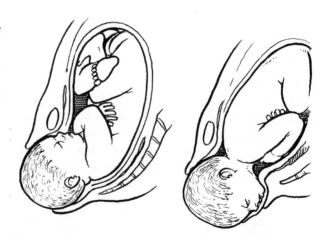

Internal rotation may be interrupted by prominent ischial spines or be restricted by reduced pelvic diameters as in the android pelvis. Delivery then has to be completed by section or, if full dilatation has been reached, by manual or forceps rotation, or by the use of the ventouse (see Chapter 14).

303

BREECH PRESENTATION

The breech is a malpresentation and occurs once in about 40 cases of labour in mature pregnancies.

AETIOLOGY

The breech is the presenting part in 25% of cases before 30 weeks, therefore prematurity is an important factor.

The legs of the fetus may be extended and interfere with flexion of the body so breech with extended legs is common especially in primigravida.

Multiple pregnancy will interfere with spontaneous version.

Other related factors are:- Fetal malformation, hydramnios, lax uterus and pendulous abdomen, abnormal shape of pelvic brim or uterus, placenta praevia.

Three types of presentation are described:-

Fully flexed fetus	Not fully flexed fetus with legs extended	One or both thighs extended

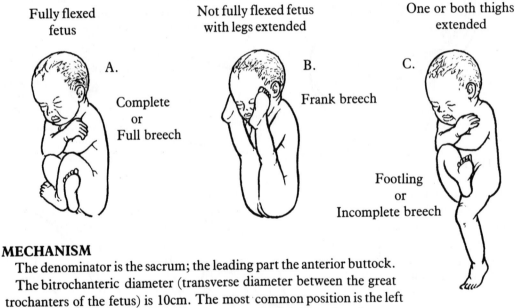

A. Complete or Full breech

B. Frank breech

C.

Footling or Incomplete breech

MECHANISM

The denominator is the sacrum; the leading part the anterior buttock.

The bitrochanteric diameter (transverse diameter between the great trochanters of the fetus) is 10cm. The most common position is the left sacro-anterior (L.S.A.). With labour there is com-paction, descent and engagement of the breech (bisiliac diameter).

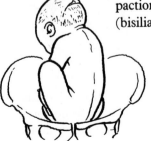

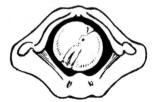

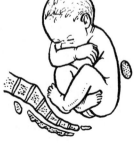

BREECH PRESENTATION

MECHANISM (continued)

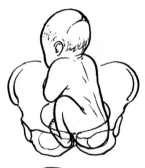

Descent continues until breech reaches pelvic floor. The anterior buttock rotates forward under the pubis (internal rotation).

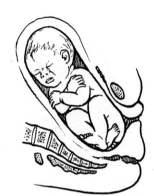

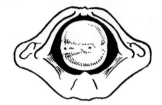

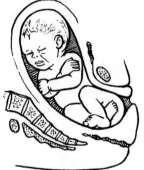

Lateral flexion of the fetal body round the pubis allows the anterior buttock to slip forward under the pubis and the posterior buttock to slip over the perineum. The breech is delivered followed by the legs. A movement of restitution of the hips takes place.

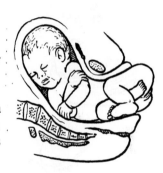

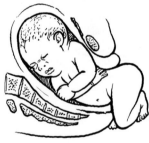

The shoulders now engage in the same pelvic diameter as the hips – the left oblique. (The bisacromial diameter of the shoulder is 11cm.)

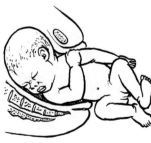

As descent continues internal rotation of the shoulders occurs in the pelvic cavity bringing one shoulder beneath the pubis and the other into the hollow of the sacrum. The anterior shoulder and arm are born first.

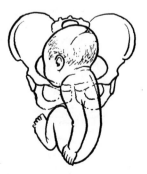

305

BREECH PRESENTATION

MECHANISM (continued)

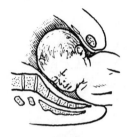

As the shoulders are being born the head enters the pelvic brim either in the transverse or left oblique of the brim. The engaging diameters of the head are the biparietal and the suboccipito-bregmatic or suboccipito-frontal.

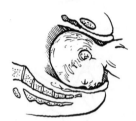

The head descends into the pelvic cavity and rotates to bring the occiput under the pubis.

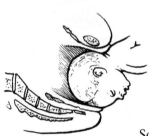

The occiput is arrested at the pubis and the head is born by flexion. The chin, face and brow are born first, and then the occiput.

Sometimes the occiput rotates posteriorly.

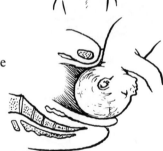

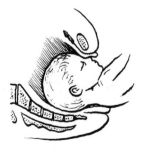

If the head is flexed the root of the nose is arrested behind the pubis and the occiput and vertex are born first followed by the face.

If the head is extended the chin is arrested above the pubis and the occiput and vertex are delivered and the face follows.

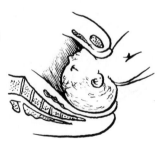

306

BREECH PRESENTATION

DIAGNOSIS

Palpation
1. Longitudinal lie.
2. Firm lower pole.
3. Limbs to one side.
4. Hard head at fundus. (Head may not be palpable at fundus because it is under the ribs – always confirm by pelvic examination.)

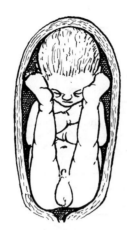

Frank breech

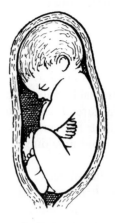

Full breech

Auscultation
The fetal heart (F.H.) is best heard above the umbilicus.

Vaginal examination
No head in pelvis. Soft buttocks felt and hard irregular sacrum. Feet may be in pelvis as leading part.

Ultrasound
Differentiation of head and breech is not always easy but the head will be readily detected by a scan.

DANGERS
(a) Ante-natal

As with other malpresentations there is an increased risk of premature rupture of the membranes and cord prolapse. This applies least to the extended breech which is a well-fitting presenting part.

(b) Delivery

The main danger in breech delivery is the speed with which the head descends through the pelvis. Rapid compression and decompression can cause intracranial injury.

Conversely, undue delay in the delivery will lead to asphyxia due to cord compression, at least from the time of delivery of the shoulders.

Traumatic injuries may occur if intervention in the delivery is required.

BREECH PRESENTATION

Risks to the fetus

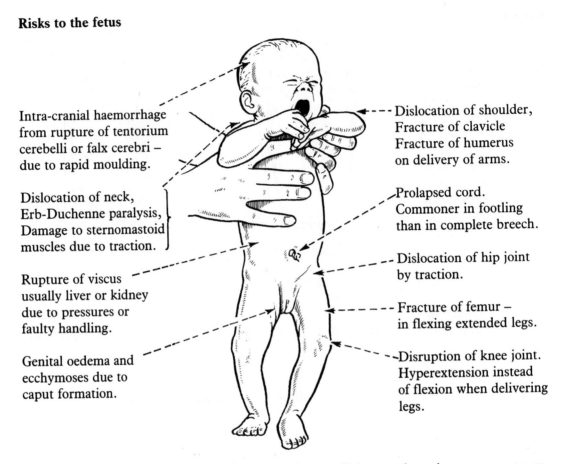

Intra-cranial haemorrhage
from rupture of tentorium
cerebelli or falx cerebri –
due to rapid moulding.

Dislocation of neck,
Erb-Duchenne paralysis,
Damage to sternomastoid
muscles due to traction.

Rupture of viscus
usually liver or kidney
due to pressures or
faulty handling.

Genital oedema and
ecchymoses due to
caput formation.

Dislocation of shoulder,
Fracture of clavicle
Fracture of humerus
on delivery of arms.

Prolapsed cord.
Commoner in footling
than in complete breech.

Dislocation of hip joint
by traction.

Fracture of femur –
in flexing extended legs.

Disruption of knee joint.
Hyperextension instead
of flexion when delivering
legs.

The placenta separates frequently in the second stage of labour as the active uterus contracts and the fetal head is in the pelvis. Apnoea is therefore a danger.

Manual assistance to complete delivery of baby is essential and may be a sudden need. Episiotomy is desirable to permit sudden interference, or complete perineal tear may result.

BREECH PRESENTATION

MANAGEMENT (Antenatal)

As already noted many babies present by the breech at 30 weeks. Most undergo spontaneous version by 32 – 34 weeks. If this does not occur the possible causes should be considered and an ultrasound scan carried out to localise the placenta and exclude fetal anomaly

External cephalic version may then be attempted. In the primigravida this will usually be done at about 34 weeks; in the parous woman it is sometimes possible much later in the pregnancy. Diazepam 10mg orally may be given as a relaxant and the mother may be placed in the Trendelenberg (head down) position to encourage the breech to rise from the pelvic brim.

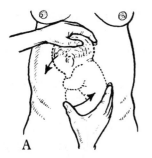 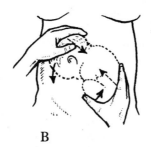 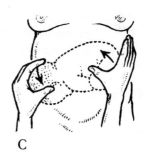

A.   The breech must be eased away from the pelvis.

B.   Pressure is applied to encourage flexion of the fetus to allow it to slip round. If the legs are flexed the baby may kick round at this point.

C.   Once past the transverse the hands simply push the fetus into position.

Complications
1. The placenta may be partly separated. The fetal heart must be checked on completion and the vagina examined for bleeding.
2. There may be unsuspected complications such as an abnormal uterus or short umbilical cord.
3. Excessive force may rupture the uterus.

Contra-Indications
1. Toxaemia (as predisposing to placental bleeding).
2. Previous scar on the uterus.
3. Multiple pregnancy or fetal abnormality.

  The commonest causes of failure are too large a fetus or too little liquor, or 'splinting' of the fetus by extended legs.

BREECH PRESENTATION

MANAGEMENT (continued)

If version is unsuccessful a decision whether to allow an attempt at vaginal delivery must be made. Some obstetricians consider vaginal breech delivery too dangerous and advocate elective Caesarean section in all cases. Caesarean section, however, carries a higher mortality and morbidity than vaginal delivery and is not necessarily atraumatic for the baby if, for example, the lower segment is not well-formed. It is reasonable, therefore to consider vaginal delivery in certain circumstances:

1. A mature pregnancy.
2. The fetal weight and biparietal diameter estimated by ultrasound have shown a baby of reasonable size (not more than 3.5 to 3.75kg).
3. Maternal pelvis is satisfactory as assessed by lateral X-ray and clinical examination.
4. Absence of other significant obstetrical complications.

BREECH DELIVERY

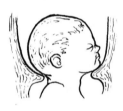

Labour should proceed normally in the breech with extended legs. In flexed and footling breeches there is an increased risk of early rupture of the membranes and cord prolapse. In these cases also, especially if premature, the breech may slip through the incompletely dilated cervix and precipitate delivery.

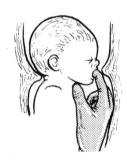

In these circumstances there is no alternative to attempting to complete the delivery by passing a hand up the fetal abdomen and inserting a finger into the baby's mouth. Traction on the jaw is applied to promote flexion and passage through the cervix.

Where labour is proceeding normally analgesia is best provided by an epidural block which will prevent premature expulsive efforts and permit controlled delivery of the head. Delivery should be in the lithotomy position to allow the baby to hang over the perineum.

Once the breech reaches the pelvic floor lateral flexion of the trunk is required to allow progress. This will be facilitated by episiotomy when the posterior buttock distends the introitus.

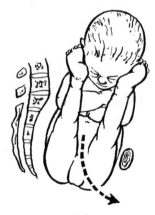

BREECH PRESENTATION

DELIVERY (continued)

If the legs are flexed they will fall out but if they are extended they should be lifted out once access can be gained to the popliteal fossa.

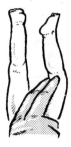
Pressure to the popliteal space to flex the knee and displace it to the side of the trunk.

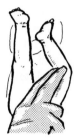
Fingers are worked along leg towards ankle to encourage further flexion of knee.

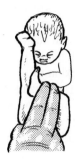
The ankle is grasped and the foot swept down over the other leg.

A loop of cord is pulled down as soon as is practicable to prevent possible tearing of it later.

When delivery of one leg is complete the delivery of the second follows quickly.

The delivery proceeds spontaneously and as the anterior shoulder blade appears the arm is delivered (1) by placing two fingers of the appropriate hand (right if right shoulder) over the clavicle and sweeping them round the point of the shoulder and down the humerus to the elbow and carrying the forearm free. (2) The ankles are then grasped and swung upwards. This permits the posterior arm being freed in a similar way. (3) The body is now allowed to hang till the head descends into the pelvis and the hair line shows.

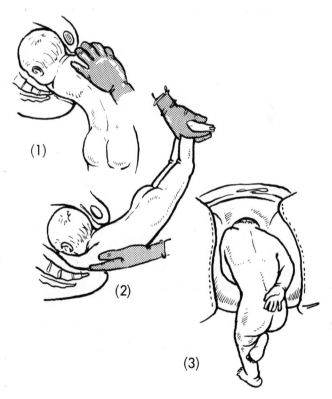

(1)

(2)

(3)

311

BREECH PRESENTATION

DELIVERY (continued)

The head may then be delivered by one of 3 methods according to the obstetrician's choice:

1. **The Mauriceau-Smellie-Veit manoeuvre**

The child is laid along the left arm and the middle finger is placed in the mouth, the index and ring fingers catch the cheek bones. Traction by these fingers will tend to promote flexion of the head. The index finger and thumb of the right hand grasp one shoulder, the middle finger presses on the occiput and the other two fingers grasp the other shoulder. Traction of the two hands will deliver the head and keep it flexed.

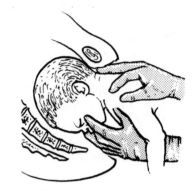

2. **Forceps**

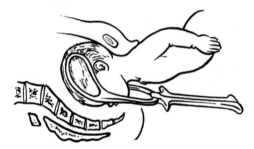

Delivery of the head may be completed by forceps. An assistant holds the baby upwards by the the feet while the blades are applied.

Traction is then in the direction of the birth canal. Forceps control and limit the moulding of the head.

3. **The Burns-Marshall method**

The feet are grasped and with gentle traction are swept in an arc over the maternal abdomen. Thus the mouth is freed and the delivery is completed slowly by further swinging over the abdomen.

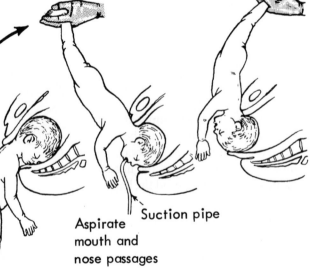

Aspirate mouth and nose passages

Suction pipe

BREECH PRESENTATION

DELIVERY (continued)

In all cases the delivery of the head should be as slow as possible to decrease the risk of damage to skull membranes by sudden compression and release. The air passages should be cleared as quickly as possible by aspirating the nose and mouth. Delivery thereafter can be slow without fear of asphyxia and it can also allow slow release of pressures and tensions on the skull. The method used to deliver the head is unimportant; what matters is the operator's experience and the achievement of a controlled delivery.

Delivery may be complicated by extension or nuchal displacement of the arms.

These complications are best managed by LØVSET's MANOEUVRE. This makes use of the inclination of the pelvic brim, the short anterior wall and the long posterior wall of the cavity. The anterior shoulder is above the symphysis while the posterior is below the promontory and if these are now reversed in position, the posterior

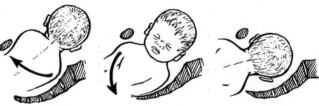

shoulder will keep below the brim and be just below the symphysis and can be easily delivered.

The Løvset manoeuvre is done by grasping the fetus by the pelvis and pulling gently while rotating to bring the posterior shoulder to the front. The direction of rotation is so that the posterior

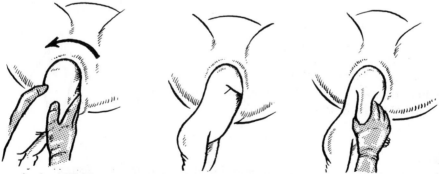

arm trails towards the chest (anti-clockwise rotation with back to mother's left and clockwise rotation with back to mother's right).

The arm is then lifted out and the rotation reversed, using the delivery arm for traction, so that the original anterior arm, which became posterior below the promontory is now swept round in the cavity to be easily picked out below the symphysis. (Often the second arm can be extracted easily without further rotation when the first arm has been delivered.)

The delivery described, where most of the baby is delivered by maternal effort and the obstetrician delivers the head (with or without Løvset's manoeuvre) is classified as an **Assisted Breech Delivery**.

313

BREECH PRESENTATION

DELIVERY (continued)

BREECH EXTRACTION is a different procedure carried out now almost exclusively to deliver a second twin after Internal Podalic Version. The twin will most commonly be lying transversely and the membranes will be ruptured (otherwise external version might be possible).

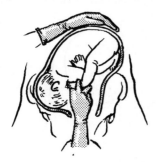

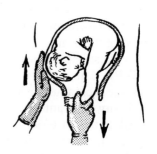

1. A hand is introduced into the uterus and the anterior foot is grasped by the heel. (Pulling on the posterior limb tends to turn the baby's back to the back of the uterus: if possible both feet should be grasped.)

2. Downward traction is made on the leg and the outside hand presses the head upwards.

3. Gentle traction is made on the delivered leg until the breech is fixed, then the other leg is extracted and the delivery completed by the obstetrician.

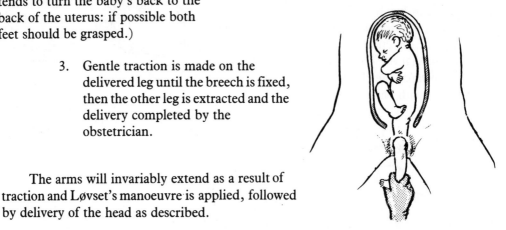

The arms will invariably extend as a result of traction and Løvset's manoeuvre is applied, followed by delivery of the head as described.

Complications

There is a risk of uterine rupture, of injury to the fetus, and of infection.

Internal version should never be attempted when the uterus has contracted down on an impacted fetus and the lower segment is thin.

FACE PRESENTATION

Face presentation is a malpresentation and occurs once in about 300 cases. The presenting part is the face and the denominator is the mentum or chin.

AETIOLOGY

Lax uterus and pendulous abdomen, polyhydramnios, flat pelvis, multiple pregnancy, prematurity, obliquity of uterus, thyroid enlargement or tumour of neck, anencephaly, spasm of the muscles of the back of the neck, dead fetus, dolichocephalic fetal skull (dolichocephalic = long headed – where breadth is less than four fifths of length).

The face may be a primary presentation, i.e. it is present before labour, but secondary face presentation is more common, i.e. it develops in labour.

Incomplete flexion with occipito-posterior vertex and marked uterine obliquity can promote extension.

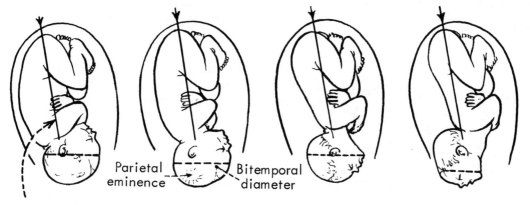

Parietal eminence — Bitemporal diameter

The action of the uterine forces, which normally tends to cause compaction, is in fact promoting extension of the head at the atlanto-occipital joint because the back of the fetus is in the same direction as the uterine obliquity.

Uterine obliquity is commonly to the right. A head presenting R.O.L. with some deflexion may also convert to a face presentation if, for example, in a flat pelvis there is partial arrest of the biparietal diameter but an easier passage for bitemporal diameter.
[Note that the brow is an intermediate presentation in these conversions to face.]

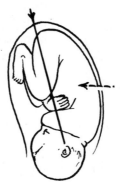

If the fetus has its back to the opposite side the same forces would cause compaction and further flexion.

315

FACE PRESENTATION

MECHANISM

The engaging diameters in a face presentation are the submento-bregmatic followed by the biparietal.

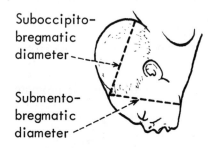

Suboccipito-
bregmatic
diameter

Submento-
bregmatic
diameter

The submento-bregmatic and suboccipito-bregmatic diameters are the same size (9.5cm). Therefore the engaging diameters are the same size as in a normal vertex presentation.

In a normal vertex the suboccipito-bregmatic and the biparietal diameters are in the same plane.

In a face presentation the submento-bregmatic and the biparietal diameters are in different planes. The submento-bregmatic and bitemporal diameters engage together.

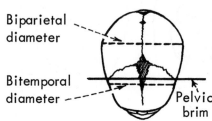

Biparietal
diameter

Bitemporal
diameter   Pelvic
                        brim

In a normal vertex presentation the engaging diameters enter the plane of the brim together.

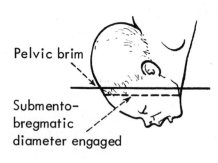

Pelvic brim

Submento-
bregmatic
diameter engaged

In a face presentation the submento-bregmatic diameter enters the plane of the brim and is followed by the other engaging diameter.

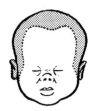

The pale areas engage first followed by the shaded areas.

Engagement is usually in the transverse diameter of the brim giving a right or left mento-lateral position. Left mento-lateral (L.M.L.) is the more common.

FACE PRESENTATION

MECHANISM (continued)

Descent continues till the pelvic floor is reached and rotation occurs.

A   Most commonly the mentum leads and rotates forward (internal rotation) to the oblique diameter – left mento-anterior (L.M.A.).

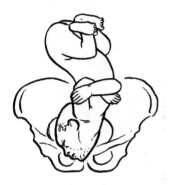

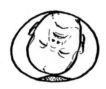

With further descent the rotation is completed to bring the mentum to the symphysis. This is the mechanism in 75% of face presentations.

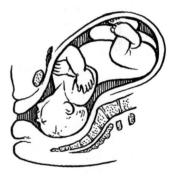

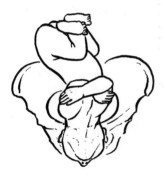

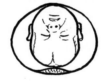

Descent continues and chin escapes from under pubis and progressive flexion allows the birth of the head.

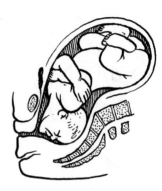

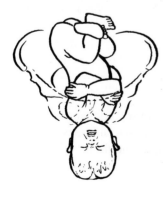

Thereafter restitution and external rotation take place and further descent delivers the baby as in a persistent occipito-posterior delivery.

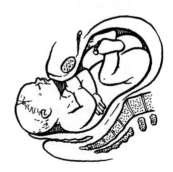

317

FACE PRESENTATION

MECHANISM (continued)

B   If the sinciput leads and rotates forward the mentum is carried to the hollow of the sacrum.

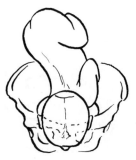

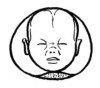

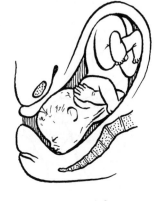

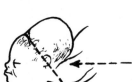

This is now a difficult mechanism because further extension of the head is necessary to negotiate the lower birth canal – and the shoulders must engage too.

A normal pelvis cannot accommodate a normal fetus because the bregmatic-sternal diameter is 18cm. Obstruction therefore occurs and delivery in the mento-posterior position will normally be by Caesarean section.

The combination of a small fetus in a roomy pelvis *may* permit birth.

A

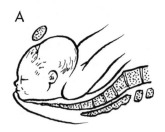

Descent continues and the occiput crushes into the shoulders till the occipital bone is behind the pubis, the perineum slips beneath the chin, the head starts to flex and the occiput is free.

The mechanism is then the same as occipito-anterior.

B

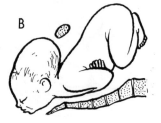

Caput formation

In face presentations the caput succedaneum is formed from the soft tissues covering the facial bones, and bruising is the rule. The mother should be assured that her baby's face will be normal in a few days.

FACE PRESENTATION

MANAGEMENT AND DELIVERY

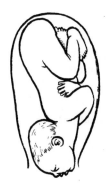

Palpation
1. Longitudinal lie.
2. Head in lower pole.
3. Groove between head and back (best felt after membranes rupture).
4. Lack of head prominence on ventral side.

Diagnosis is difficult by palpation.
(X-ray will confirm.)

Ausculation

Fetal heart best heard at front of fetus.

Vaginal examination

Malar processes

Nose – rubbery – saddle shaped
Mouth – hard areolar ridges
Supra-orbital ridges
Frontal suture and anterior fontanelle

The face is ill-fitting at first, so contractions may be poor and irregular and early rupture of membranes occurs with risk of prolapsed cord.

Labour may proceed normally thereafter when caput has formed. Engagement of the biparietal diameter and rotation of the head occurs only when the mentum is deep in the pelvis. If the chin rotates anteriorly spontaneous delivery can occur. It is therefore reasonable to wait and watch when face presentation is detected early in labour.

If the chin rotates posteriorly interference is required to procure delivery. Caesarean section is the method. In exceptional circumstances (very small head or anencephaly) delivery may be spontaneous.

If the second stage is reached and delay occurs, delivery can be completed using forceps. If the head is arrested in the transverse position, rotation manually or by Kielland's forceps is possible.

319

BROW PRESENTATION

A brow presentation is unstable and tends to convert to a vertex or face presentation.

The aetiology is similar to that of face.

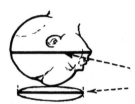

There is no mechanism for brow presentation given a normal sized fetus and pelvis, because the engaging diameters are the mento-vertical and biparietal.

The mento-vertical diameter is 14cm and the largest pelvic diameter is 12.5cm.

If the head is small or the pelvis roomy moulding takes place and engagement occurs with descent.

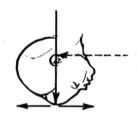

The uterine forces thrust down. The head is roughly equal in size in front of and behind the brow. Thus the leverage to encourage flexion or extension is equal.

Unequal resistance of the pelvic parts or oblique direction of thrust will tend to create flexion or extension of the head, thus leading to vertex or face presentation.

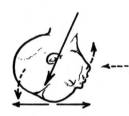

Oblique thrust and
equal resistance will tend to cause flexion.
Thrust in the other oblique would cause extension.

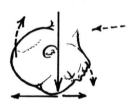

Straight thrust and
unequal resistance will tend to cause extension.
Opposite inequalities of resistance would cause flexion.

Oblique thrust and unequal resistance may augment or neutralise each other.

If conversion to a vertex or face presentation does not occur then moulding reduces the occipito-mental and increases the occipito-frontal diameters.

BROW PRESENTATION

MECHANISM

This is only possible when the baby is very small in relation to the pelvis.

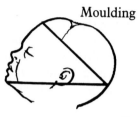

Moulding

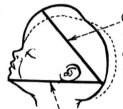

Occipito-frontal diameter increases

Occipito-mental diameter decreases

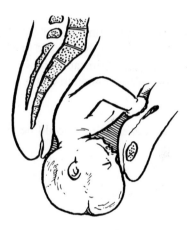

CERVIX

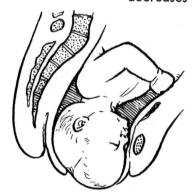

The brow slowly descends to pelvic floor and turns forward under the symphysis.

Flexion then follows and the brow, vault of the skull and occiput are born.

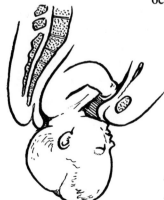

The head drops back over the perineum and the face and chin are born.

The mechanism thereafter is the same as O.P.

321

BROW PRESENTATION

MANAGEMENT

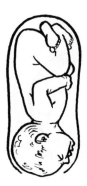

Palpation

This feels like normal vertex except that the head feels unduly large, due to palpation across the mento-vertical diameter. Head appears disproportionate.

Auscultation Fetal heart site not significant.

Vaginal Examination Head is high because of disproportion. Membranes rupture early in labour. Brow is palpated through cervix and is identified by:-
1. Anterior fontanelle and frontal suture leading to
2. Supra-orbital ridge and root of nose.

The brow is ill-fitting so the membranes can rupture early and labour may be poor at the beginning. There is a risk of cord prolapse. With a normal baby and pelvis labour is impossible. The presentation is unstable, however, and it is therefore reasonable to observe initially in labour to see if conversion to vertex or face occurs. Caesarean section will, however, usually be required.

A Brow presentation should be suspected when a parous woman has unexpected dystocia.

COMPOUND PRESENTATION

This means the prolapse of a limb alongside the presenting part. It is a rare complication and head-and-arm are most often seen although head-and- foot and breech-and-hand have been described.

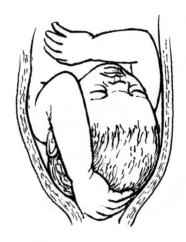

Predisposing Causes

It occurs with an ill-fitting presenting part – malposition, malpresentation, disproportion, small infants are therefore its associated conditions. It is also seen in the multipara whose lax abdomen allows the head to remain high; and the cord may prolapse as well.

Treatment

Usually nothing need be done. If the hand is palpated in front of the head and appears to be causing delay, it should be pushed up out of the way. It is important to distinguish hand from foot by identifying the presence or absence of the heel.

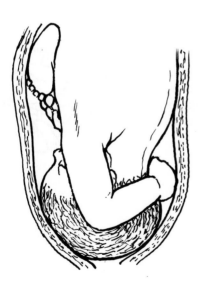

Nuchal Displacement of the Arm

This will prevent delivery and should be looked for when forceps delivery is unsuccessful for some unrecognised reason. When the arm is palpated, an attempt can be made to restore it to the front of the fetus after dislodging the head; but section may well be necessary.

323

SHOULDER PRESENTATION

Shoulder presentation is a malpresentation and occurs in 1 out of 250–300 cases. It is more common in multipara than in primipara and in premature than in mature labours.

AETIOLOGY

This is similar to other malpresentations. Twins, polyhydramnios, placenta praevia, contracted pelvis, anything preventing engagement of the head in the pelvis may encourage shoulder presentation. Unusual fetal shape (due to some abnormality) or an abnormal uterine shape, e.g. subseptate uterus, are occasional causes. The commonest cause, however, is laxity of the uterine and abdominal wall muscles in parous patients.

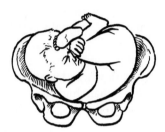

The Lie is transverse or oblique.

The head may be to right or left and the back may be anterior or posterior.

The Denominator is the shoulder.

Vaginal examination reveals an empty pelvis, and an unusual presenting part. The shoulder might be mistaken for the breech but the ribs have a characteristic feel.

When the fetus and pelvis are of normal size there is obstruction and no mechanism.

If the pelvis is large and the baby small spontaneous evolution can occur, ending in breech delivery; but if the baby is viable, delivery by Caesarean section is to be preferred.

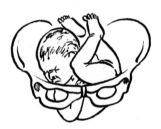

Occasionally, when the child is dead, it may be expelled with the shoulder leading and the rest of the baby doubled up and following (corpore conduplicato). This is spontaneous expulsion.

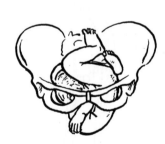

SHOULDER PRESENTATION

MANAGEMENT

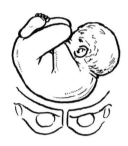

Palpation

1. Fundal height is less than expected.
2. Uterine breadth is greater than expected.
3. Head in one flank and breech in opposite side.
4. Lie may be transverse or oblique.

Auscultation

Site of fetal heart not significant (best heard through fetal back).

Vaginal Examination

Prior to labour and in early labour, pelvis is empty. Hand, arm or elbow may be in pelvis, or ribs, tip of shoulder or iliac crest may be felt.

When encountered antenatally causes such as placenta praevia should be excluded by ultrasound scan. The condition will commonly be seen as part of an unstable lie (see Chapter 10).

In early labour, if the membranes are intact, external version to a vertex or breech can be attempted. If the membranes have ruptured and the liquor has drained, the uterus wraps round the fetus and manipulation is very dangerous. Caesarean section is therefore the treatment of choice, even with a dead baby. The lower segment may be poorly-formed and Classical section may occasionally be required.

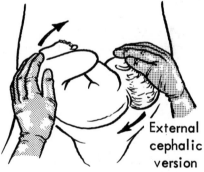

External cephalic version

ABNORMALITIES OF THIRD STAGE OF LABOUR AND OF PLACENTA AND CORD

The **Third Stage** of labour remains the most unpredictable and dangerous stage of labour from the mother's point of view.

The first part of this chapter describes two relatively common third stage complications:

Retained Placenta – incidence 1–2% and
Primary Post Partum Haemorrhage (PPH) – incidence 3–4%;
and the rare but very grave complication
Inversion of the Uterus

RETAINED PLACENTA

When Syntometrine has been given as described in Chapter 11, with the crowning of the head or the delivery of the anterior shoulder, separation of the placenta will usually occur within a few minutes of the delivery of the baby. Certainly, if the placenta is undelivered at 20 minutes it should be considered to be 'retained'.

CAUSES

1. **Placenta separated but undelivered**

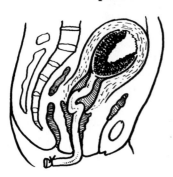
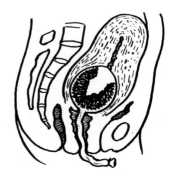

In such cases there have usually been signs of placental separation — bleeding, alteration of the shape of the uterus, lengthening of the cord. If the signs have been missed bleeding into the uterine cavity will occur because the uterus cannot retract fully until it is empty. The fundus will therefore appear broad and boggy, thus disguising the fact that separation has occurred. Failure to recognise the signs of separation is one of the commonest forms of mismanagement of the third stage.

In this situation the fundus should be rubbed up to make it contract and the placenta removed by the *Brandt-Andrews method*. The cord is pulled gently, and the other hand presses the uterus upwards so as to prevent inversion. A slight see-sawing motion is imparted by both hands, and provided separation has occurred the placenta should be delivered.

RETAINED PLACENTA

CAUSES (continued)

2. **Placenta partly or wholly attached**

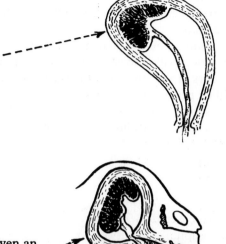

   If the placenta fails to separate at all there will be no bleeding. A cornual implantation of the placenta may cause this.

   Partial separation will cause bleeding but the fundus will remain broad because the placenta still occupies the upper segment. Needless handling of the uterus during the third stage is thought to encourage partial separation.

   Where oxytocics have been given an hour glass constriction may develop in the lower segment and the cervix begins to close down.

Placenta Accreta is a rare cause of retained placenta. There is abnormal adherence of the placenta to the uterine muscle due to a defect of decidual formation. It is usually partial, and presents by partial separation accompanied by bleeding. On rare occasions it is complete, and bleeding is absent. Attempts at manual removal open the blood sinuses causing severe bleeding, and hysterectomy may be necessary.

Placenta accreta should be suspected when the operator has difficulty in finding the line of cleavage when attempting manual removal. The placenta may be left in utero if there is no bleeding, but infection is inevitable. Probably, in this rare condition, hysterectomy is the safest course.

RETAINED PLACENTA

TREATMENT

Intervention becomes necessary either because of bleeding or when 20 minutes have elapsed.

An attempt should be made to remove the placenta by rubbing up a contraction and applying cord traction as described previously. If the placenta remains adherent the cord may break. If this occurs or the attempt is unsuccessful manual removal of the placenta under anaesthesia should be performed.

This should not be delayed because of the risk of haemorrhage from partial separation. The procedure itself, however, is not without risk from infection and damage to the uterus.

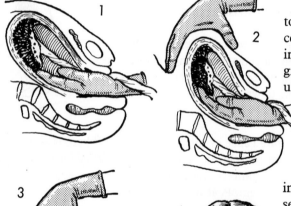

The hand covered with antiseptic cream is introduced into the vagina, following the cord.

The fingers begin to separate the placenta from the uterine wall. Never grasp the placenta until it is separated.

Note that the abdominal hand presses the uterus into the placenta and prevents tearing of the lower segment.

The placenta is inspected at once to see that it is complete and, if there is any doubt, the uterus is re-explored. Ergometrine or oxytocin is then given and the uterus rubbed up to make it contract.

PRIMARY POST-PARTUM HAEMORRHAGE (PPH)

Primary Post-Partum Haemorrhage is blood loss from the birth canal of 5dl or more within 24 hours of delivery. After 24 hours abnormal bleeding is classed as Secondary Post-Partum Haemorrhage.

CAUSES

1. **Uterine Atony** — the uterus, although empty, fails to contract and control bleeding from the placental site. This is the commonest and potentially most dangerous cause.

    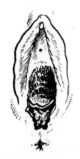

    Uterus failing to contract

    Predisposing Causes
    (a) Excessive uterine distension (twins, polyhydramnios, large baby)
    (b) Multiparity (fibrosis in uterine muscle).
    (c) Prolonged labour (uterine inertia).
    (d) Labour augmented with Syntocinon.
    (e) General anaesthesia.
    (f) Placenta praevia — lower segment does not contract well enough to stop bleeding.
    (g) Abruptio placentae — the 'Couvelaire' uterus may not contract. In addition a coagulation defect may develop.

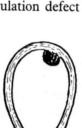
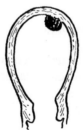

2. **Partial Separation of the Placenta** – uterus is prevented from contracting.

3. **Retention of Placental Fragments**

4. **Trauma** (uterus, cervix, vagina, episiotomy).

CONSEQUENCES OF PPH

1. Bleeding may be very rapid, causing circulatory collapse leading to shock and death.
2. Puerperal anaemia and morbidity.
3. (Very rarely) damage to the pituitary blood supply, leading to pituitary necrosis — Sheehan's syndrome.
4. Fear of further pregnancies. Haemorrhage is terrifying for the mother.

331

PRIMARY POST-PARTUM HAEMORRHAGE

TREATMENT
1. **Measurement of blood loss**

    Blood spilt on bed linen and dressings is often ignored and only blood actually collected in a bowl is measured. The estimated loss is therefore invariably lower than the actual loss and the mother's response will be governed by her haemoglobin level.

2. **Use of Oxytocic Drugs**

    Two are used: Ergometrine 0.5mg and oxytocin 5 units. Syntometrine is a proprietary combination of both these drugs.

    Ergometrine produces tonic contractions of the uterus and is also vasoconstrictor. It may therefore cause elevation of the blood pressure especially if given intravenously. Its action affects the uterus for 2–3 hours.

    Synthetic oxytocin produces rhythmic contractions of the uterus. It is virtually free from systemic effects in therapeutic dosage and its action lasts for 20–30 minutes. In an emergency either can be given intravenously with almost immediate effect.

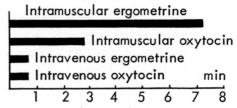

Time between injection and action of oxytocin.

3. **Plan of Treatment**

    The aim is to stop the patient bleeding.

    (a) Give an oxytocic intravenously.

    (b) Rub up a contraction of the uterus to control bleeding and if the placenta is undelivered attempt removal by cord traction.

    (c) Rapid assessment of the mother's condition; set up an I.V. line and send blood for cross-match.

    (d) Treat the cause

    (i) If the placenta has been delivered check for completeness. If in doubt exploration of the uterus must be carried out.

    (ii) If the uterus appears well-contracted and bleeding continues, damage to the cervix or vagina should be suspected. Proper assessment of this will require exploration under anaesthesia.

    (iii) If both these causes have been excluded uterine atony is diagnosed.

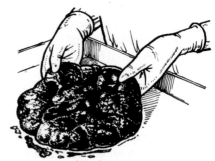

Placenta examined on a flat surface to demonstrate any missing lobe.

PRIMARY POST-PARTUM HAEMORRHAGE

TREATMENT OF UTERINE ATONY

Having excluded an incomplete placenta and trauma to the genital tract by thorough exploration, the uterus is compressed between the hands to control bleeding and stimulate contraction.

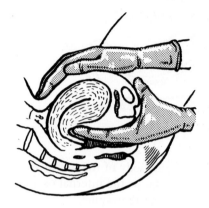

The fingers of one hand are pressed into the anterior fornix. If a good pressure is not obtained, as the vagina is lax, the whole fist can be inserted.

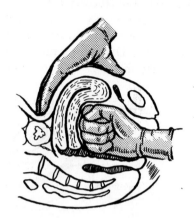

If this is not effective the uterus should be packed firmly with gauze. The packing usually remains in position for at least 12 hours. If contraction is still not obtained hysterectomy must be carried out. By this time the patient is likely to be in a serious condition and a decision to operate, difficult as it is, must not be made too late. In cases of persistent bleeding the presence of a clotting defect should be excluded.

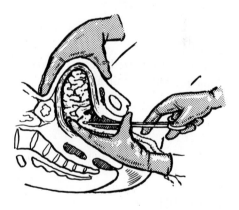

ACUTE INVERSION OF THE UTERUS

Acute inversion of the uterus is a very rare condition in modern practice but important because of its serious consequences.

First Degree (Incomplete) - - - - - - - - - →

The inverted fundus reaches the external os. Diagnosis is made by vaginal examination.

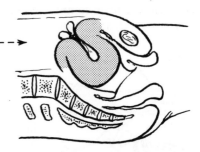

←- - - - - - - **Second degree** (Complete)

The whole body of the uterus is inverted as far as the internal os and protrudes into the vagina.

Third Degree - - - - - - - - - - - →
   Prolapse of inverted uterus, cervix and vagina outside the vulva.

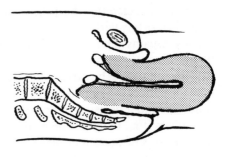

CAUSATION

1.   Most commonly due to a too vigorous attempt to deliver the placenta by cord traction in the presence of an uncontracted uterus.
2.   It is favoured by laxity of the uterine muscles as in women of high parity, and by fundal attachment of the placenta. It can be brought on by any sudden bearing down effort.

CONSEQUENCES

1.   Usually very severe shock and perhaps bleeding. Death may follow if untreated.
2.   Sepsis is common and the shock may be followed by anuria and renal failure.
3.   Inversion may become chronic.
4.   The uterus may strangulate and slough off.

334

ACUTE INVERSION OF THE UTERUS

TREATMENT

If the doctor is present when inversion occurs he should at once attempt to replace the uterus by hand. He must not use too much force, and if not immediately successful, he should simply replace the inverted uterus in the vagina and institute treatment for shock. It is probably safer to leave the placenta if it is attached; removal might precipitate severe haemorrhage.

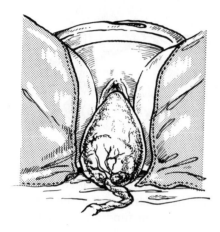

Reduction by taxis

Under general anaesthesia an attempt is made to reduce the inversion by gradual replacement of the uterus, pressing first on that part of the corpus which was inverted last. The most difficult part to reduce is the retraction ring between upper and lower segments.

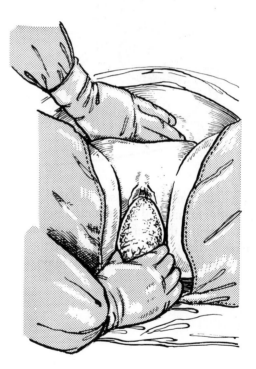

Once reduced, the hand is kept inside the uterus until ergometrine or oxytocin has produced a firm contraction.

335

ACUTE INVERSION OF THE UTERUS

Reduction by hydrostatic pressure

If taxis fails, O'Sullivan's hydrostatic method should be attempted.

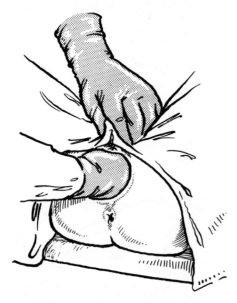

A douche nozzle is passed into the posterior fornix, and an assistant closes the vulva around the operator's wrist. Warm saline is run in (up to 2 gallons) until the pressure gradually restores the position of the uterus.

Reduction by the abdominal route

If other methods fail, the abdomen should be opened.

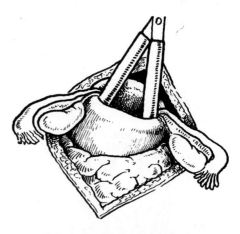

The constricting ring is stretched. Then the posterior part of the ring is divided and the fundus hooked up and resutured.

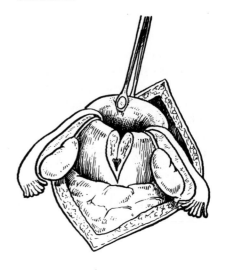

ABNORMALITIES OF THE PLACENTA

The placenta develops from the chorion frondosum, the part in contact with the most vascular decidua. Any developmental abnormality may have a clinical significance.

Placenta Membranacea (syn: Diffusa)

More or less the whole chorion develops functional villi and the placenta occupies the greater part of the uterine wall. This may cause retention in the third stage. Antepartum haemorrhage may also occur.

Another variety is placenta annularis in which the placenta surrounds the chorion like a wide ring. This is normal in the dog, while membranacea is normal in the pig.

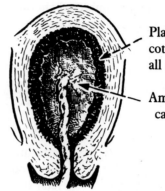

Placental cotyledons all round

Amniotic cavity

Placenta Bipartita

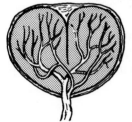

The placenta is partly divided into two lobes, with connecting vessels.

Placenta Duplex

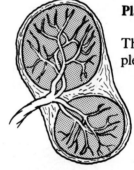

The placenta is completely divided into two lobes, with vessels uniting to form the cord.

Placenta Succenturiata
('substitute')

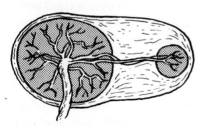

(A variant of Duplex)

Sometimes the placenta is partly or completely divided into two or more lobes (multipartita, multiplex). In placenta succenturiata there is a vascular connection between main and accessory lobes. This may be torn at delivery, and torn vessels may be seen at the edge of the membranes. In such cases the accessory lobe is retained and must be manually removed.

337

ABNORMALITIES OF THE PLACENTA

Placenta Circumvallata. The membranes appear to be attached internally to the placental edge, and on the periphery there is a ring of thick whitish tissue which is in fact a fold of infarcted chorion. This abnormality has an association with antepartum and postpartum haemorrhage.

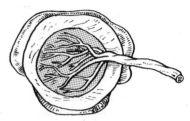

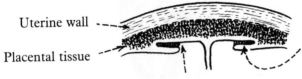

Uterine wall

Placental tissue

Attachment of membranes to fetal surface

Reduplicated and infarcted chorion

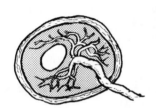

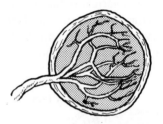

Placenta Fenestrata

A defective area appears in the middle of the placenta. It may be wrongly taken for the site of a missing lobe.

Battledore Placenta

Sometimes the cord has a marginal instead of a central insertion. This has no clinical significance.

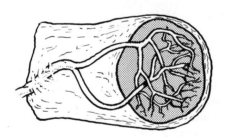

Placenta Velamentosa. The placenta has developed some distance away from the attachment of the cord and the vessels divide in the membranes. If they cross the lower pole of the chorion a condition arises called vasa praevia. Rupture of the membranes will then precipitate haemorrhage which will exsanguinate the fetus.

Placental Infarcts are areas of degeneration showing hyaline and often calcareous change. Their aetiology is unknown and they have no clinical significance unless so large as to interfere with fetal nutrition.

Placental Tumours are exceedingly rare and the haemangioma is the only one of any significance. It is often accompanied by hydramnios.

338

ABNORMALITIES OF THE CORD

Cord Round the Neck

One or two loops of cord are quite often seen round the baby's neck at vertex delivery and normally do no harm. As soon as the neck is visible at the vulva the loop should be clamped and divided before delivery of the shoulders and trunk.

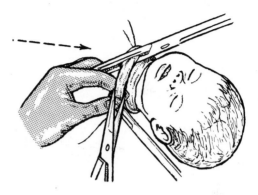

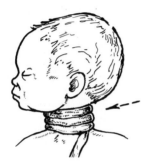

Much less frequently six or seven loops are drawn tightly round the neck. As the fetus descends the cord tightens, the blood supply is interrupted and the baby is stillborn. This is one cause of sudden acute fetal distress.

Abnormal Length of Cord

The average length is 50cm but extremes of 15cm and 150cm have rarely occurred. Prolapse and looping round the neck seem more likely with lengthy cords, while delayed fetal descent and premature placental separation may occur with very short ones. A cord of normal length may become relatively short because of multiple looping round the neck.

Knots in the Cord

True knots are seen quite often, but Wharton's jelly usually prevents actual obstruction by kinking. False knots are protuberances of connective tissue matrix, sometimes containing varices.

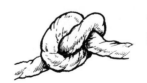

True knot

Single Umbilical Artery

This finding is sometimes associated with congenital abnormalities in the fetus.

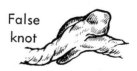

False knot

CHAPTER 14

OBSTETRICAL OPERATIONS
AND MATERNAL INJURIES

EPISIOTOMY

EPISIOTOMY (Gr. A cutting of the pubic region)

Making an incision in the perineal body at the time of delivery.

Indications

1. To prevent a perineal tear or excessive stretching of the muscles. A tear is less controllable and may involve the anal sphincter, and overstretching will predispose to prolapse in later years.

2. To protect the fetus if it is premature or is being forced repeatedly against an unyielding perineum which is obstructing delivery.

3. To prevent damage from an abnormal presenting part — occipitoposterior positions, face presentations, after-coming head in breech deliveries, all instrumental deliveries. In such cases it may be done before the perineum is distended. The obstetrician must himself put the tissues on the stretch before cutting.

Types of Incision

1. The median incision is easiest to make and to repair, but in the event of extension it does not give any protection to the anal sphincter.

2. The posterolateral incision is more difficult to repair as the edges retract unequally. Anatomical apposition is, therefore, sometimes difficult to achieve. It gives the best protection against sphincter damage, and best answers the purpose of the operation.

3. The 'J-shaped' incision is a theoretical compromise which becomes a posterolateral incision in practice.

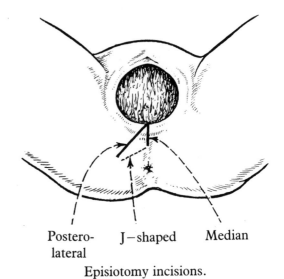

Postero-   J—shaped   Median
lateral

Episiotomy incisions.

EPISIOTOMY

Anaesthesia

In the conscious patient the best method is to inject 10 ml of lignocaine 1% along the track of the proposed incision. Time should be allowed for this to take effect.

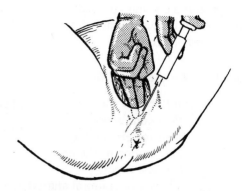

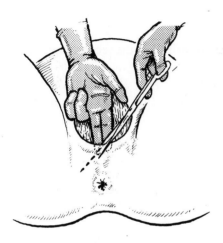

Technique

Two fingers are placed as shown to protect the fetal head, and a long clean cut is made with scissors. It is important to start from the fourchette, otherwise anatomical apposition will be difficult when the repair is undertaken. Too long an incision will open up the ischiorectal fossa and fatty tissue will be seen, but provided there is no infection this does not affect healing.

The timing of an episiotomy must be learnt by experience. If done too soon, blood loss will increase, if delayed too long, a tear of the vagina or deep perineal muscles will occur.

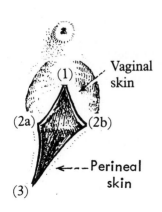

Repair

The repair is done in 3 layers using absorbable material:

1. Vaginal skin — a continuous suture starting at (1) and ending at the hymen, bringing together points (2a) and (2b).
2. Muscle — interrupted sutures, burying the knots under the muscle layer.
3. Perineal skin — continuous or interrupted sutures burying the knots under the surface.

343

FORCEPS DELIVERY

This remains a common procedure in British obstetric practice, although the incidence has tended to fall in recent years. A forceps delivery rate of approximately 15% is common in many British centres.

Indications for the use of forceps

1. Delay in the second stage of labour. This may be due to:
   - Poor contractions,
   - Poor maternal effort,
   - Malrotation of the head,
   - Perineal rigidity,
   - The use of epidural anaesthesia.

   Where epidurals are employed some obstetricians will allow the second stage to last much longer than normal.

2. Fetal distress:

3. Maternal distress:
   Hypertension,
   Cardiac disease,
   Maternal exhaustion,
   Over-stressed emotionally.

Conditions for forceps delivery

1. The cervix must be fully dilated.

2. A suitable presenting part:
   Vertex,
   Face,
   After-coming head in breech.

3. Head *at least* engaged and no significant mechanical problem.

   These are fundamental requirements and failure to observe them will lead to fetal and/or maternal injury. To them may be added:

4. The bladder should be empty,

5. Suitable anaesthesia.

OBSTETRIC FORCEPS

The obstetric forceps is designed to grasp the fetal head when it is in the vagina and effect delivery by traction and guidance without causing injury to mother or fetus.

A forceps consists of two arms which can be articulated.

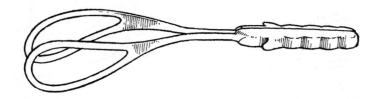

The blades have two curves.

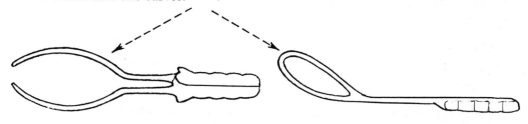

The cephalic curve is adapted to provide a good application to the fetal head.

The pelvic curve allows the blades to fit in with the curve of the birth canal.

There are several kinds of lock:-

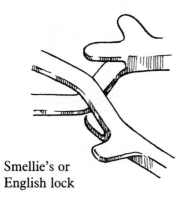

Smellie's or English lock

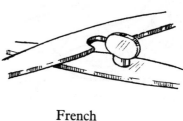

French lock

OBSTETRIC FORCEPS

Forceps operations are of two kinds:

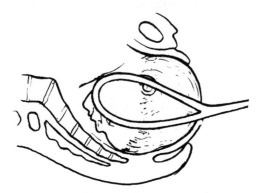

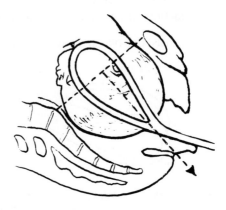

Low Forceps

The fetal head has reached the perineal floor and is visible at the vulva.

Mid Forceps

Engagement has taken place and the leading part of the head is below the level of the ischial spines.

Application of the forceps when the head is not engaged is known as 'high forceps'. In this situation the pelvic axis necessitates traction 'round the corner', so some forceps have detachable handles on rods which allow traction in the pelvic axis.

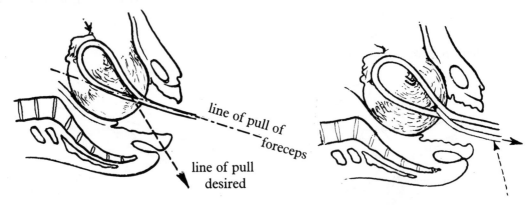

Axis traction rod pulling in axis of pelvic curve.

This technique of axis traction should be unnecessary in present-day practice when a difficult forceps delivery is avoided by Caesarean section.

OBSTETRIC FORCEPS

There are very many different patterns. The forceps shown here are all well known and are identified with the three main operations — the low forceps, the mid forceps, and the rotation-extraction forceps delivery.

Wrigley's Forceps

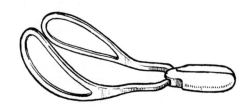

Wrigley's Forceps is designed for use when the head is on the perineum and local anaesthesia is being used. It is a short light instrument with pelvic and cephalic curves and an English lock.

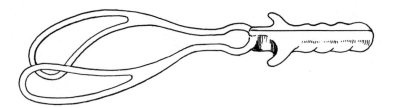

Anderson's (Simpson's) Forceps

This forceps is suitable for a standard mid-forceps delivery with the sagittal suture of the head in the antero-posterior axis. It has cephalic and pelvic curves but the shanks and handle are longer and heavier than Wrigley's.

Kielland's Forceps

This forceps was originally designed to deliver the fetal head at or above the pelvic brim, lying in the transverse axis of the pelvis and rotating it when it had reached the pelvic cavity. The forceps is used today for rotation and extraction of the head which is arrested in the deep transverse or occipito-posterior position.

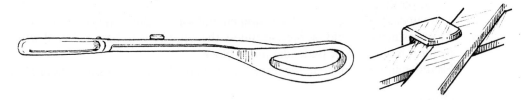

The blades have very little pelvic curve and are virtually an axis traction forceps. A large episiotomy is needed. The shallowness of the curve allows safe rotation in the vagina. Downward traction encourages rotation of the head.

347

OBSTETRIC FORCEPS

Kielland's Forceps(continued)

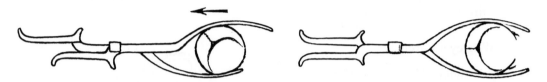

The claw lock allows the blades to slide on each other and correct or encourage asynclitism of the the fetal head as required.

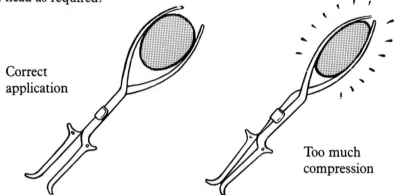

Correct application

Too much compression

This range of movement allowed by the lock makes it possible to apply lethal compression to the fetal head if the instrument is used improperly.

TECHNIQUE OF FORCEPS DELIVERY

Preparations

1. The patient will usually be in the lithotomy position although some operators prefer the left lateral position.
2. The vulva should be cleaned and draped and aseptic precautions observed.
3. An anaesthetist should be present unless the delivery is to be conducted with only local perineal infiltration or pudendal nerve block.
4. Facilities and personnel for the resuscitation of the baby, if necessary, should be available.

Anaesthesia

1. Low forceps delivery, using Wrigley's blades, requires only the *local infiltration* necessary to make an episiotomy.
2. Anaesthesia for mid-cavity forceps delivery is usually a combination of *local infiltration* and *pudendal nerve block*. Lignocaine 1% without adrenaline is satisfactory and up to 50 ml may be used with safety.

TECHNIQUE OF FORCEPS DELIVERY

Anaesthesia (continued)

Local infiltration

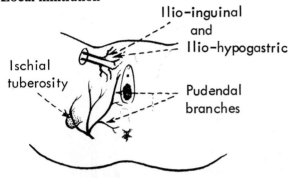

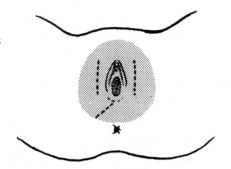

Principal nerves supplying vulva and perineum.

Area of vulva and perineum which should be infiltrated.

Pudendal Nerve Block

The forefinger is placed on the ischial spine (behind which runs the pudendal nerve) and a long needle is passed via the ischiorectal fossa. When needle point, spine and finger are in conjunction, 5 ml of lignocaine are injected. It is advisable to withdraw the plunger before injecting to make sure that the needle is not in a blood vessel. The needle, preferably a guarded one, can be passed per vaginam if the operator finds it easier.

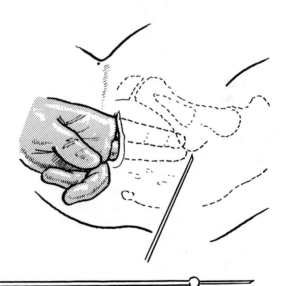

A transvaginal guarded needle.

3. *Epidural block* is widely used and suitable for all types of vaginal delivery, (see Chapter 11).

349

FORCEPS DELIVERY

Anaesthesia (continued)

4. *Spinal anaesthesia* may sometimes be used for speed, when a full block is needed and an epidural is not already in situ.

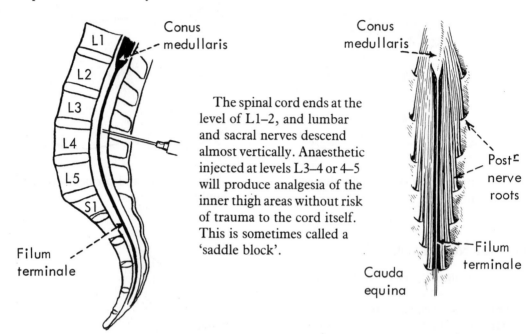

The spinal cord ends at the level of L1–2, and lumbar and sacral nerves descend almost vertically. Anaesthetic injected at levels L3–4 or 4–5 will produce analgesia of the inner thigh areas without risk of trauma to the cord itself. This is sometimes called a 'saddle block'.

Physiology of Spinal Anaesthesia

The effect is that of 'chemical sympathectomy'. The pre-ganglionic autonomic fibres are blocked first, followed by those serving temperature, pain, touch, motor and proprioceptive function in that order. Skeletal muscle action may still be possible when sensory blockade is complete.

Circulatory Effects

Paralysis of the pre-ganglionic fibres leads to arterial dilatation with a fall in venous return and cardiac output. Blood loss at operation may aggravate this and cause an acute and serious fall in blood pressure.

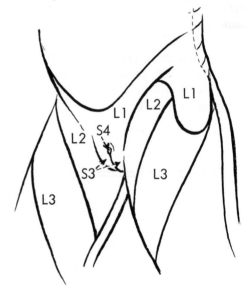

Areas affected by a saddle block

350

FORCEPS DELIVERY

LOW FORCEPS DELIVERY

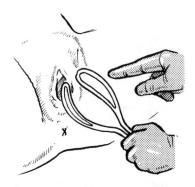

1. Choosing the left blade.

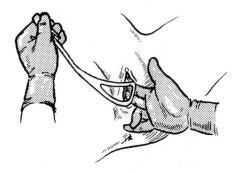

2. Applying the left blade.

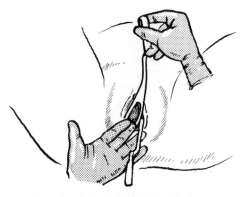

3. Applying the right blade.

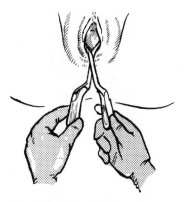

4. Locking the blades.

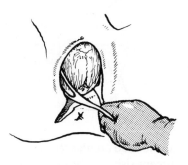

5. Gentle traction with an episiotomy at crowning.

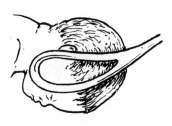

6. The correct cephalic application (in the mento-vertical line).

351

FORCEPS DELIVERY

MID FORCEPS DELIVERY

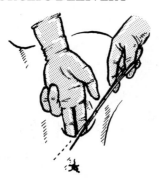

1. Making a large episiotomy before starting.

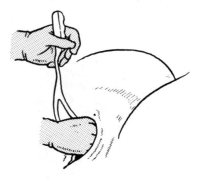

2. Applying the left blade. Hand protects vagina from damage by careless insertions of blade.

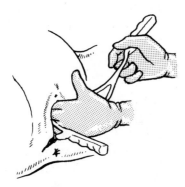

3. Applying the right blade.

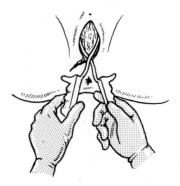

4. Locking the handles.

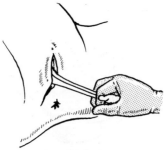

5. Traction, maintaining downward pressure to keep in the line of the birth canal.

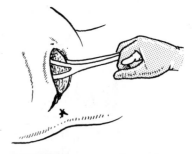

6. As the head crowns the handles of the forceps rise and the head is lifted over the perineum.

FORCEPS DELIVERY

DELIVERY WITH KIELLAND'S FORCEPS

The position of the occiput must be known and is here taken as R.O.L.

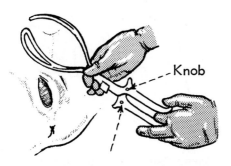

1. Holding forceps with the knobs directed towards fetal occiput.

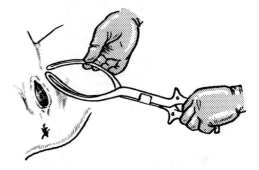

2. The anterior blade is selected to be applied first (some obstetricians prefer to apply the posterior blade first).

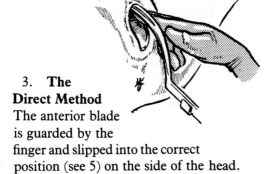

3. **The Direct Method** The anterior blade is guarded by the finger and slipped into the correct position (see 5) on the side of the head.

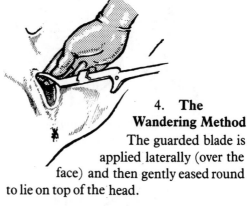

4. **The Wandering Method** The guarded blade is applied laterally (over the face) and then gently eased round to lie on top of the head.

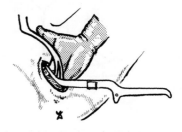

5. It now lies with the concavity of the blade applied to left (uppermost) side of the fetal head.

6. The posterior blade is applied directly to the right (lower) side of the head. The vagina is protected by the guiding hand.

FORCEPS DELIVERY

Delivery with Kielland's Forceps   (continued)

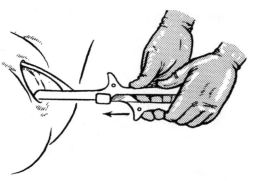

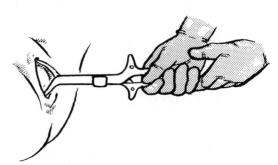

7. The forceps are locked. Note how their position shows asynclitism.

8. Asynclitism is corrected and the forceps blades are opposite each other.

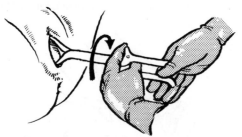

9. The head is gently rotated to the OA position. Varying asynclitism and gentle traction help to rotate into the pelvic axis. A large episiotomy is needed.

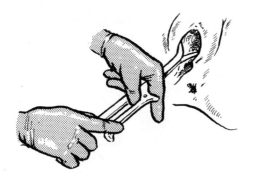

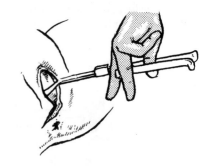

10. To prevent over compression of the baby's head, a thumb is kept between the handles.

11. As the head extends, the direction of pull must be altered upwards.

FORCEPS DELIVERY

MANUAL ROTATION

This may be used as an alternative to rotation with forceps and delivery is then completed with Anderson's blades.

First determine the exact position by palpating the anterior fontanelle. This may be extremely difficult to detect if there has been much moulding or caput formation.

An ear may be palpable. The root of the pinna must be identified to distinguish left from right.

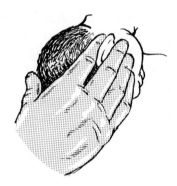

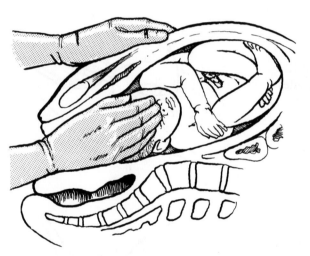

The right hand then grasps the head, while the left hand through the abdominal wall pushes the shoulder forward. The head may have to be dislodged slightly to achieve this, and once round it must be held in position until the forceps blades are applied.

FORCEPS DELIVERY

OTHER APPLICATIONS of FORCEPS

1. Delivery of the head in the occipito-posterior position.

    This may be the easiest and best method of delivering a fetus with the head in the direct OP position, pro—vided the head is low in the pelvis. Little traction should be required and the fetus is spared the risk of manipulation. A large episiotomy is necessary.

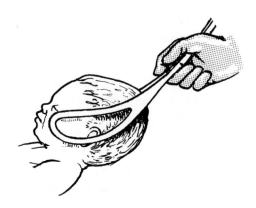

2. In a breech presentation the forceps can be applied to the head once it has entered the pelvis. Anderson's blades are preferred because of their length.

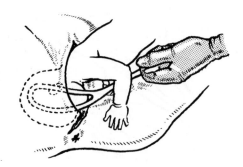

3. In a face presentation (mento-anterior) the forceps may be applied direct. (Mento-posterior positions must be rotated.)

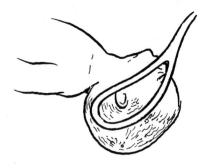

FORCEPS DELIVERY

COMPLICATIONS of FORCEPS DELIVERY

Lacerations

1. Perineal tears are inevitable unless episiotomy is done at the right time.

2. Vaginal wall may be split, especially if compressed between ischial spine and fetal head or forceps inserted carelessly.

3. Cervical and vaginal tears may be caused during a Kielland's rotation. After delivery the vagina and cervix should be carefully inspected and all damage repaired.

Haemorrhage

Except from lacerations, haemorrhage is no more likely than after spontaneous delivery. Many obstetricians give an intravenous oxytocic with the delivery of the anterior shoulder of the baby when conducting a forceps delivery. This allows speedy completion of the third stage of labour by cord traction.

Injury to baby

If the blades have been properly applied, the fetal head should be protected by the rigid case of the forceps blades. Where excessive traction force has been applied, there may be bruising, facial nerve palsy or depression fracture of the skull.

TRIAL OF FORCEPS

This term is used when delivery is indicated but the obstetrician remains uncertain whether safe vaginal delivery is mechanically possible.

The procedure requires the presence of an experienced operator and the delivery is conducted in an operating theatre with the staff and facilities to proceed to Caesarean section. Careful re-examination in theatre may convince the operator that delivery is not possible. If still uncertain, however, he may proceed to apply the forceps blades and even exert traction. If application of the blades is difficult or no descent of the head occurs with reasonable traction, Caesarean section is performed. The operator's mental approach to the procedure is important, that is to say the possibility of Caesarean section being required has been clearly acknowledged.

VACUUM EXTRACTOR (Ventouse)

The vacuum extractor is a traction instrument used as an alternative to the obstetric forceps. It adheres to the baby's scalp by suction and is used in the conscious patient to assist the maternal expulsive efforts.

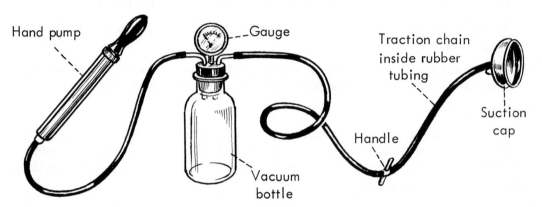

The suction cup obtains its grip by raising an artificial caput. The original Malmström instrument consisted of a metal cup and hand pump. Negative pressure is raised by $0.2kg/cm^2$ every two minutes to a maximum of 0.8. The patient is usually in the lithotomy position and the same aseptic precautions are observed as for forceps operations. Probably the most convenient anaesthetic is a pudendal nerve block, but sometimes only inhalational analgesia or sufficient local anaesthetic for an episiotomy is required.

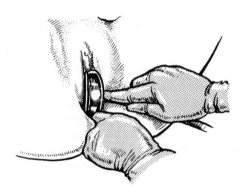

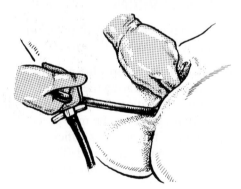

1. The cup is insinuated into the vagina. When applying it to the scalp, the fontanelles and sutures should be avoided if possible.

2. Traction is made downwards with the right hand while the left hand presses the cup against the fetal head.

358

VACUUM EXTRACTOR

3. As the head is delivered an episiotomy may be necessary.

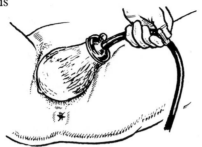

4. The artificial caput made by suction cup immediately after delivery

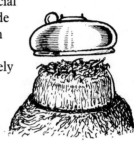

Recently a new vacuum extractor, with a malleable silicone cup and an electrical pump has become popular. The advantages of the new instrument are that it produces a much less marked 'chignon' on the fetal scalp and the speed with which the vacuum can be raised.

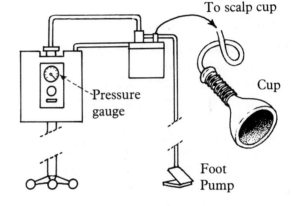

The Place of the Vacuum Extractor

1. This instrument was introduced as a means of avoiding difficult forceps delivery or even Caesarean section in patients in whom there was delay in labour with the cervix not quite fully dilated. It may still occasionally be used for this purpose, but it is mainly used as the instrument of choice by obstetricians who prefer it even when forceps delivery would be easy.

2. Like the forceps, it should normally be applied only when the head is engaged and there is no question of disproportion. An exception to this rule may be in the case of a second twin where the head remains at a relatively high level. In these circumstances the application of the vacuum extractor may be simpler and safer than the use of forceps.

Precautions in Use

1. Care should be taken, in applying the cup to the fetal scalp, to exclude vaginal skin from the edges of the cup.

2. Prolonged or excessive traction should not be used. Traction for more than 10 minutes will increase the risk of scalp damage, cephalhaematoma or more serious sub-aponeurotic bleeding.

SYMPHYSIOTOMY

Symphysiotomy means the cutting of the fibres of the symphysis pubis to allow vaginal delivery in the presence of moderate disproportion. The procedure has a place in obstetrical practice in developing countries when facilities for Caesarean sections are not available, or in order to avoid the risk of rupture of a Caesarean section scar in a subsequent pregnancy in women being confined by unskilled attendants in remote areas.

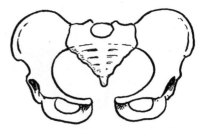

The transverse diameter can be enlarged up to 3 cm and the pubic angle widened, but there is little increase in AP diameters.

Principles of Operation

1. The head should be two-fifths or more in the pelvis.
2. The cervix should be at least 8 cm dilated in a primigravid or 6 cm in a multipara.
3. The legs are held in abduction by assistants (stirrups are not used) to prevent excessive stretching of the vaginal tissues when the joint is divided.
4. A catheter is placed in the bladder and one finger in the vagina pushes the urethra to the side to protect it from injury.
5. The symphysis pubis and perineum are infiltrated with local anaesthetic.
6. A stab incision with a scalpel is made into the centre of the joint. The blade is moved to divide the fibres of the symphysis.

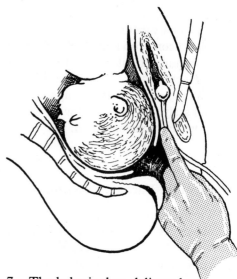

7. The baby is then delivered spontaneously or by vacuum extractor aided by an episiotomy.
8. The mother's legs are strapped together for 12 hours post-operatively and ambulation is gradually introduced.

Complications

1. Soft tissue damage and fistula during operation and later stress incontinence.
2. Subsequent pelvic joint pain and difficulty in walking.

The incidence of these complications will obviously be reduced by an experienced surgeon, but very few obstetricians in the United Kingdom are familiar with the operation which has been completely replaced by lower segment section.

CAESAREAN SECTION

Caesarean section means the delivery of the baby through incisions in the abdominal wall and uterus. The operation has been performed more frequently in the United Kingdom in the last decade and rates of 10–15% are now common in British hospitals. Caesarean section has replaced complicated operative vaginal delivery and it is used increasingly in the management of the 'at risk' fetus, especially if premature.

It must be remembered, however, that the morbidity and mortality of Caesarean section are considerably greater than for vaginal delivery, and the patient's management in a subsequent pregnancy is likely to be dominated by the fact that her uterus is scarred.

INDICATIONS

The decision to deliver by Caesarean section will often be based on a combination of factors or circumstances. The following list gives the common indications for Caesarean section but should not be regarded as comprehensive:

In Labour	Fetal distress in the first stage of labour, Delay in the first stage of labour due to disordered uterine action or suspected disproportion.
Other Emergencies	Cord prolapse, Fulminating pre-eclampsia, Abruption of the placenta where the baby is alive.
Elective	Placenta praevia, 2 previous Caesarean sections, and in some cases of Intra-uterine growth retardation, Bad obstetric history, Maternal diabetes, Breech presentation (especially if premature).

ANAESTHESIA

Epidural block has become the preferred method of anaesthesia for Caesarean section in many hospitals.

Advantages:	Avoids the dangers of general anaesthesia (failed intubation, inhalation of gastric contents). Improved retraction of the uterus. Permits the mother (and her partner) to see and hear the baby at birth. Rapid post-operative recovery.

The preparation of an epidural anaesthetic for Caesarean section may be time-consuming, and if time is short and it is wished to avoid general anaesthesia, a spinal anaesthetic may be given.

General anaesthesia is still commonly used, however, especially in cases where there may be severe haemorrhage e.g. placenta praevia. Some woman may be frightened by the prospect of abdominal delivery while remaining awake and request a general anaesthetic.

361

CAESAREAN SECTION

LOWER SEGMENT SECTION

In this procedure a transverse incision is made in the lower uterine segment. It is the operation of choice. Although slightly more complicated to perform, repair of the uterus is usually simple, the scar heals well and subsequent rupture is uncommon.

The lower segment may be approached through either a midline sub-umbilical abdominal incision or a transverse suprapubic incision.

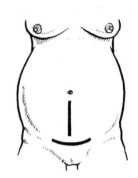

Technique of Lower Segment Section

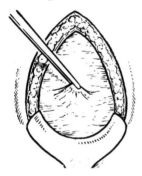

The loose uterovesical peritoneum is picked up.

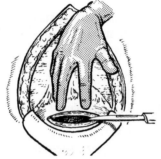

Peritoneum is cut to expose lower segment, and a small transverse incision is made.

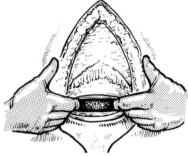

The uterine incision is widened with the fingers.

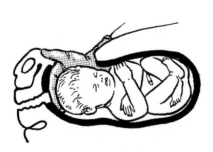

The operator's right hand is passed into the uterus to lift the baby's head, while the assistant presses on the fundus to push the baby out.

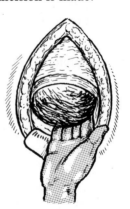

Sometimes it is necessary to extract the head with forceps.

362

CAESAREAN SECTION

Technique of Lower Segment Section (continued)

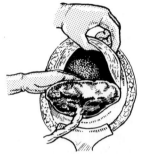
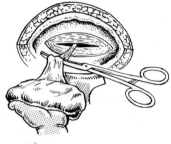
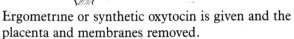

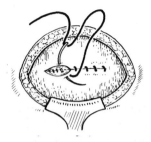

Ergometrine or synthetic oxytocin is given and the placenta and membranes removed.

The uterine wound is closed with 2 layers of catgut and the peritoneum re-sutured.

CLASSICAL CAESAREAN SECTION

This means a longitudinal incision in the upper uterine segment.

The operation is quick and easy but it is an abdominal procedure rather than a pelvic one and more often followed by peritonitis and ileus. The involution of the uterus may not allow sound healing and the scar may rupture in a subsequent pregnancy.

The operation is still, however, occasionally indicated:

1. Some cases of placenta praevia with an ill-formed lower segment.
2. Transverse or unstable lie with poor lower segment.
3. Very premature delivery where the lower segment has not formed.
4. Fibroid distorting the uterus.
5. When an inexperienced surgeon is operating in an emergency.

Technique of Classical Section

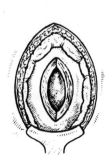

Abdominal contents are packed off and the uterus is opened in the midline. If the placenta is anterior (40% of cases) it is cut through or pushed aside at once. Bleeding is ignored.

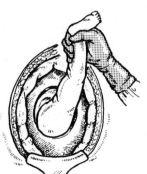

The easiest way to remove the baby is to pull it out gently by the legs.

The placenta is delivered as before and the wound closed in 3 layers.

363

CAESAREAN SECTION

COMPLICATIONS

Haemorrhage

Caesarean section is a vascular operation and the blood loss is commonly between 500 and 1000 ml. Cross-matched blood should, therefore, always be available and an intravenous drip set up. Increased bleeding is to be anticipated in cases of placenta praevia or multiple pregnancy where there may be impaired retraction of the placental site.

If the lower segment incision tears at the angles during the extraction of the baby, the large uterine vessels may be torn and haemorrhage will be severe. The patient can very quickly become shocked. The blood loss can usually be controlled by suturing, but if this proves impossible the operator may need to resort to removal of the uterus. Identification of the cervix is not always easy and a sub-total hysterectomy may be carried out.

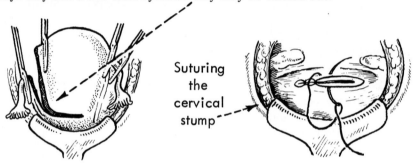

Suturing the cervical stump

Post-Operative Distension

Gaseous distension of the bowel is common after Caesarean section, but the lax condition of the abdominal muscles, although it accentuates the swelling, reduces the pain of distension. There may be reduced bowel sounds and an absence of flatus for the first 24–48 hours. If this 'incipient ileus' does not resolve quickly, gastric suction and parenteral fluids should be started.

Wound Dehiscence and Infection

Because of the abdominal distension a longitudinal sub-umbilical incision is under tension and dehiscence is commoner than after other abdominal operations. For this reason a transverse abdominal incision is much to be preferred. A Pfannenstiel incision rarely dehisces but haematoma formation is relatively frequent and careful attention to haemostasis is important.

Pulmonary Embolism

The risk of this serious complication is increased with Caesarean section compared with vaginal delivery. The risk is reduced by early ambulation and this is aided by the use of epidural anaesthesia.

DESTRUCTIVE OPERATIONS

These procedures were designed to reduce the bulk of dead or grossly abnormal fetuses to allow vaginal delivery. Nowadays Caesarean section will usually be preferred.

The only procedure likely to be employed in practice today is perforation of the head of a hydrocephalic fetus. This may be done in the second stage of labour to allow vaginal delivery.

CRANIOTOMY — Perforation of the skull to allow drainage of CSF and collapse of the skull. Any pointed instrument will serve, such as a wide-bore trocar and cannula.

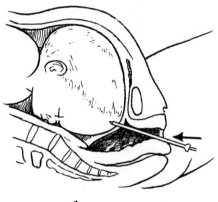

Head presentation

The skull sutures are perforated per vaginam, and an assistant must press the head downwards to prevent rupture of the lower segment as the operator forces the trocar upwards.

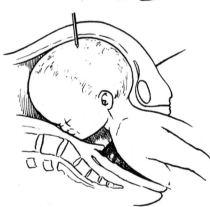

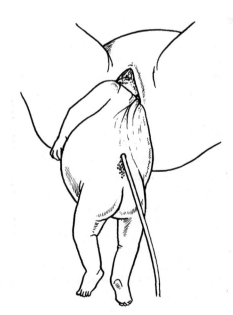

Breech Presentation

The trocar is passed through the abdominal wall. If a meningocele is present it is possible to drain a hydrocephaly by passing a straightened male catheter up the spinal canal.

365

STERILISATION

This in practice means interruption of the continuity of the fallopian tubes. The patient's convenience is best suited by doing it in the immediate post-natal period but as the operation has a slight but recognised association with thrombo-embolism, as does the early puerperium, it is wiser to delay for at least two months. A further reason for delay is to allow the patient time to reconsider her decision free from the pressures of pregnancy.

TUBAL LIGATION

A loop of tube is ligated with catgut and the top of the loop is excised.
When the catgut absorbs the divided areas will spring apart leaving a defect in the tube. This is known as the Pomeroy method of sterilisation.

TUBAL OCCLUSION

The fallopian tubes can be occluded by rings or clips applied under laparoscopic vision.

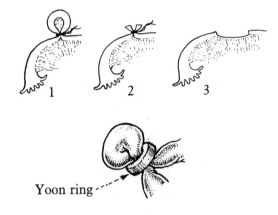

Yoon ring

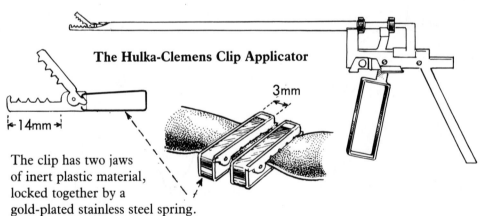

The Hulka-Clemens Clip Applicator

3mm

14mm

The clip has two jaws of inert plastic material, locked together by a gold-plated stainless steel spring.

The patient should understand that the operation is designed to be permanent, and although patency can sometimes be restored, normal function leading to conception can by no means be guaranteed.

There is a very small risk of failure with any method — 3–4/1000. Ligated tubes can become patent through a fistulous opening, and clips and rings may be defective.

TERMINATION OF PREGNANCY

Termination of pregnancy prior to the time when the fetus is considered viable has been made legal in the United Kingdom if the continuation of pregnancy would involve a greater risk:

1. To the mother's life.
2. To the mother's physical or mental health.
3. To the existing child(ren)'s physical or mental health or,
4. If there is a substantial risk of serious mental or physical abnormality in the baby.

At present the legal age of viability is 28 weeks but this is likely to be reduced, possibly to 24 weeks, in the near future. Very few abortions are carried out after 24 weeks but there remain a significant number between 20 and 24 weeks, often associated with the late detection of fetal abnormality.

In Scotland in 1986 there were approximately 9500 legal abortions and the number in England and Wales in the same year exceeded 170,000. In Scotland more than 90% of the terminations were carried out under Clause 2 and three-quarters of the women were either unmarried, separated, divorced or widowed.

VACUUM ASPIRATION

This is the best method up to 12 weeks' maturity.

Plastic curettes of various design are commonly used and are less likely to damage the uterus than metal instruments.

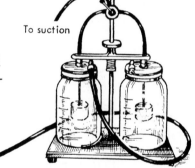

To suction

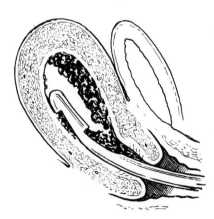

Complications

1. The main disadvantage is the likelihood of incomplete evacuation if the pregnancy is more advanced than was expected. Forceps may be needed to remove fetal parts which resist suction.

2. Perforation is possible although unlikely but if it happens, a laparotomy must be carried out.

3. Sepsis. If incomplete evacuation is suspected, antibiotic cover should be provided and a repeat curettage done after 48 hours.

4. The more advanced the pregnancy, the greater the blood loss. At 12 weeks, 2.5 – 5 dl loss may be expected.

367

TERMINATION OF PREGNANCY

PROSTAGLANDIN TERMINATION

The oxytocic action of prostaglandins can be made use of to terminate pregnancy at any stage.

The name prostaglandin was given in 1935 to a substance found in human seminal fluid which caused smooth muscle contractions, and was thought to be a hormone secreted by the prostate. It is now known to consist of at least 13 related compounds which are synthesised from fatty acids by an enzyme system of prostaglandin synthetases found in all tissues. Prostaglandins act as 'local hormones' at the site of formation, and are released during any tissue breakdown.

The nomenclature of prostaglandins based on prostanoic acid

5-carbon (cyclo-pentane) ring   2 hydrocarbon side chains

PGE2 (Dinoprostone). This is the prostaglandin commonly used in the United Kingdom. It is 10–20 times more potent than PGF2α.

Note the different group attached to the cyclopentane ring.

PGF2α

The metabolising of natural prostaglandins is rapid and begins at carbon atom 15. The attachment of a methyl group at 15 produces the analogy 15-methyl-PGF2α which is more resistant to degradation in lung and liver, and is therefore longer acting.

TERMINATION OF PREGNANCY

Prostaglandin Termination (continued)

PGE2 can be given intravenously, intra-amniotically, or extra-amniotically through the cervix. The extra-amniotic route produces fewest side-effects and has become established as the most commonly used technique.

A 12 gauge Foley's catheter is passed into the cervix and connected to a 50ml syringe containing 5 mg of PGE2 in 50 ml of saline (100 micrograms/ml). The pump delivers at a very slow rate usually beginning at 1 to 2 ml per hour, which may be increased. Further stimulation by intravenous oxytocin is commonly employed and in most patients abortion will occur in 12–18 hours. In many cases the abortion will be incomplete and surgical evacuation of the uterus is required.

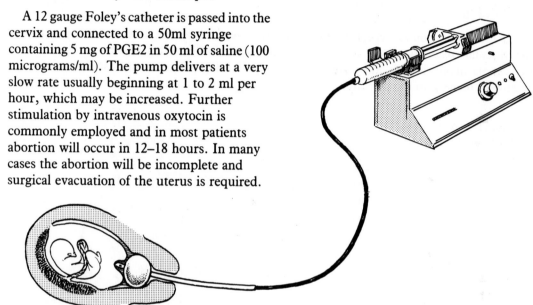

Complications of Extra-Amniotic PGE2

1. Nausea and vomiting may occur.

2. Pallor, rigors and intense uterine pain may occur if the solution is introduced directly into the circulation.

3. Over-stimulation of the uterus can occur and cases of uterine rupture and cervical damage have been reported.

4. The presence of an intra-uterine catheter for a prolonged period carries a risk of introducing infection.

Medical induction of abortion is psychologically more distressing to the patient than a surgical operation, and probably a more unpleasant experience. Clinically it is an obstetric procedure, calling for a knowledge of midwifery in the attendants.

TERMINATION OF PREGNANCY

INTRA-AMNIOTIC INJECTION

The intra-amniotic injection of hypertonic urea will kill the fetus and initiate uterine contractions. Prostaglandin E2 is commonly combined with the urea and provides a powerful stimulus to the uterus. The use of hypertonic saline or glucose injection has been abandoned because of their greater risk.

The mode of action of hypertonic solution is not yet understood, but a mild degree of intravascular coagulation is known to occur, with a rise in fibrin degradation products and a fall in plasma fibrinogen and platelet counts. The level of progesterone also falls probably because of damage to the placenta.

Technique

The patient may be pre-medicated and with full aseptic precautions 150 ml of liquor are withdrawn using a 50 ml syringe and a broad bore needle, and 80 g urea in 140 ml saline are injected. 2.5 mg of prostaglandin may be added.

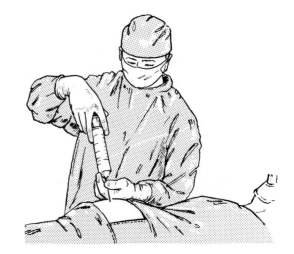

Disadvantages

1. The uterus has to be at least 16 weeks' size to be technically suitable, and delaying to this stage may distress the patient, especially if she begins to feel movement.

2. As with extra-amniotic prostaglandins, over-stimulation of the uterus is possible. Oxytocin infusion should be used with caution and the possibility of uterine or cervical damage must be borne in mind.

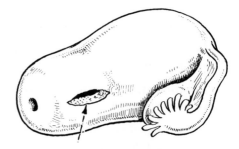

3. Retained placenta and haemorrhage may occur and an obstetric unit is the most suitable place for this procedure.

4. Cervical tears and even fistulae may occur, and the cervix should be inspected on completion.

TERMINATION OF PREGNANCY

ABDOMINAL HYSTEROTOMY

The introduction of extra-amniotic prostaglandins has made this an uncommon operation. It would not normally be performed nowadays unless accompanied by sterilisation. Hysterotomy with sterilisation is still probably the most humane treatment for the older parous woman who is certain that she wants no more children and wishes to avoid the unpleasant experience of an induced abortion.

The main disadvantages of the procedure are the risks of any abdominal operation — general anaesthesia, sepsis and thrombosis, and the slight risk of uterine rupture in a subsequent pregnancy.

A small suprapubic incision is made and a finger, hooked through a stab wound, delivers the uterus. Quite a large uterus can be delivered through a small incision.

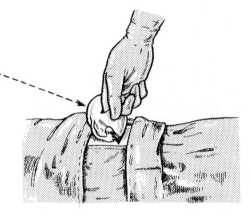

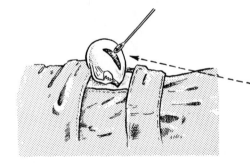

After extrusion of the fetus and placenta, the uterus is curetted. It is very important to avoid spilling decidual tissue on the abdominal wound, as endometriosis of the wound is a common sequel.

MATERNAL INJURIES

INJURIES TO THE VULVA

Haematoma of the Vulva

Rupture of vaginal veins (after prolonged or operative delivery) may produce a very large effusion of blood, extending downwards into the labium majus. If acute and extensive it causes great pain and this with blood loss soon causes shock.

Haematoma may not develop until after perineal repair.

Treatment

1. Analgesia and blood transfusion as required.

2. The haematoma may contain itself but if it continues to extend it will require evacuation under general anaesthesia. The cavity will require suture and possibly packing.

3. Antibiotics may be given.

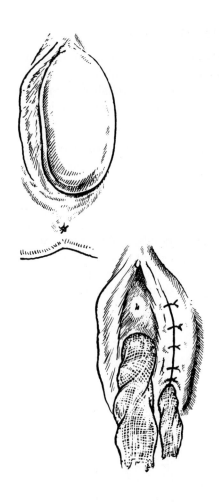

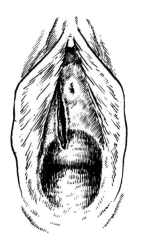

TEARS of the VESTIBULE

These are not common and arise from over-distension during delivery (see Perineal tears). They may bleed freely, especially if the clitoral artery is approached, and should be sutured. If the tear passes close to the urethral meatus a catheter should be inserted and continuous drainage with antiseptic cover continued for 48 hours.

MATERNAL INJURIES

PERINEAL TEARS

These are more common in primigravidae who have more rigid perinea. Probably the most important factors are the width of the pubic arch (and hence the amount of room available) and the size and position of the fetal head. All malpresentations increase the amount of distension of the perineum.

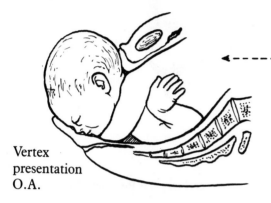

– – – – – – – In the normal O.A. position the sub-occipito-frontal diameter (10.0cm) distends the vulva, and the widest part of the head is under the bony arch.

Vertex
presentation
O.A.

When the position is O.P. the occipito-frontal diameter (11.5cm) distends the vulva, and the widest part of the head distends the perineum. – – – –→

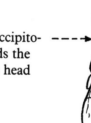

Vertex
presentation
O.P.

Face
presentation
M.A.

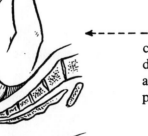

← – – – – – –When the face is presenting, once the chin is delivered, the submento-vertical diameter (13.5cm) will distend the vulva, and again the widest part of the head passes over the perineum.

373

MATERNAL INJURIES

Perineal Tears (continued)

1st degree Perineal Tear

Vaginal and perineal skin are torn, but the perineal muscles are intact.

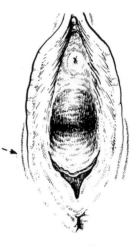

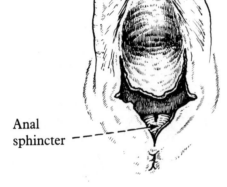

Anal
sphincter

2nd degree Perineal Tear

The perineal body is torn right down to (and sometimes partly involving) the anal sphincter. The vaginal tears often extend up both sides of the vagina.

3rd degree Tear —'Complete Tear'

The whole anal sphincter is torn apart, and there may be a tear of the rectal wall. Note how the ends of the sphincter muscles tend to retract.

This injury, if not repaired, leaves the patient with faecal incontinence.

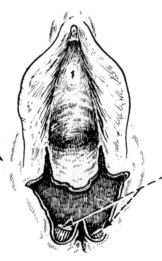

Torn ends
of anal
sphincter

374

MATERNAL INJURIES

PERINEAL TEARS — REPAIR

Perineal damage should be repaired very soon after delivery. Blood loss will be lessened, the chance of infection reduced, and the patient is usually relaxed and euphoric.

First and Second Degree Tears

The repair is done under aseptic conditions with the patient in the lithotomy position under a good light. 20–30 ml. of 1% lignocaine are injected into the muscles and under the skin.

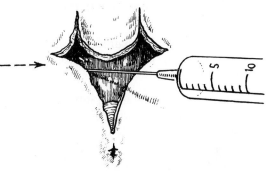

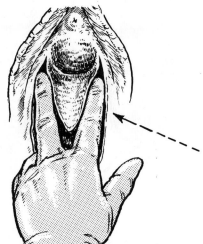

Correct anatomical apposition is essential. Bleeding must be controlled and swabs used freely to expose the tissues. The upper limits of the tear must be demonstrated by stretching apart with the fingers so that suturing may begin there.

1. Close vaginal tears with continuous No. 1 catgut.
2. Suture perineal muscles together with interrupted No. 1 catgut.
3. Close skin over muscles with catgut or non-absorbable material.

Sutures tied too tight will cause pain. Be sure the vagina admits 2 fingers easily when the repair is completed.

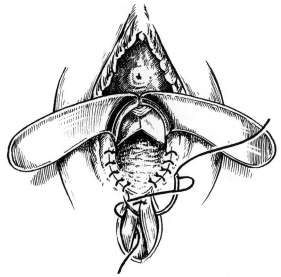

375

MATERNAL INJURIES

PERINEAL TEARS — REPAIR

Third Degree Tears

Such tears heal much better if repaired at the time rather than months or years later. The operation is best performed with the patient under general anaesthesia.

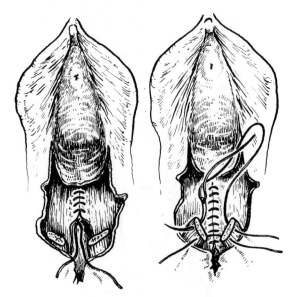

1. The rectal wall is repaired with fine chromic catgut sutures, tied inside the rectum.

2. The two ends of the anal sphincter are picked up in tissue forceps and apposed with 2 or 3 No. 1 catgut sutures. (The anus should then accommodate the little finger).

3. The repair is continued as for a 2nd degree tear. The skin of the anal margin should be closed with fine catgut.

Post operative treatment

1. Low residue diet for a week.

2. The bowel is contained for several days and a softening agent should be given.

3. If no bowel movement, an olive oil enema may be given.

   If the repair breaks down, it should be left for 3 months before a second repair is attempted.

   If pregnancy follows a well-healed complete tear, section might be considered. Certainly a large episiotomy would be needed.

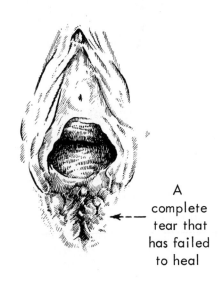

A complete tear that has failed to heal

376

MATERNAL INJURIES

VAGINAL TEARS

Colporrhexis (Rupture of the vaginal wall)

This is an uncommon but serious injury. The most usual site is the posterior or lateral fornix and the cervix may be involved. Tearing may result from obstructed labour, but it is more often due to improper application of the forceps, especially when attempts at delivery have been made before the cervix is fully dilated.

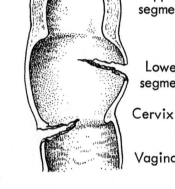

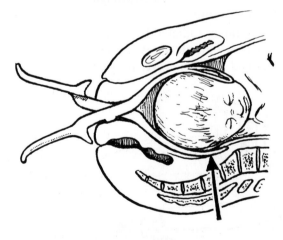

In obstructed labour the pathological retraction ring (Bandl's ring) is a sign of excessive traction on lower segment and cervix. Rupture may occur in the lower segment or at the cervico-vaginal junction (see Uterine rupture).

If the posterior blade of Kielland's forceps is not properly guided by the hand, the tip of the blade may perforate and tear the posterior fornix.

Treatment

If the examining finger passes completely through the vaginal tear, laparotomy is necessary to check on the extent of the damage. The symptoms are those of rupture of the uterus, and bleeding is usually considerable. A blood transfusion will probably be needed and hysterectomy may be the quickest and easiest way of stopping the haemorrhage.

377

MATERNAL INJURIES

VAGINAL FISTULAE
Vaginal fistulae are uncommon injuries in present day obstetrics.

Vesicovaginal Fistula
This is caused by direct trauma e.g. in operative delivery or by prolonged compression of vaginal wall and bladder between fetal head and maternal symphysis pubis.

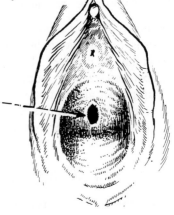

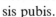

If fistula is due to trauma, urine appears at once, but sloughing takes about 5 days, and fistula will not appear until then.

Repair of Vesicovaginal fistula
If observed at delivery it should be closed forthwith, using fine chromic catgut (interrupted through-and-through, then a continuous suture).

Continuous catheter drainage preferable with suction is instituted for a week and antibiotic cover provided.

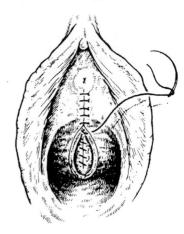

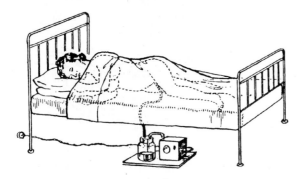

The patient should be encouraged to lie on her side or front as much as possible to keep urine from collecting on the bladder base.

If the fistula is a result of a sloughing wound and does not appear for 5 days after delivery, drainage must be prolonged for several weeks to allow every chance of spontaneous closure or at least shrinkage. Repair is then a gynaecological procedure.

MATERNAL INJURIES

Vaginal Fistulae (continued)

Rectovaginal Fistula

This type of fistula nearly always occurs after the imperfect healing of a repair of complete tear.

Repair

No attempt at re-repair should be made for at least 3 months, and the operation is then performed in a gynaecological ward. It is usual to break down the perineum to some extent so that the rectum may be mobilised before suture.

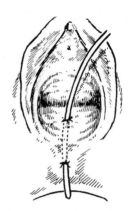

INJURIES TO THE CERVIX

Lacerations

The cervix is always torn to some extent during delivery. This causes the appearance of the parous os. Severe tears may follow strong contractions on a rigid cervix, or arise from a previous cervical operation. The commonest cause is surgical trauma following forceps or breech delivery.

A tear is suspected when bleeding is heavy although the uterus is firmly contracted. The cervix must be examined and this may be difficult because of the bleeding and friability of the tissues.

Several pairs of ring forceps and at least one assistant are needed and, once demonstrated, the tear should be sutured with interrupted catgut sutures.
By the time the operation is completed, if not before, the patient may need a blood transfusion.

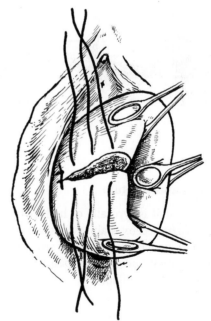

Annular Detachment of the Cervix

This rare laceration usually occurs in a primigravida in whom strong contractions are driving the vertex against a rigid cervix. The vaginal cervix gradually develops a pressure necrosis, and the sloughed cervix separates and is delivered in front of the head. There is little bleeding and the cervical stump heals well.

379

MATERNAL INJURIES

RUPTURE OF THE UTERUS

Rupture of the uterus is an uncommon injury in the United Kingdom and it is nearly always due to rupture of a previous Caesarean section scar. It may however arise, particularly in a parous patient, from obstructed labour due to cephalopelvic disproportion or malpresentation.

Rupture of a Classical Caesarean Scar

This may occur in late pregnancy or early labour. Bleeding is often slight because the fetus and placenta are extruded into the peritoneal cavity and the uterus retracts. There is acute abdominal pain and this may be accompanied by shock.

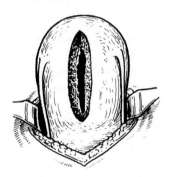

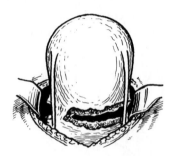

Rupture of Lower Segment Scar

This is not always easily detectable as the rupture is initially extra-peritoneal. Dehiscence of a lower segment scar may cause virtually no bleeding or shock and the rupture is discovered only on section for delay in labour. If, however, the tear extends there will be intraperitoneal bleeding with severe pain and shock.

Spontaneous Rupture

The patient is typically of high parity, and labour has been obstructed by malpresentation or disproportion. Contractions have been strong and rupture begins in the lower segment and is accompanied by pain, bleeding, haematuria and collapse.

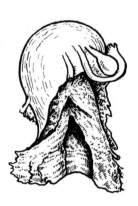

MATERNAL INJURIES

Rupture of the Uterus (continued)

Diagnosis and Treatment

The diagnosis is sometimes obvious but may be impossible without laparotomy. Persistent abdominal pain, a rise in pulse rate and fresh vaginal bleeding should be looked for. Rupture is followed by cessation of contractions.

Intra-Abdominal Hemorrhage

This may cause rapid collapse. The blood may be confined retroperitoneally as a broad ligament haematoma. Accidental haemorrhage must be considered in the diagnosis.

Alteration in Shape of Abdominal Swelling

If the fetus is wholly or partly extruded into the abdominal cavity the uterus will contract and may be detectable as a separate mass in the abdomen. Vaginal examination reveals an empty pelvis.

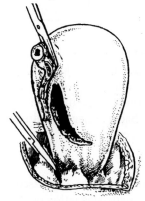

Once the diagnosis is reached laparotomy must be carried out with blood transfusion set up.

Hysterectomy is usually the safest treatment, but this decision will depend on the extent of the damage and the patient's parity. If the tear is small the simplest procedure may be repair and conservation of the uterus.

If hysterectomy is decided on, the tear will in most cases have half completed the operation. Subsequent steps in the operation are indicated below. If bleeding is severe this will be an operation in which speed is of importance.

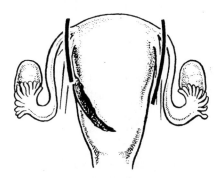

Division of the fallopian tubes and broad ligaments, leaving behind the ovaries and part of the tubes.

After incision of the peritoneum at the site of rupture the bladder is stripped from the uterine wall and a sub-total hysterectomy performed.

381

MATERNAL INJURIES

HAEMATOMA OF THE RECTUS SHEATH

A rare condition occurring mostly in multiparous woman as a result of coughing or sudden expulsive effort. Muscle fibres and branches of the deep epigastric veins are torn.

It is a condition most likely to be diagnosed on the history of sudden effort followed by pain.

If rupture occurs below the umbilicus, blood can track anywhere along transversalis fascia and is virtually retroperitoneal. If above the umbilicus the haematoma is more likely to be localised.

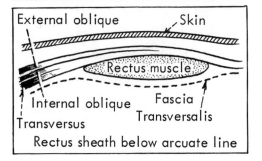

Rectus sheath above arcuate line

Rectus sheath below arcuate line

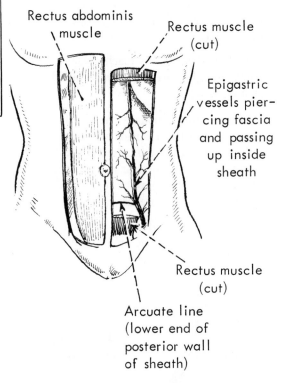

There is pain, possible peritonism, and a vague abdominal swelling. If blood loss is large there may be collapse. The condition must be distinguished from accidental haemorrhage, rupture of uterus, ovarian cyst.

Treatment. If small and localised, the haematoma may be left to absorb, but usually operation is required, with evacuation of clot, ligation of any bleeding points, and closure with drainage.

MATERNAL INJURIES

TRAUMATIC NEURITIS (Syn. Obstetric Palsy)

Traumatic neuritis is a rare condition in which one or both legs show signs of motor and/or sensory nerve damage shortly after labour.

The lateral popliteal nerve which divides into the musculocutaneous and anterior tibial nerves is most commonly affected.

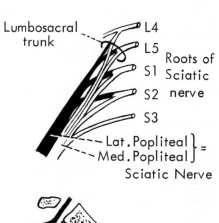

Theories of Causation

1. Prolapse of an intervertebral disc (L.4–5 or L.5–S.1). Disc prolapse is a flexion injury and may be caused by the exaggerated lithotomy position used for forceps delivery.

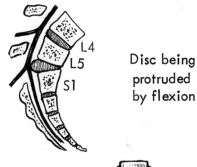

2. The fetal head may compress the lumbo-sacral trunk as it crosses the sacro-iliac joint (especially when pelvis is flat). The 5th lumbar nerve is the largest root of the sciatic nerve.

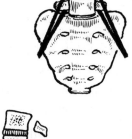

3. The sacrum may rotate back a little in labour, and put traction on the lumbo-sacral trunk.
   Forceps delivery has a definite association with neuritis.

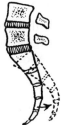

4. The popliteal nerve may be compressed between the head of the fibula and the lithotomy stanchion if no padding is used.

TRAUMATIC NEURITIS

Pain is felt in the sciatic region (L.5 may contribute to the cutaneous supply to the back of the thigh) and there may be a tingling sensation in the lower leg.

Muscular wasting may be slight or extend so far as to involve the glutei (L.4,5 : S.1,2). Tension reflexes are variable but the ankle jerk is usually diminished and the knee jerk brisk.

Foot drop varies from weak dorsiflexion to complete paralysis of the peronei, tibialis anterior and extensor digitorum longus. The patient may be unable to flex her foot or extend her toes.

Sensory impairment: Hyperalgesia (increased sensitivity to pinprick) and hypo-aesthesia are demonstrated on the skin area over the dorsiflexors and peronei, usually to a minor degree.

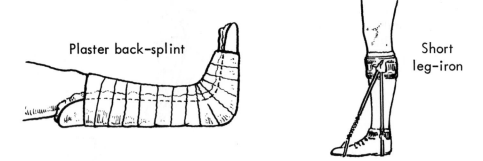

Plaster back-splint

Short leg-iron

Treatment: If disc prolapse is diagnosed or suspected, the patient is nursed with fracture boards under the mattress. Traction may be necessary to relieve the pain. The foot drop is protected by a blanket cage and a plaster back-splint. When walking begins a short leg iron may be required for several months until full function returns.

An episode of traumatic neuritis might be regarded as an indication for delivery by section in a subsequent pregnancy.

Backache associated with limping might result from sacro-iliac strain following parturition, or even from sacro-coccygeal strain (coxalgia); but in such cases there will be no evidence of a lower motor neurone lesion.

CHAPTER 15

THE PUERPERIUM — NORMAL AND ABNORMAL

THE PUERPERIUM

The puerperium is the period following childbirth when the woman is returning as nearly as possible to her pre-gravid state.

For the purposes of notification of infections the puerperium is defined, in law, as the 14 days (England and Wales) or 21 days (Scotland) following confinement.

A midwife is required to attend a puerperal woman for a period of not less than 10 days after her confinement.

The uterus contains a raw bleeding surface –
– a wound. *Infection* must be prevented.

The newborn baby requires careful nursing and observation.

Breast feeding must be initiated (or lactation properly suppressed).

Muscles are of poor tone and ligaments slack after pregnancy and labour. Systematic exercises should be given to help prevent chronic postural defects, hernia and prolapse.

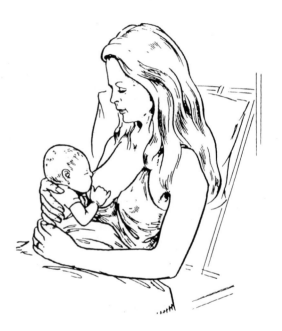

The mother's mood is unstable: she must be given sympathy and support.

Better physical and emotional preparation for childbirth, shorter and less tiring labours and early ambulation have led to a decrease in puerperal morbidity. Less nursing care is needed and many women can return to their families after only a short period of recovery in hospital. This is a desirable situation and requires an effective and well-integrated community midwifery service.

PHYSIOLOGICAL CHANGES

The process by which the uterus returns almost to its pre-gravid state is known as *Involution* — a dramatic example of atrophy due to withdrawal of the support of the placental hormones.

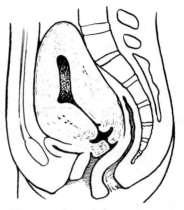

Uterus after delivery

Involution is caused by the phenomenon of *Autolysis* — enzymatic digestion of excess cytoplasm — and thrombosis and hyaline degeneration of vessels; but traces of fibro-elastic tissue remain as evidence of pregnancy. The endometrium is regenerated by the 10th day, except at the placental site, where it takes 6 weeks.

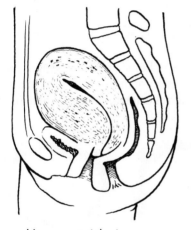

Uterus at 6th day

The *Lochia* (the discharges of childbirth) consist mainly of blood and necrotic decidua. They persist for about 2–3 weeks, gradually becoming colourless and scanty. They are sterile to begin with but by the 3rd–4th days the inside of the uterus is said to be colonised by vaginal commensals (non- haemolytic streptococcus, E. coli, etc.).

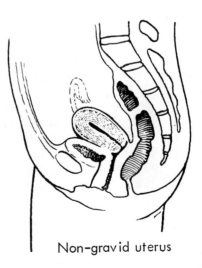

Non-gravid uterus

PHYSIOLOGICAL CHANGES

The uterus reduces to about 1/25 of its size in about 6 weeks although it never returns exactly to its nulliparous proportions.

Muscle fibres from uterus

Pregnant

Puerperal

Non-pregnant

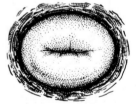

Body

Cervix

Nulliparous uterus

Parous uterus

This reduction in size is achieved partly by the removal of blood and blood vessels, and partly by digestion of a large part of the cell cytoplasm. The number of muscle cells is probably not much diminished, but the individual fibres are very much shorter and thinner than during the pregnancy.

The cervix never returns to its pristine appearance and although completely healed will always give evidence of parturition.

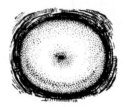

Nulliparous cervix

Parous cervix

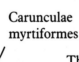

Carunculae myrtiformes

The vagina and vulva, considerably stretched during labour, have returned almost to their pre-gravid size by the 3rd week. Rugae appear in the vagina, and the labia regress to a less prominent and fleshy state than in the nulliparous condition. Only small sessile tags of hymen are left (carunculae myrtiformes — 'pieces of flesh in the shape of myrtle') and, like the parous cervix, are evidence of previous pregnancy.

CLINICAL ASPECTS

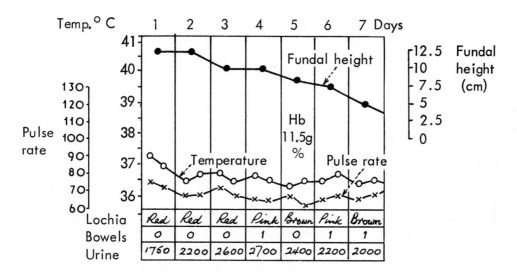

Fundal height is measured each day. The bladder must be empty and the uterus is rubbed up to contract and the height of the fundus above the symphysis is measured. Failure of involution suggests retained placental tissue.

Pulse tends to be slower, about 60–70 per minute, probably because the woman is resting completely after the exertion of labour.

Temperature may be slightly elevated during the first 24 hours, but thereafter should remain within normal limits. Persistent pyrexia requires investigation (see page 394).

Constipation is the rule for some days. Progesterone continues to inhibit smooth muscle motility. Haemorrhoids are a common, troublesome complication.

Urine — There is a diuresis during the 2nd to 5th days and urinary nitrogen is much raised. The body is getting rid of the excess fluid retained during pregnancy, and the high nitrogen excretion is a direct result of the autolytic process at work in the uterus. Urinary retention is relatively common especially after instrumental delivery. It may be due to oedema of the bladder neck as a result of stretching or bruising or due to the pain of perineal sutures.

Lochia should gradually change colour from red to pale yellow over 10 days. There are great variations in this due to the fluctuations in the amount of blood being lost during this period. Excess fresh lochia suggest retained products.

Blood — The haemoglobin level is important and should be stable by the 5th day, when normal haemoconcentration is approached.

389

LACTATION AND BREAST FEEDING

Prolactin from the anterior pituitary gland causes the lacteal glands to secrete milk. *Oxytocin* from the posterior pituitary acts on the myo-epithelial cells surrounding the glands and causes the milk to be secreted into the lactiferous ducts and thence to the nipple. Oxytocin also stimulates the output of more prolactin.

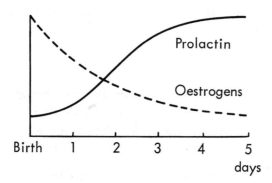

Sensory stimuli to pituitary gland

Prolactin

Oxytocin

The 'milk let-down' reflex
The 'draught' reflex
The 'milk ejection' response

The conditioned reflex set off by the stimulus of the baby's mouth at the nipple (or even by preparations for feeding) which results in lactation.

Prolactin

Oestrogens

Birth 1 2 3 4 5

days

Placental oestrogens inhibit the secretion of prolactin; and it takes 3 or 4 days for this effect to wear off completely. Normal milk is not being secreted until that time. While oestrogens still dominate (during pregnancy and immediately after delivery) *colostrum* is secreted.

Colostrum is a yellowish fluid, containing a much greater quantity of protein than normal milk, plus quantities of desquamated endothelial cells. Its function is not known; but its high gamma-globulin content may be a provision for the supply of antibodies which the baby must acquire in the first months. Dairy farmers always feed the colostrum to their calves as a protection against disease.

	Colostrum	Human milk
Protein	6%	1%
Fat	2.5%	3.5%
Carbohydrate	3%	7%

LACTATION AND BREAST FEEDING

SUPPLEMENTARY FEED

A supplementary feed is given in place of a breast feed. It might be required when the breast is being rested because of cracked nipples; or in the case of twins taking turns at breast and bottle.

COMPLEMENTARY FEED

A complementary feed is given at the end of a breast feed if the baby is not contented or is not gaining weight. The time at the breast is shortened to 5 minutes at each breast (most of the milk is taken in that time) and the baby is offered 30–50 ml of artificial feed.

INHIBITION OF LACTATION

The mother should decide before delivery whether or not she intends to breast-feed. If the baby is to be bottle-fed, the breasts should be firmly supported following delivery and in most women no medication will be required to prevent lactation.

If the breasts fill or if suppression of lactation is required after starting to breast-feed, Bromocriptine 2.5 mg twice daily for 2 weeks is the drug of choice. Oestrogens should be avoided because of the increased risk of venous thrombosis.

WEANING

Weaning is the gradual change from breast feeding to completely artificial feeding or mixed feeding (milk and semi-solids). Three months might reasonably be the recommended age for beginning. The mother should begin by giving a bottle instead of the 2 p.m. feed and continue over a week. The 6 a.m. feed will be the last to be given up as the breasts tend to be fullest at that time, after a night's rest.

The supply of milk should decrease step by step with demand; but if the weaning is done abruptly medication with Bromocriptine may be required.

LACTATION AND BREAST FEEDING

PROBLEMS WITH BREAST-FEEDING

Any pathological condition in the mother will adversely affect breast-feeding at once.

Not enough milk

The only way to prove this is by weighing the baby before and after each feed for 24 hours. If the mother is not producing at least 60 ml per feed, and the baby is not gaining weight, she must eat and drink more and generally lead as placid an existence as possible. There are no drugs known to increase lactation.

Too much milk

This is suspected if the baby passes undigested stools — bulky and offensive, sometimes bloodstained — or leaves the breast unemptied. It may also regurgitate milk and may even vomit during or immediately after a feed. Such babies are usually strong, voracious feeders and the treatment is to reduce the time at the breast to lessen stimulation and give sterile water if the baby will not sleep.

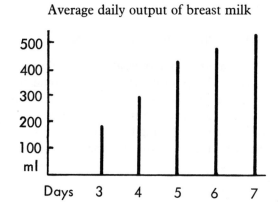

Average daily output of breast milk

Painful Nipples

Cracks and fissures of the nipples are caused by too vigorous sucking by the baby in an effort to get the nipple properly into its mouth. It is because of this that nipple protraction should be encouraged in the antenatal period. Treatment is to use a nipple shield through which the baby sucks, or to rest the nipple for 24 hours using breast expression to prevent engorgement. A protective cream or spray may be applied.

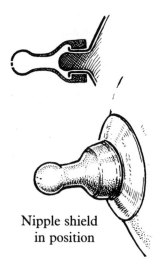

Nipple shield
in position

POSTNATAL EXERCISES

During the latter half of pregnancy ligaments are softened and slackened (probably a consequence of the fluid retention caused by placental hormones), muscles are stretched, posture changed to compensate for the increasing weight of the gravid uterus. During parturition, the pelvic floor is always stretched and may be damaged.

Postnatal exercises are given (1) to prevent the development of hernia, pelvic floor prolapse and postural defects such as sacro-iliac strain; (2) to prevent circulatory stasis and reduce the risk of thrombosis and embolism.

Besides early ambulation, the patient should be instructed in a systematic course of exercises designed to restore tone in the different muscle groups, especially the lumbo-dorsal, abdominal and perineal. The following are examples:-

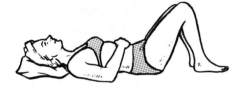

Patient's hands press on abdominal muscles. First, thoracic breathing is done, then abdominal.

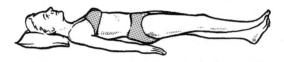

Both knees straight and legs crossed, buttocks and thighs are contracted and relaxed. Anus and perineum are drawn in as if trying to prevent micturition.

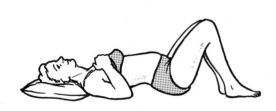

Lying on back with knees bent, rock abdomen and buttocks backward. Forward rocking aggravates sacro-iliac discomfort.

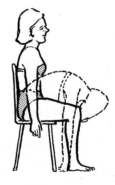

Sitting in a chair, slowly bend forward to touch toes, and slowly sit up and straighten shoulders.

393

SECONDARY POST-PARTUM HAEMORRHAGE

Secondary Post-Partum Haemorrhage means abnormal bleeding from the genital tract from 24 hours after delivery until the completion of the puerperium.

Causes
1   Retained placental tissue. This inevitably leads to infection.
2.   Intra-uterine infection with or without retained products.
3.   Slow involution of the uterus or inadequate drainage of the lochia sometimes lead to fresh bleeding later than expected.

Management

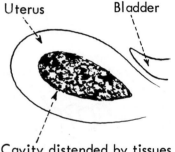

Uterus   Bladder

Cavity distended by tissues

1.   Ultrasound scan to detect retained products.
2.   Antibiotics (broad spectrum + anti-anaerobe e.g. Metronidazole).
3.   Evacuation of uterus if products seen.

This can be a treacherous condition and bleeding sometimes persists after evacuation.   Occasionally packing the uterus and even hysterectomy are required.

PUERPERAL PYREXIA

Puerperal pyrexia means a temperature of 38°C, maintained for or recurring within 24 hours, within 21 days (14 days in England) of childbirth or abortion. This definition derives from the time when notification of puerperal pyrexia (whatever the cause) was a legal obligation. This is no longer the case in Scotland.

Puerperal pyrexia may be due to an infection, genital or extra-genital.

1.   Genital tract —
          Perineum, Vagina, Cervix, Uterus, Adnexa.
2.   Breasts.
3.   Urinary system (see Chapter 7).
4.   Superficial thrombo-phlebitis or deep vein thrombosis (see Chapter 7).
5.   Respiratory system —
          Common cold, Influenza, After general anaesthesia.

Puerperal pyrexia requires, therefore, a complete physical examination and bacteriological examination of urine specimen, throat swab or sputum, high vaginal swab and in some cases blood culture.

GENITAL TRACT INFECTION

Synonyms: Puerperal Fever, Puerperal Sepsis, Childbed Fever.

Infection can occur during labour, especially if associated with prolonged rupture of the membranes. Vaginal examination in labour, even with proper care and aseptic precautions, can encourage the transfer of organisms from the vagina to uterine cavity. The most worrying organism, which can be found in the normal, healthy vagina, is the beta-haemolytic streptococcus.

Until the middle of this century infection in childbirth was a major cause of maternal mortality and morbidity. The development of antibiotics provided a means of treating this but better care in labour, the improvements in hospital facilities and the avoidance of overcrowding have all contributed to reduce the incidence of genital tract infection.

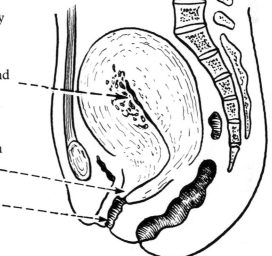

In the puerperium infection may enter through one or more of these wounds:

The *Placental* site is a raw wound with gaping veins occluded by thrombi
— a good culture medium.

The *Cervix* is nearly always torn even in normal parturition.

The *Vagina* is often torn, or involved in an episiotomy.

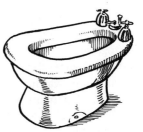

In the puerperium the mother should be encouraged to be mobile as quickly as possible and to bath or use a bidet at least twice daily.

395

GENITAL TRACT INFECTION

1. ENDOMETRITIS

Endometritis is the most common and usually mildest form of genital infection.

4 Classical Signs:–

1. Pyrexia 37.8°–39°C.
2. Pulse 100–120.
3. Fundal height not falling — poor involution.
4. Lochia remain red and have characteristic offensive smell.

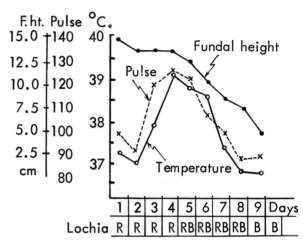

Lochia	R	R	R	R	RB	RB	RB	RB	B	B
Days	1	2	3	4	5	6	7	8	9	

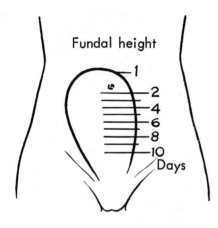

Normal Involution

Investigations

Vaginal and cervical swabs are taken via a sterile speculum. If the diagnosis is uncertain, a throat swab and MSSU are also sent.

Treatment

A broad spectrum antibiotic such as a Cephalosporin, together with Metronidazole to treat anaerobic infections is given while awaiting the bacteriology reports. Treatment should be maintained for at least 5 days. Blood culture may be advisable.

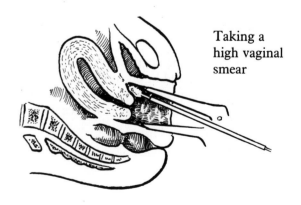

Taking a high vaginal smear

GENITAL TRACT INFECTION

2. PARAMETRITIS (Syn. Cellulitis)

Infection may spread from the uterus, from a cervical laceration, or even from thrombophlebitis or peritonitis into the loose areolar connective tissue, setting up a *Parametritis*. The infection may extend retroperitoneally in any direction, commonly between the leaves of the broad ligament, round the vagina or rectum, or even up to the loin. Sometimes infection spreads along the round ligament and might then point above the inguinal ligament, near the inguinal ring.

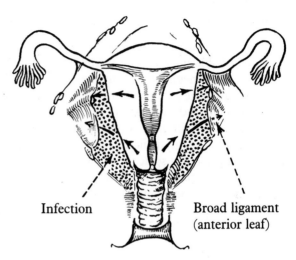

Infection   Broad ligament (anterior leaf)

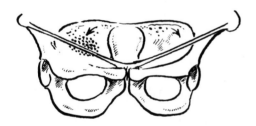

The condition occurs later than endometritis, usually in the second week and presents with fever and malaise. Pelvic examination reveals a large, often very hard mass and the lochia are red and heavy. Pain is less than might be expected.

Treatment

The appropriate antibiotic is given usually for 2 or more weeks, until the pelvis feels normal. If collections of pus appear they must be drained. A poor response to treatment calls for a search for spread: and the possibility of subphrenic abscess must be remembered.

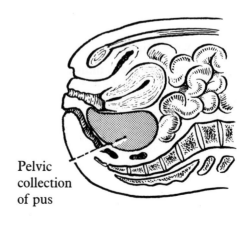

Pelvic collection of pus

397

GENITAL TRACT INFECTION

3. PERITONITIS AND SALPINGITIS

These two conditions are almost indistinguishable and neither is common. The pelvic peritoneum may be involved in the same way as the parametrium and also be spread along the fallopian tubes. A generalised peritonitis may occur with the development of paralytic ileus; and very rarely the infection is so acute and fulminating that the condition of 'septic' or 'irreversible' shock is met with.

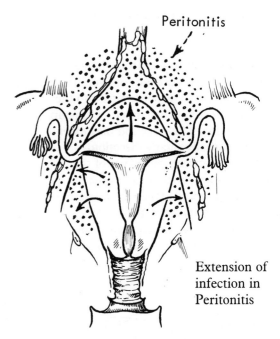

Extension of infection in Peritonitis

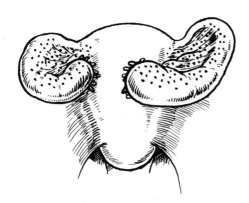

Acute Salpingitis
Permanent blockage is unusual.

Diagnosis and Treatment

In some cases it may be impossible to exclude acute appendicitis without an exploratory laparotomy; but otherwise treatment is along the same lines as described for parametritis. If laparotomy is carried out and only acute salpingitis found, the abdomen should be closed without drainage.

ENGORGEMENT OF THE BREASTS

As the circulating oestrogens fall the anterior pituitary output of prolactin rises. If milk secretion outstrips milk removal (as with a weak or lethargic baby) the breasts become overfull, the venous and lymphatic drainage is obstructed and the breasts become oedematous, swollen, painful and too tender even to allow expression of milk. Engorgement may also be due to blocking of the ducts with inspissated colostrum or sebaceous matter during the antenatal period. The treatment is to *Rest* the breasts, *Support* them with a firm brassière or binding and *Express* the milk as soon as tenderness is relieved.

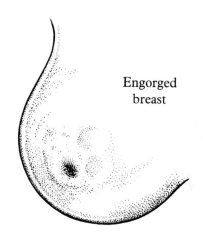

Engorged breast

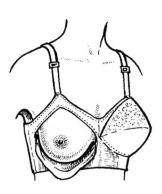

Nursing brassière which gives good support

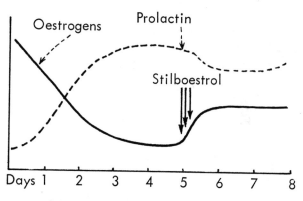

Stilboestrol inhibits prolactin secretion

Engorgement is an extremely painful condition and analgesics may be required. Reduction in fluid intake, or the administration of diuretics may have a marginal effect but, in spite of the already noted objection, it may be justifiable to give Stilboestrol 15 mg 8 hourly for 24 hours to reduce lactation briefly.

BREAST INFECTION

Mastitis is a disease of lactation.

Infection (nearly always Staph. aureus) enters through a cracked and abraded nipple, and sets up a local inflammation of parenchyma and interstitial tissue, which proceeds to abscess formation.

The presenting symptom is usually pyrexia. Then a painful area is felt and a 'flush' appears on the breast, usually radial in outline, red and tender but not fluctuant or swollen. At this stage an antibiotic should be given empirically. Cloxacillin or Flucloxacillin are good choices as the organism is probably a penicillin-resistant staphylococcus. The breast is supported and lactation may be suppressed temporarily or permanently. In many cases the infection will now subside.

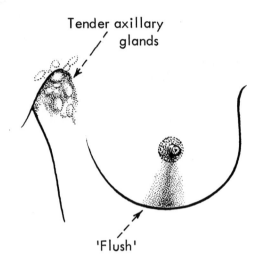

Tender axillary glands

'Flush'

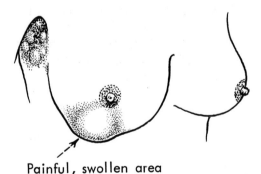

Painful, swollen area

The next stage is overt inflammation — a brawny, swollen, painful breast which probably contains pus although not yet fluctuant. If definitely not ready for incision, a kaolin poultice or other source of heat may be applied for a day; but it is better to incise early than late. Lactation must be suppressed at this stage.

BREAST INFECTION

Under general anaesthesia, a radial incision is made and all pockets of pus broken down. A drain must be left in for 3 days and pus sent for culture and antibiotic sensitivity.

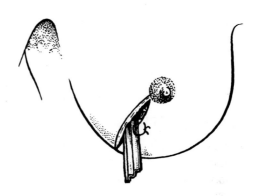

Acute breast infection may also occur when weaning is begun. In such cases infection is probably already present, and when the drainage provided by the flow of milk is stopped the usual inflammatory reaction occurs. Treatment is the same as for lactational mastitis.

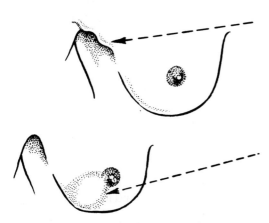

There is occasionally an extension of mammary tissue into the axillary tail, which becomes swollen and painful during lactation. It should soon regress but sometimes discomfort is so great that lactation has to be suppressed.

Galactocele This is an accumulation in a lobe of the breast whose duct is blocked by inspissated secretions. It is usually absorbed and should be left alone unless discomfort is severe.

(These two conditions must be distinguished from inflammation).

The lactating woman's chance of developing a breast infection is much reduced if she is properly instructed in the care of the breasts and nipples during the pregnancy and if engorgement is avoided in the early puerperium. If the patient has decided against breast feeding, lactation should be inhibited from the start.

401

SEPTIC SHOCK

(ENDOTOXIC OR BACTERAEMIC SHOCK: GRAM-NEGATIVE SEPTICAEMIA)

This grave complication occasionally follows puerperal infections. It means severe circulatory failure due to the toxins of bacteria. These cause vascular damage leading to increased capillary permeability; or widespread arteriolar and capillary thrombosis (Disseminated Intravascular Coagulation; DIC). The condition has a mortality of over 60% and may be a sequel to any operative procedure as well as puerperal infection.

INFECTING BACTERIA

Gram-positive
  Staphylococcus
  Streptococcus
  Clostridium

Gram-negative
  Escherichia coli
  Bacteroides fragilis
  Pseudomonas pyocyanea

Any organism including viruses and fungi can cause shock. They release foreign polysaccharides or proteins in the blood stream either as specific exotoxins or by release of endotoxins after breakdown (as in the case of gram-negative bacteria), which activates the immune system. This leads to the release of vaso-active agents such as serotonin, prostaglandins and histamine and kinins (polypeptides).

Pathology

Ischaemia of organs	Caused at first by a protective spasm as a means of preserving circulatory volume, and then by DIC.
Low cardiac output	First there is an acute fall in circulating blood volume due to peripheral vasodilatation and then myocardial failure as a result of endotoxins.
Cerebral damage	There is hypoxia which increases vasospasm, and leads to anxiety, confusion and coma.
Lungs	Low tissue perfusion follows the fall in circulatory volume, but even after this is corrected, the capillary damage may lead to pulmonary failure ('shock lung').
Liver and Spleen	Endotoxins inhibit the phagocytic (Kupffer) cells of the liver and the reticulo-endothelial system generally, which is important in disposing of microthrombi.
Kidney	Low perfusion leads to renal failure, metabolic acidosis and further hypoxia.

SEPTIC SHOCK

SIGNS AND SYMPTOMS

Early Hyperdynamic Phase

The body's first reactions to sepsis are pyrexia and local vasodilatation to improve perfusion of the affected area. The fall in peripheral resistance is countered by an increased heart rate and there may even be polyuria. At this stage the patient, although mildly hypotensive, is usually warm, alert and anxious.

Circulatory Failure Phase

The onset of this phase may be very sudden simulating amniotic fluid embolism or myocardial infarction. The patient becomes comatose, and extreme vasoconstriction produces cold cyanosed hands and feet. Blood pressure and pulse become almost unrecordable, blood tests for DIC become positive, and signs of failure of the different organs gradually make their appearance.

TREATMENT

Early recognition of the problem is vital and as treatment of the condition is complex and highly specialised it should take place in an Intensive Care Unit.

Infection: Until bacteriological guidance is available the antibiotic cover must be empirical:

> E.g. lincomycin 600 mg 8-hourly i.m.
> gentamycin 80 mg 6-hourly i.v.
> metronidazole 500 mg 8-hourly i.v.

Any septic focus must, if possible, be dealt with surgically. The body's normal defence against bacteria is phagocytosis, which is inhibited in shock, and the use of antibiotics to kill bacteria in the blood stream carries a risk of increasing the amount of circulating endotoxin.

Circulation

The principles are to obtain an increase in cardiac output and circulating blood volume so that tissue perfusion is restored.

Blood, plasma proteins, Dextran or polygeline (Haemaccel) are given in sufficient quantity to maintain the haematocrit at about 30%.

Myocardial contractility is improved by the use of catecholamines such as isoprenaline or dobutamine, which increase cardiac output and reduce the peripheral vasospasm by dilating arterioles.

Coagulation

Tests for DIC include:–
Prothrombin Time (PT)
  12–14 secs.
Partial Thromboplastin Time (PTT)
  30–40 secs.
Thrombin Clotting Time (TCT)
  8–11 secs.
Fibrin Degradation Products (FDP) less than 10μg/ml.

Some degree of DIC is inevitable, and if there is an inadequate response to whole blood, fresh frozen plasma must be given.

SEPTIC SHOCK

TREATMENT   (continued)

Lung

After the initial resuscitation there is a latent period of hyperventilation which may be followed by gradual pulmonary insufficiency leading to the adult respiratory distress syndrome (ARDS) which is the lung's response to prolonged vascular damage and DIC. The only treatment is ventilation through an endotracheal tube.

Kidney

Oliguria is the rule, and if the serum osmolarity approaches 1 (normal is over 2) a mannitol infusion should be given.

Haemodialysis may be required.

Vasoconstriction

Vasodilators may be required to overcome this. E.g: thymoxamine (Opilon) 30 mg given with extreme care, because of the effect of sudden vasodilation on the central venous pressure.

Corticosteroid therapy

Two doses of dexamethasone 30 mg are given at 8-hourly intervals. Corticosteroids combat vasoconstriction and acidosis, but they also depress inflammatory responses including phagocytosis. Their use in shock conditions is debated.

Naloxone

Naloxone hydrochloride (Narcan), an opiate antagonist, has been used with good effect in cases of shock with persistent hypotension. It counteracts the effect of the endogenous opiate beta-endorphin which is released in quantity in conditions of stress and is a hypotensive agent as well as an opiate. Such treatment is likely to uncover pain which will require exogenous analgesia.

MENTAL ILLNESS IN THE PUERPERIUM

Severe puerperal depression is uncommon nowadays and the delirious states due to toxic absorption have virtually disappeared as obstetric standards improve. Nevertheless latent or pre-existing mental illness is likely to be aggravated by the stress of pregnancy and labour, and apart from the common mild depression, both depressive neurosis and psychosis are occasionally met with. The incidence is about 1 in 2000.

MILD POSTPARTUM DEPRESSION   ('4th Day Blues')

About the third or fourth day the woman may be found weeping for no ascertainable reason, and displaying excessive anxiety about some trivial condition in the baby or herself. This is a common occurrence and the cause is uncertain. Clearly tiredness, perineal pain, feeding difficulties and a sense of anticlimax following the birth can be contributing factors. With sympathetic reassurance and support, most of these mothers will be normal within 48 hours About 10% of this group will subsequently manifest further depressive symptoms such as irritability, fatigue and backache, inability to cope with the baby or other children, and loss of sexual interest, and it may be as much as a year before they recover their normal energies. A few of these women will eventually need psychiatric support.

DEPRESSIVE NEUROSIS

This is a more severe degree of depression likely to be seen in a patient with a tendency to obsessional neurosis or hysteria, and should not simply be classed as 4th day blues. These patients need psychiatric treatment but respond well.

PSYCHOTIC DEPRESSION

Depression or schizophrenia are likely to occur in psychotic patients during the puerperium, and the obstetric staff must constantly be on the watch for symptoms of delusion. There may be confusion and disorientation in time and space; paranoid delusions ('The nurses are trying to poison me'); or an aversion to the baby. Unless the patient is unmanageable (abusive, dirty, offensive to the other patients) she may be nursed in a single room in the obstetric unit, in the charge of a psychiatrist. Severe depression leads to suicide and infanticide which must be guarded against, although the baby should be left with its mother as much a possible to achieve 'bonding'. Antidepressive drugs will be given, and if there is no improvement within a week, the patient should be transferred to a psychiatric unit.

EFFECT ON THE MOTHER-CHILD RELATIONSHIP

Anything but the most short lived depression is bound to interfere with the development of this relationship, and subsequent baby battering is commoner, especially when the mother has a disturbed personality and is of subnormal intelligence.

POSTNATAL EXAMINATION

This is usually made about 6 weeks postpartum:

1. To assess general well-being and especially the blood pressure in women who have been hypertensive.
2. To make sure that the genital tract has returned to normal.
3. To make sure that lactation is satisfactory (or that it has been satisfactorily suppressed, and that the baby is thriving).
4. To offer birth control advice if asked for.
5. To discuss future pregnancies especially if there have been complications e.g. Caesarean section or stillbirth.

RETURN OF MENSTRUATION

In lactating women menstruation is suppressed for about three months after which it may return even if breast feeding is continued. If menstruation is occurring, so probably is ovulation. Ovulation may return before menstruation and has been reported as early as 7 weeks.

In the non-lactating women endogenous oestrogen builds up in the endometrium. When it falls irregularly, as it does in the puerperium, the endometrium cannot be maintained and breaks down. This may be reported as continuation of the lochial discharge. Ovulation may occur from 5 weeks onward.

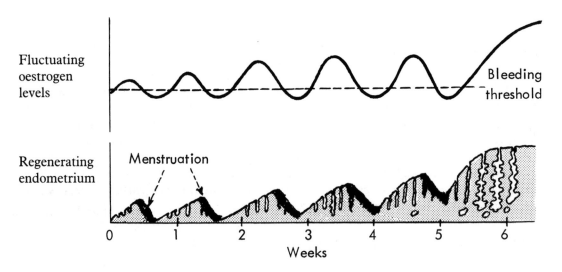

Wide variations in this pattern are met with. On rare occasions, a new pregnancy may be diagnosed at the postnatal visit.

POSTNATAL EXAMINATION

CLINICAL EXAMINATION

Involution should be complete by 6 weeks. The size, shape and mobility of the uterus are noted, and vaginal and cervical lacerations palpated to make sure there is no potential source of dyspareunia.

The uterus may be found to be retroverted. This means posterior displacement of the uterus with the corpus leaning backwards instead of forwards. It should be ignored unless causing symptoms such as backache or dyspareunia. If the position is thought to be producing symptoms it can be corrected and a Hodge pessary inserted.

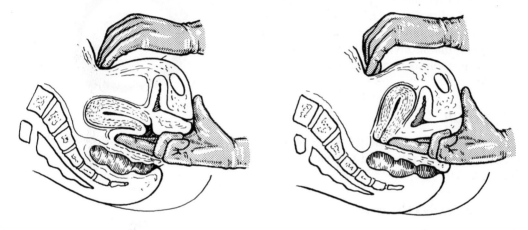

Correction of retroversion is called 'Basculation': the manipulating hand 'rocks' the uterus forward. (Fr. bascule, a cradle.)

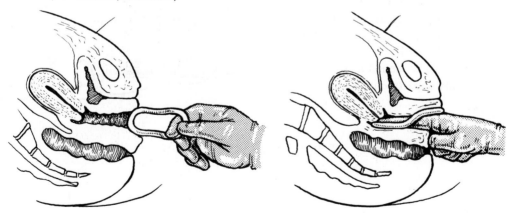

Inserting a Hodge pessary

The pessary should be maintained in position for a month. It should not be felt by the patient after a day or two and should not interfere with any pelvic function, including intercourse.

POSTNATAL EXAMINATION

A speculum is passed and the cervix examined.

A cervical smear can be taken if this examination has not been done within the last 3 years.

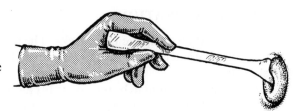

The cervix may show an ectopy, an outgrowth of endocervical epithelium. This requires no action unless producing symptoms e.g. excessive discharge. Any action (cryocautery, diathermy) should be delayed to allow squamous metaplasia to occur spontaneously.

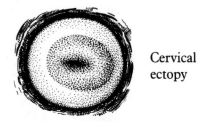

Cervical ectopy

DISCHARGE

Slight discharge is the rule at 6 weeks postpartum. If profuse and irritating, bacteriological specimens must be taken and treatment instituted.

STRESS INCONTINENCE

This occasionally occurs even when there is no sign of prolapse and no history of difficult delivery. It nearly always responds to simple physiotherapy (such as conscious contraction and relaxation of the levator ani muscles) but sometimes vaginal faradism is needed in a physiotherapy department.

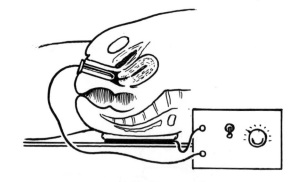

CHAPTER 16

THE NEWBORN BABY

THE NEWBORN BABY

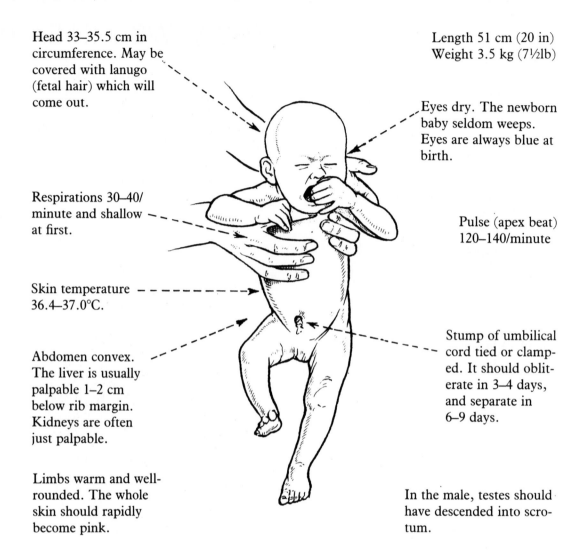

Head 33–35.5 cm in circumference. May be covered with lanugo (fetal hair) which will come out.

Length 51 cm (20 in)
Weight 3.5 kg (7½lb)

Eyes dry. The newborn baby seldom weeps. Eyes are always blue at birth.

Respirations 30–40/ minute and shallow at first.

Pulse (apex beat) 120–140/minute

Skin temperature 36.4–37.0°C.

Abdomen convex. The liver is usually palpable 1–2 cm below rib margin. Kidneys are often just palpable.

Stump of umbilical cord tied or clamped. It should obliterate in 3–4 days, and separate in 6–9 days.

Limbs warm and well-rounded. The whole skin should rapidly become pink.

In the male, testes should have descended into scrotum.

The baby is covered in utero with a sebaceous secretion called 'vernix caseosa' (L.,a cheese-like coating). This protects the skin against maceration while in the liquor amnii and has antibacterial properties.

MANAGEMENT OF THE NEWBORN BABY

WIPING THE EYES

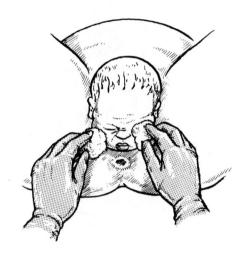

The eyes may be swabbed with sterile cotton wool to remove any infective secretion such as the gonococcus, although this is no longer done routinely in many centres. In some countries there may be a legal obligation to instil prophylactic antibacterial agents.

The cord is clamped and divided as soon as pulsations have ceased.

CLAMPING and LIGATING the CORD

If ligation is done carelessly, the baby may lose a great deal of blood very quickly.

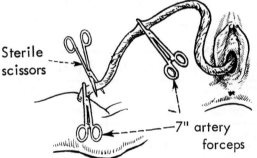

Sterile scissors

7" artery forceps

It is then ligated with a special clamp or rubber bands or tapes.

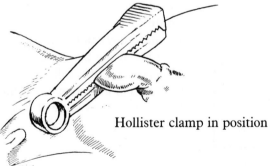

Hollister clamp in position

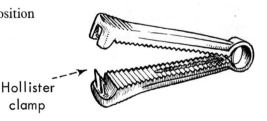

Hollister clamp

MANAGEMENT OF THE NEWBORN BABY

All mucus, blood and meconium must be sucked out before the baby has a chance to inhale them. This may be done by a mouth-operated mucus extractor as shown, or by means of a syringe or mechanical suction.

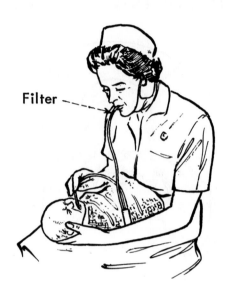

Filter

Assessment of the baby's condition at birth

Sign	0 points	1 point	2 points
Skin colour	Cyanosis Pallor	Periph. Cyanosis	Pink
Muscle tone	Flaccid	Moves Limbs	Good
Resp. effort	None	Gasps	Good
Heart rate	None	<100	>100
Response to stimulus	None	Slight	Good

The Apgar scoring system is universally accepted, and evaluation is made at one minute after delivery and again at five minutes. A score above seven indicates good condition. A score of 3 or less at one minute indicates the need for active, full resuscitation including intubation and ventilation. A score of 6 or less at 5 minutes suggests perinatal asphyxia.

412

APNOEA NEONATORUM

There are two sources of stimuli to which the fetal respiratory centre responds.

1. Blood gas changes (high CO_2, low O_2) which develop during the second stage and delivery, *provided that the period of hypoxia is not prolonged.*

2. Sensory stimuli brought about by the change from the warm watery conditions in the uterus to the colder temperature of the outside world in which the fetus is at once touched and handled.

A relatively high negative pressure is required to overcome lung resistance to expansion, but lung compliance increases thereafter, and progressively less effort is needed. The first breath is all-important, and if it does not occur within one minute of delivery a state of apnoea is considered to exist.

DEGREES OF APNOEA

1. **Primary Apnoea**
   (the old 'asphyxia livida')
   Cyanosed, with some muscle tone and a heart beat over 100. Efforts at breathing are made and gasping occurs.

2. **Secondary Apnoea**
   (the old 'asphyxia pallida')
   This is sometimes called terminal apnoea because if not soon corrected brain damage or death will follow. The skin is greyish-white, there is no muscle tone and the heart beat is less than 100.

It is often difficult in practice to decide on the degree of apnoea, especially when drug-induced depression is present.

CAUSES OF APNOEA

Antenatal

Any condition leading to fetal hypoxia, such as placental insufficiency, pre-eclampsia, abruptio placentae.

Natal

Prolonged hypoxic labour, traumatic delivery, opiate drugs, anaesthesia. (Even epidural anaesthesia if prolonged).

Postnatal

Immaturity, cerebral trauma, congenital abnormalities such as diaphragmatic hernia.

APNOEA NEONATORUM

MANAGEMENT OF PRIMARY APNOEA

1. Any liquor, mucus, meconium etc. must be gently sucked out of the nose and mouth. This is unlikely to relieve any obstruction in the airways if one exists, but it often provides sufficient stimulus to make the baby gasp.

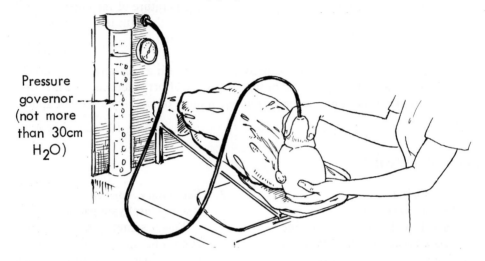

Pressure governor (not more than 30cm H_2O)

2. The baby is gently dried to reduce heat loss by evaporation, and covered with a warm towel.

3. An oxygen mask is held over the face. The object is not to insufflate lungs, but to enrich any breaths that are taken.

4. Drug-induced Depression

    Drugs such as morphine, pethidine and pentazocine which are commonly used in labour, all cross the placental barrier and cause some degree of respiratory depression and hence asphyxia (an increase in pCO_2 and a lowering of the oxygen saturation) and pethidine has been shown to have a more prolonged effect and to retard the development of feeding and other reflexes. If drug depression is suspected, naloxone hydrochloride (Narcan Neonatal) 40 micrograms in 2 ml should be injected via the umbilical vein or intramuscularly.

SECONDARY APNOEA

MANAGEMENT

If the baby is born in this condition, or if there is no response to simple treatment, oxygen must be given by effective bag and mask ventilation or, after intubation, with an endotracheal tube. This technique requires practice and is best done by an anaesthetist or paediatrician, but the obstetrician and midwife should have some experience. It is vital to remove any meconium visible in the upper airway and larynx before attempting assisted ventilation.

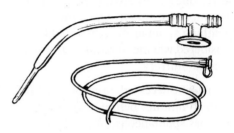

Bag and mask ventilation

A special endotracheal catheter is used, with shoulders near the tip to prevent its being inserted too far. The mucus aspirator also shown is small enough to pass through the catheter.

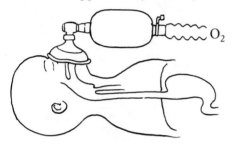

Straight bladed laryngoscope

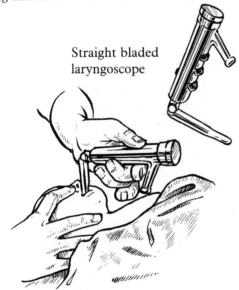

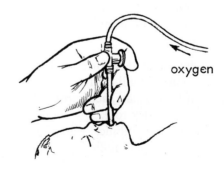

oxygen

The neonatal larynx lies opposite C.3 and 4. The tip of the laryngoscope catches the epiglottis and pulls it forward to allow clear view of the vocal cords.

Once the catheter is inserted, pressure is regulated by a finger on the escape hole. It is usual for the oxygen to pass through a water manometer which 'blows off' above a pressure of 30 cm of water.

415

APNOEA – RESUSCITATION

This method of giving oxygen is known as intermittent positive pressure respiration (IPPR) and its administration requires experience.

The first sign of recovery is a quickening and strengthening of the fetal heart, followed by attempts at respiration and improved colour. Once the baby is breathing spontaneously it should be considered whether it requires transfer to a special nursery.

It may be necessary to employ IPPR for up to 20 minutes before respiration becomes spontaneous, or death is recognised as inevitable.

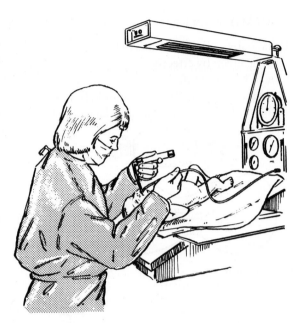

OTHER MEASURES

Cardiac massage

If the heart rate falls below 50, rhythmic pressure should be applied over the sternum, at the rate of about 5 compressions to one inflation of the lungs.

Acidosis should be corrected by the injection of 5 milli-equivalents/kg of molar bicarbonate, accompanied by 5 ml of 10% dextrose. This should be given via the umbilical vein after insertion of an umbilical catheter.

Hypothermia

An apnoeic baby loses heat very quickly, especially if it is immature and the recommended labour room temperature of 25°C is too low. Local heat must be provided by warm towels, and preferably by a 400 W radiant heater attached to the resuscitation table.

Drugs

Except for naloxone (Narcan) which reverses the depressive effect of opiates, there is little place for drugs in resuscitation.

HEAT LOSS IN THE NEWBORN

If the skin temperature falls below 36.5°C the baby loses heat more quickly than it can be produced. As the central (core) tempreture falls the metabolism slows down and hypothermia develops. Pre-term babies with a deficient fat layer, and babies which have had difficult deliveries are particularly exposed to this hazard.

Heat production

1. Energy from diet.
2. Metabolic activity mainly in the muscles. (Babies have no protective shivering reflex).
3. Breakdown of fat. Fat in certain areas such as the perirenal capsule (brown fat) can be catabolised very quickly.

Heat loss from the skin

1. Radiation.
2. Evaporation from wet skin exposed to air.
3. Convection.
4. Conduction.
   Small amounts of heat are lost through respiration and in urine and faeces.

Clinical Features of Hypothermia (Cold Injury)

This is rare and avoidable.

The baby is difficult to rouse, cold to touch, lethargic and unwilling to feed. There is oedema of the hands and feet and eyelids, and a hardening of the subcutaneous tissues. The redness of cheeks and extremities and the absence of crying give a misleading appearance of healthiness. As the metabolism slows down, the baby becomes hypoglycaemic and death occurs.

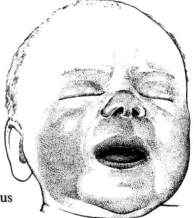

Note oedema of face

Shaded areas represent redness and subcutaneous sclerema

Treatment

Hypothermia is very difficult to reverse, and the only effective treatment is complete prevention.

1. The labour room temperature should be above 25°C.
2. All resuscitative procedures should be carried out under an infra-red heater.
3. The baby should be dried at birth and covered with a dry towel. It must be well wrapped up if it is staying in the ward.
4. If transfer to a Special Care Unit is necessary this must be done in a heated cot. Once in an incubator the paediatrician's object is to maintain a temperature of 37°C, and very small babies may require an ambient temperature as high as 37°C.

417

INSPECTION FOR CONGENITAL DEFECTS

Certain of the commoner defects should be noted at birth.

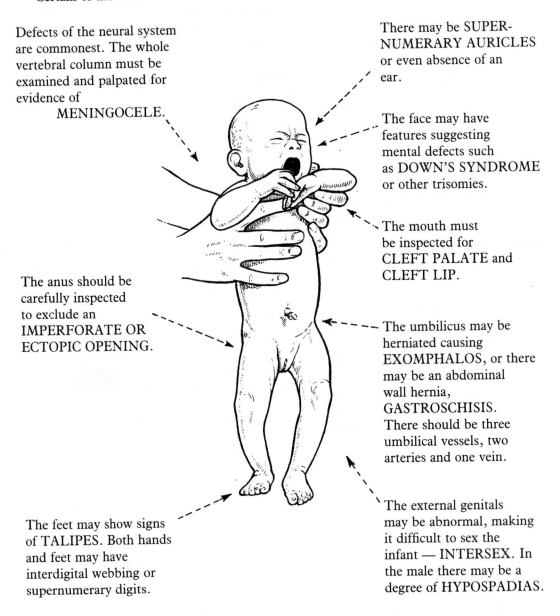

Defects of the neural system are commonest. The whole vertebral column must be examined and palpated for evidence of
MENINGOCELE.

There may be SUPER-NUMERARY AURICLES or even absence of an ear.

The face may have features suggesting mental defects such as DOWN'S SYNDROME or other trisomies.

The mouth must be inspected for CLEFT PALATE and CLEFT LIP.

The anus should be carefully inspected to exclude an IMPERFORATE OR ECTOPIC OPENING.

The umbilicus may be herniated causing EXOMPHALOS, or there may be an abdominal wall hernia, GASTROSCHISIS. There should be three umbilical vessels, two arteries and one vein.

The feet may show signs of TALIPES. Both hands and feet may have interdigital webbing or supernumerary digits.

The external genitals may be abnormal, making it difficult to sex the infant — INTERSEX. In the male there may be a degree of HYPOSPADIAS.

418

ROUTINE SCREENING TESTS

CONGENITAL DISLOCATION OF THE HIP (CDH)

The term CDH includes various degrees of instability of the hip joint. Ideally diagnosis should be made on the first day of life for the best outcome of treatment, but X-rays at this stage are difficult to interpret because so much of the hip joint is cartilaginous.

In the normal baby the flexed hip joints should be capable of 90 degree abduction with the baby supine.

Ortolani's Test

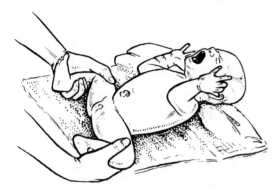

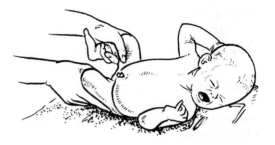

Limitation of abduction would be an indication for continued investigation and observation.

The flexed legs are grasped with the forefingers lying along the thigh. If the joint is dislocated, forced abduction will cause a 'click' as the femoral head slips into articulation.

ROUTINE SCREENING TESTS

PHENYLKETONURIA (PKU)

PKU is the best known of a numerous but rare group of congenital metabolic disorders, in which the baby inherits an inability to convert the amino-acid phenylalanine (PH) to tyrosine. There are at least three varieties of the disease which is more properly called 'hyperphenylalaninaemia'. 'Classical' PKU (97% of cases) is due to Phenylalanine hydroxylase (PHE) deficiency. This can be completely controlled by diet.

PKU in the BABY

Every baby is screened by the Guthrie test which demonstrates abnormal blood levels of PH after feeding is well established (7-10 days).

The disc impregnated with blood from a heel stab is placed in an outline of B subtilis in which there is a special inhibitor. If PH is present in abnormal concentration the inhibitor is neutralised and growth of B subtilis occurs.

```
┌──────────────────────────────────┐
│  Patient's Name  ...............  │
│  Address .....................    │
│  Date.......................      │
│  Date first feeding.............. │
│  Bottle ☐  Breast ☐  Both ☐      │
├──────────────────────────────────┤
│  FILL ALL CIRCLES WITH BLOOD      │
│   ◯    ◯    ◯    ◯               │
└──────────────────────────────────┘
```

If the test is positive the baby must be subjected to complex tests to establish the type of PKU.

PKU in the MOTHER

Transmission is by a recessive gene and it has been estimated that about 1:50,000 mothers have undiagnosed PKU. The following 'at risk' group should be screened: —

1. Mothers with a family history of PKU.

2. Mothers of low intelligence.

3. Mothers who have had infants with microcephaly (This has an association with PKU).

Screening is complicated by the wide diurnal variation in PH levels and several tests are needed.

A woman with PKU *must*, if she becomes pregnant, return to a rigorous low PH diet, and she should not breast feed the baby since her milk will have high PH concentrations.

The PKU problem is going to increase as more babies are diagnosed at birth and achieve normal maturity as a result of diet control.

In the common type I, the diet must be low-phenylalanine until maturity. Failure to control PKU results in mental retardation and progressive neurological deterioration.

The Guthrie test blood can also be used to exclude HYPOTHYROIDISM, by measurement of thyroxine levels or thyroid stimulating hormone.

NURSING CARE

MANAGEMENT OF THE NEWBORN BABY

Most infants are given vitamin K (1 mg) intramuscularly immediately after birth as protection against haemorrhagic disease.

About 6-8 hours after delivery the baby is cleansed of any vernix, blood or meconium by gentle wiping with swabs soaked in sterile water, and then dressed in a gown and napkin, and placed in a cot in room temperature between 18° and 20°C.

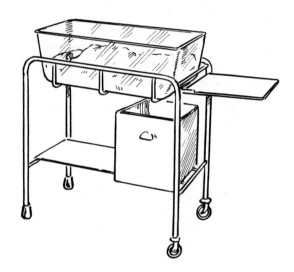

The ideal cot for the newborn should be draught proof and easily cleaned. It should be possible to raise and lower the head, and there should be a box for the toilet materials provided separately for each baby.

MOTHER AND CHILD RELATIONSHIP

Babies which have been separated from their mothers because of immaturity or illness are more at risk of being rejected later on by the mother and physically ill-treated. Child abuse is an increasingly recognised social problem in this country, and either or both parents may be guilty. The social factors are more difficult to deal with — the mother is typically young, emotionally disturbed, of low intelligence and living in poverty — but the importance of 'bonding' the mother and child is now recognised.

Bonding is encouraged by nursing mother and child in the same room, with the cot alongside the bed so that there may be intimate contact. The father should have been present throughout the labour and the baby placed in the mother's arms as soon as the cord has been cut. If admission to the special care nursery is required, facilities should be provided to allow both parents to make frequent visits.

BREAST FEEDING

The infant should be put to the breast as soon as possible after birth. He should be carefully observed during this feed for evidence of inhalation or difficulty with swallowing. If 'mucousy', oesophageal atresia should be excluded.

The baby should be put to the breast frequently. The mother must be comfortable and be able to hold the baby in such a way that both are relaxed and at ease.

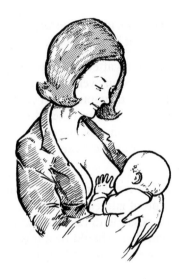

The baby may have to be taught to 'fix', i.e. to take a good grip of the breast.

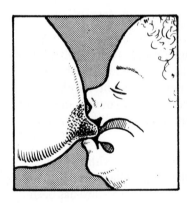 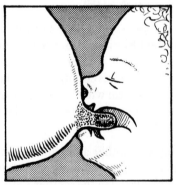 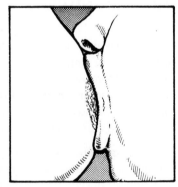

The baby feels the nipple at its lips.

The nipple is 'fixed' — nipple and areola are sucked into the mouth.

The baby's lips are in contact with the areola.

BREAST FEEDING

Once established on the breast, the baby requires 110 cal/kg/day and this is available from 150 ml of milk/kg/day. Most infants take 6–8 feeds per day, taking 10 minutes at each breast, with a short rest between to bring up swallowed air. After the initial loss (before lactation is completely established) weight gain should be about 30 g per day.

The baby should be put to the breast when it wants it and this stimulates lactation. An attempt at a 3–4 hourly schedule should be made.

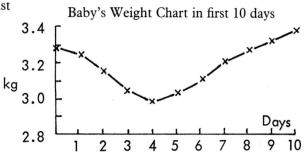

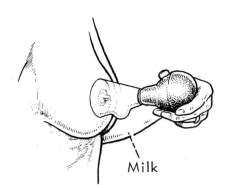

Milk

If, for whatever reason, the baby is unable to suck from the breast, it may be necessary to empty the breast artificially to maintain lactation and avoid engorgement. This may be done by a manual pump or 'breast reliever', which is simple and easy to use.

Alternatively the mother may use a mechanical breast milker, driven by an electric motor, which produces a gentle, interrupted suction stimulating closely the sensation of normal suckling.

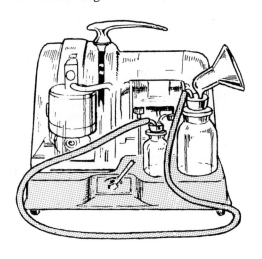

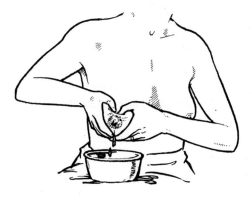

Some mothers prefer manual expression.

ADVANTAGES OF BREAST MILK

1. Chemical Composition

All mammalian animals feed their young on a unique milk adapted by nature to their needs. Human milk fats are much better absorbed than the butter fat in unmodified cow's milk which combines with calcium in the gut to reduce the absorption of calcium. Neonatal hypocalcaemia is associated with convulsions and perhaps with dental enamel hypoplasia and subsequent caries.

2. Protection against Infection

Human milk contains a large amount of IgA, including specific antibodies to E. Coli and respiratory syncytial (RS) virus. It is resistant to digestion in the stomach and reaches the intestine undamaged, where it acts on pathogenic organisms and inhibits their multiplication.

Human milk also by some means encourages the bacillus bifidus to colonise the gut and reduce pH so that the growth of pathogens is inhibited in the same manner as in the adult vagina.

The action against bacteria is strengthened by the high proportion of unsaturated iron-binding protein (lactoferrin) in human milk. Once in the intestine it reduces the amount of free iron far below the level necessary for bacterial growth.

3. Energy

Bottle – fed babies may imbibe more calories and are more often overweight than breast-fed babies. If the feed is too highly concentrated the excessive sodium content makes the baby cry from thirst, and this is mistaken for hunger and more milk is given. If rehydration does not occur, the very high plasma sodium levels (hypernatraemia) may cause brain damage. This is avoided by the use of appropriately prepared modified cow's milk formula.

4. Maternal Bonding

Physical closeness seems to be a factor in bonding, and the critical time is the first few weeks of life. Mothers who breast feed may have a more intimate relationship with their infants and handle them more affectionately.

DRUGS IN BREAST MILK

Nearly all drugs taken by the mother will be found in some concentration in the breast milk, and will be absorbed by the baby. The concentration depends on various pharmacological factors such as plasma level, pH and degree of dissociation of the drug, and the means by which it becomes incorporated in the milk. The clinician should therefore allow the lactating patient only those drugs which are absolutely necessary, but most commonly used drugs will reach the baby in insignificant dosage.

ANTIBIOTICS

Sulphonamides displace bilirubin from its albumin binding and may precipitate or increase jaundice.

Tetracyclines may discolour the baby's teeth.
Gentamycin and Kanamycin can damage hearing.
Penicillins and Cephalosporins are generally safe.

SEDATIVES AND ANTICONVULSANTS

Benzodiazepines and Barbiturates should be avoided.
Phenytoin may be used.

ANTICOAGULANTS

Heparin is not transmitted in milk and hence is safe.
Warfarin is bound to maternal proteins and is present in insignificant amounts in breast milk.

ANTITHYROID DRUGS

It appears that Propylthiouracil is probably safe as long as the infant's thyroid status is monitored.
Carbimazole should not be used.

OTHER DRUGS TO BE AVOIDED

Laxatives
Lithium
Opiates
Cytotoxics
Immunosuppressives.

ARTIFICIAL FEEDING

Artifical feeding is by modified cow's milk, usually made up from dried or evaporated concentrates. Cow's milk has three times as much protein as breast milk, but much less carbohydrate. Because of this carbohydrate (lactose) is often added.

	Human milk	Cow's milk
Protein	1.0%	3.5%
Fat	3.5	3.5
CHO	7.0	4.5
Cal/dl	67	65

An infant's calorie and fluid requirements rise over the first few days of life. Initially they are 50cal/kg/24 hour (approximately 70 ml/kg/day), and rise steadily over the first week. The calorie requirements are approximately 110 cal/kg/day from day 5 onwards. This is usually provided by 150 ml/kg/day of artificial formula. For example, a 3.5 kg infant requires approximately 525 ml/day i.e. 80-90 ml per feed x 6/day.

HOW TO MAKE UP A FEED

(This is a STERILE procedure)

1. Volume of boiled cooled water in bottle.

2. Add appropriate number of scoops of powder (avoid over-packing) — 1 scoop to 30 ml water.

3. Fix teat.

4. Test temperature.

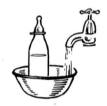

Cool the milk in cold water and …

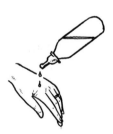

…test its temperature on the back of the hand. It should be at body heat.

In hospitals the milk is now supplied in sterile disposable 120 ml bottles with disposable teats. This very much reduces the risk of infection.

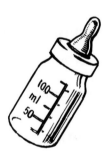

ARTIFICIAL FEEDING

After each feed all utensils must be cleaned and STERILIZED either by boiling or storing in antiseptic.

Boiling method

Boil bottle and teat for 5 minutes in a pan big enough to cover them with water. Leave in pan, with lid on.

Antiseptic method (Hypochlorite is tasteless and harmless to the baby, e.g. 'Milton').
(after cleaning)

1. Make up, every day, a supply of the antiseptic as instructed. Immerse bottle and teat, making sure bottle is full, and leave for at least 3 hours.

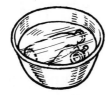

2. When feed is due, remove bottle and teat and pour in feed WITHOUT RINSING. Place cap on teat until ready to feed.

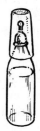

Feeds may be batch prepared and refrigerated.

PHYSIOLOGY OF THE NEWBORN BABY

PHYSIOLOGICAL JAUNDICE

occurs in about one third of normal babies between the 2nd and 5th days. It is due in part to the immaturity of the liver cells and the hyperbilirubinaemia caused by destruction of red cells. (Hb. level falls from 20 g % at birth to about 11 g by third month).

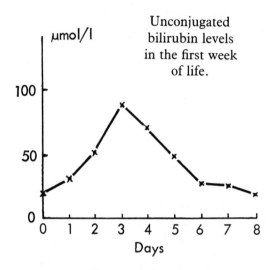

Unconjugated bilirubin levels in the first week of life.

STOOLS

Meconium — mainly cast-off cells, mucus and bile pigment — is passed for the first 2–3 days. It should appear within 36 hours of birth. The bowel is sterile at birth but is colonised by bacteria within a few hours. Formed stools appear on the 5th day, usually light yellow in colour, with the odour of faeces. Breast-fed babies may pass less faeces than bottle-fed ones.

URINE

The fetus swallows liquor and the kidneys excrete in utero. Urine should be passed within 24 hours of birth.

The passage of urine and faeces must be recorded — they are evidence of normal function.

RESPIRATORY SYSTEM

The fetal lungs are airless and filled with lung fluid and amniotic fluid. The fetus exists at an arterial oxygen pressure of approximately 30–35 mmHg. This changes quickly to adult levels with the establishment of respiration. The rate is about 30/minute and there may be much irregularity.

GENITAL SYSTEM

Manifestations of oestrogen withdrawal may occur, known as the 'genital crisis' (consequent on cessation of placental circulation). There is sometimes swelling of the breasts and even a little colostrum secretion ('witches' milk'). The female may bleed a little from the vagina and the male may develop a transient hydrocele. No treatment is required.

428

PHYSIOLOGY OF THE NEWBORN BABY

CARDIOVASCULAR SYSTEM

With the first breath the lungs expand and the constricted pulmonary vessels increase in size. The *ductus arteriosus*, which has a very muscular coat, actively contracts and all the right ventricular blood passes to the lungs. This will increase the left atrial pressure while the right atrial pressure is reduced by cessation of placental flow. Blood now tends to flow from left to right through the *foramen ovale* and this will cause its closure.

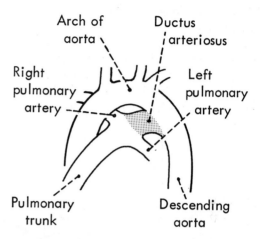

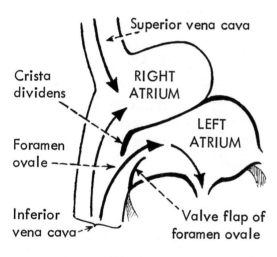

Following the clamping of the cord the *umbilical arteries* thrombose and persist as the obliterated hypogastric arteries. The *umbilical vein* obliterates by the 4—6th day and persists as the ligamentum teres of the liver. The *ductus venosus* obliterates a little later and persists as the ligamentum venosum.

The *ductus arteriosus* closes functionally almost at once and is obliterated by the 6th week. The *foramen ovale* closes gradually and may take months, but is functionally closed once the left atrial pressure is greater than the right.

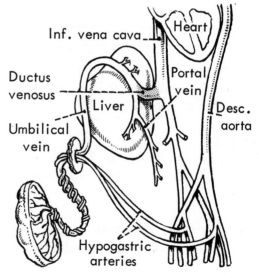

ROUTINE OBSERVATIONS

Baby charts must be kept in meticulous detail. A baby's condition can deteriorate very quickly.

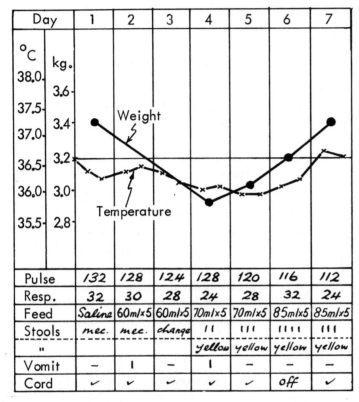

Day	1	2	3	4	5	6	7
Pulse	132	128	124	128	120	116	112
Resp.	32	30	28	24	28	32	24
Feed	Saline	60ml×5	60ml×5	70ml×5	70ml×5	85ml×5	85ml×5
Stools	mec.	mec.	change	II	III	IIII	III
"				yellow	yellow	yellow	yellow
Vomit	–	I	–	I	–	–	–
Cord	✓	✓	✓	✓	✓	off	✓

WEIGHT usually falls in first 3–4 days, even with artificial feeding. Birthweight should be regained within 10 days.

TEMPERATURE — about 36.7°C but some minor instability is usual in the first week.

PULSE is taken by auscultating the apex beat. It is usually 120–150/minute.

RESPIRATION — about 30 per minute at first and becoming slower. Irregularity is common in the first week.

FEEDS   The first feed is often boiled water in case the baby should inhale some fluid because of a congenital defect (but see page 422).

STOOLS   Meconium should give way to normal, formed stools by the 4th day. They should be yellow with a faecal odour, and may be less frequent in breast-fed babies.

VOMIT — Vomiting is a non-specific sign in infants. It should alert staff to the possibility of other illness such as infection. Bile-stained vomiting is a danger sign and may indicate a bowel obstruction. It must always be investigated.

RELUCTANCE TO FEED   Infants who are reluctant to feed should be carefully observed to detect any signs of significant illness e.g. infection, hypoglycaemia etc.

430

LOW BIRTHWEIGHT BABIES

THE LOW BIRTHWEIGHT BABY

This means a baby weighing 2.5 kg or less, at birth. The cause can be either preterm labour or failure to thrive in utero — intra-uterine growth retardation. A baby can be both preterm and growth-retarded.

The PRETERM BABY

A baby born before the 37th week. It is possible for such a baby to weigh more than 2.5 kg but it is still disadvantaged by its immaturity.

The GROWTH-RETARDED BABY

A baby whose birthweight is below the tenth percentile for its gestational age. Such a baby is almost always less than 2.5 kg, and the prognosis depends on the cause of the failure to thrive.

Although identification and treatment of these babies requires paediatric skills their diagnosis is of extreme importance to the obstetrician. The skin of the growth-retarded baby tends to be dry and even wrinkled. The umbilical cord may be thin with little Wharton's jelly. The growth-retarded baby is usually alert and active while the preterm baby is more likely to be hypotonic.

Complications

Preterm	Growth-retarded
Hypothermia	Hypothermia
Respiratory distress syndrome	Hypoglycaemia
Jaundice	Hypocalcaemia
Infection	
Cerebral haemorrhage	

431

ESTIMATION OF GESTATIONAL AGE

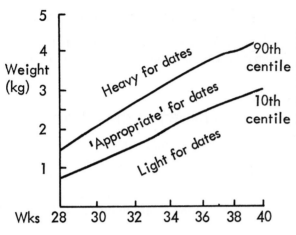

Estimating the gestational age of the new born can be as difficult as estimating the maturity during pregnancy. The weight is unreliable — the baby can be light, heavy or 'appropriate' for dates — and the method of evaluation used by the paediatrician is based on the system of Dubowitz et al. (J.Pediat. 1970,77,1).

EXTERNAL CRITERIA

There are ten external signs each with a varying score.

Examples:–

EXTERNAL SIGN	SCORE				
	0	1	2	3	4
1 Oedema	Obvious oedema hands and feet.	No obvious oedema hands and feet.	No oedema.		
2 Lanugo	No lanugo.	Abundant; long and thick over whole back.	Hair thinning especially over lower back.	Small amount of lanugo and bald areas.	At least half of back devoid of lanugo.
3 Ear firmness	Pinna soft, easily folded, no recoil.	Pinna soft, easily folded, slow recoil.	Cartilage to edge of pinna, but soft in places, ready recoil.	Pinna firm, cartilage to edge, instant recoil.	

NEUROLOGICAL CRITERIA

There are ten tests of posture and reflex, each with a varying score. They depend on the infant's state of alertness and freedom from asphyxia.

Examples:–

NEURO-LOGICAL SIGN	SCORE					
	0	1	2	3	4	5
1 Posture						
2 Head lag						
3 Ventral suspension						

The maximum score is 70, and the gestational age can be calculated from a table. A mature baby (over 37 weeks) should score over 45.

IDIOPATHIC RESPIRATORY DISTRESS SYNDROME (IRDS)

IRDS is one of the commonest causes of neonatal mortality. The management of affected babies is in the hands of paediatrician, but the prevention of IRDS and a reduction of its severity is largely the responsibility of the obstetrician.

Definition

Respiratory
rate > 60/minute
Indrawing of
sternum
Expiratory
grunting

Developing within 4 hours of birth and persisting for at least 24 hours.

Cause

A deficiency of surfactant in the alveoli.

Surfactant is a mixture of lipids (mainly a lecithin, dipalmitoyl phosphatidylcholine) which is continuously secreted by type II pneumocytes in the alveolar wall. It forms a monolayer over the watery surface of the alveolus and so lowers the surface tension, making the lung easier to expand. During expiration it is believed that the surfactant solidifies under pressure, and 'like an archway of bricks' splints the alveolus and prevents atelectasis.

Pathology   Immature (or damaged) lungs do not secrete enough surfactant so that more force is needed to expand them than the baby possesses. The lungs become atelectatic, and the alveoli are lined with a fibrinous exudate called hyaline membrane.

Clinical features

As tachypnoea develops, the increased respiratory effort is marked by the indrawing of the chest wall. The baby begins to grunt as air is forced through partly closed glottis in an attempt to keep the alveoli open for as long as possible.

Atelectasis and hypoxia lead to pulmonary vasoconstriction and cyanosis appears, which is aggravated by a right-to-left shunt through the foramen ovale and the ductus arteriosus. The CO_2 tension rises, and hypoglycaemia and hypocalcaemia develop. Hypoproteinaemic oedema which is usually present in immature babies is increased.

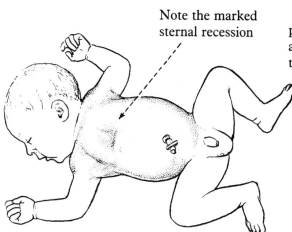

Note the marked sternal recession

IDIOPATHIC RESPIRATORY DISTRESS SYNDROME

Predisposing factors

1. Immaturity
   Surfactant is first produced at about 22 weeks and rises sharply to a mature level between 34 and 36 weeks.

2. Acute intrapartum hypoxia
   (Chronic hypoxia as in pre-eclampsia and non-lethal placental infarction, appears to stimulate surfactant secretion, possibly as a response to stress.)

3. Postpartum hypoxia as when the baby is born in a shocked condition.

Differential diagnosis

1. Transient tachypnoea of newborn ('Wet lung')
   This is a generally mild condition occuring in mature babies.

2. Meconium Aspiration.
   Meconium will have been observed at delivery, and aspirated from the baby's pharynx and trachea.

3. Pneumonia.   Occurs after prolonged rupture of membranes.

4. Cardiac abnormalities.

5. Diaphragmatic hernia. The heart is displaced to one side, usually the right, and the abdomen is scaphoid. An X-ray picture will give the diagnosis.

Prevention

1. The avoidance, as far as possible, of pre-term labour (see Chapter 10).

2. Monitoring in labour; avoidance of hypoxia; readier resort to section for pre-term babies; effective and immediate resuscitation; avoidance of hypothermia.

3. Administration of glucocorticoids to the mother to stimulate surfactant secretion. Betamethasone has been claimed to be beneficial between 30-32 weeks. It must be given for at least 48 hours before delivery (see Chapter 10).

IDIOPATHIC RESPIRATORY DISTRESS SYNDROME

Treatment

This is undertaken in a special care baby unit (SCBU) and demands considerable paediatric skill. The principles are:

1. Avoid unnecessary handling.

2. Avoid heat loss. A naked immature baby must be nursed at 36°C.

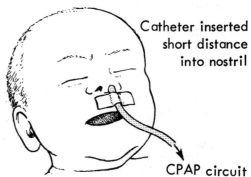

Catheter inserted short distance into nostril

CPAP circuit

3. Provide a higher concentration of oxygen. The ordinary incubator cannot maintain a concentration above 30% and a headbox may be required. If there is no improvement, continuous positive airways pressure (CPAP) must be provided.

This means the passage of oxygen to the lungs under pressure, either by mask, nasal catheter or endotracheal tube. The principle risk of CPAP is pneumothorax. Infants deteriorating may require intermittent positive pressure ventilation (IPPV).

4. Correction of Acidosis.

Molar solutions (7.4%) of bicarbonate have long been used to correct metabolic acidosis, but there have been suggestions that the sudden injection of relatively large amounts of alkali may contribute to the risk of intraventricular haemorrhage. It is safer to use a 4.2% solution and to inject slowly; but acidosis must not be allowed to persist.

5. Maintenance of blood pressure.

6. Replacement of Surfactant.

This is currently being actively investigated and a number of preparations for tracheal instillation have shown promise.

JAUNDICE IN THE NEWBORN

Jaundice is quite common in mature infants (physiological jaundice), especially when breast-feeding is initiated, and it is almost the rule in immature infants. Excessively high concentrations of unconjugated (fat soluble) bilirubin can cause damage to the brain particularly in immature babies.

Physiology   Unconjugated bilirubin which comes from the breakdown of haemoglobin is either:

CONJUGATED in the liver........or........ DECOMPOSED in the skin by
blue light (photodecomposition).

Fat-soluble ⟶ Water-soluble
bilirubin (toxic) ↑ bilirubin (non-toxic)
glucuronyl
transferase

Fat-soluble ⟶ Water-soluble
bilirubin ↑ dipyrroles (non-toxic)
blue light

Jaundice develops if the liver function is inadequate. It is non-obstructive in type — much the commonest. If excretion from the liver is impaired, the jaundice is obstructive — not common.

Causes of non-obstructive jaundice

1. Immaturity.
2. Intrapartum hypoxia.
3. ABO or Rh incompatibilty (Haemolysis — intravascular).
4. Extravasated blood from bruising (Haemolysis — extravascular).
5. Infection.

There are many other uncommon conditions which give rise to jaundice, outwith the responsibility of the obstetrician.

Investigations

The ABO and Rhesus groups of mother and infant should be determined together with the Coombs' test. The baby's haemoglobin and reticulocyte count should be determined and serial estimations of the level of unconjugated bilirubin are required.

Treatment

1. Prevention, as far as possible, of immaturity.
2. Adequate fluid intake.
3. Phototherapy — An artificial light source of fluorescent tubes is used to encourage photodecomposition. It is given when the infant's serum bilirubin rises above $200\,\mu$mol/l. The eyes must be bandaged during exposure.
4. Exchange transfusion (p. 167) may be necessary if there is no response to phototherapy.

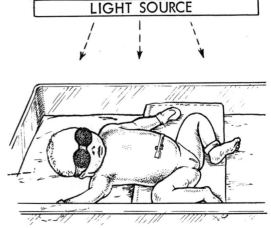

LIGHT SOURCE

INTRACRANIAL HAEMORRHAGE

This is often lethal and surviving infants are often brain–damaged. It can occur in the ventricles, in the substance of the brain, in the subdural space, or as a consequence of a tear of the dura mater.

SUBEPENDYMAL/INTRAVENTRICULAR HAEMORRHAGE

Bleeding starts in the subependymal vessels overlying the caudate nucleus in the wall of the lateral ventricle. The bleeding can stop at this stage or progress either into the substance of the brain or into the whole of the ventricular system.

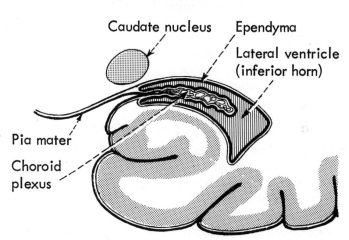

Clinical features

It occurs most commonly in preterm infants, usually within the first three days of life. The infant may become limp and unresponsive, and within 12 hours cyanotic attacks and seizures may occur. As the haemorrhage proceeds, the infant becomes comatose and death may occur or hydrocephalus develop. The condition can now readily be recognised by cranial ultrasound.

Aetiology

The cause is unknown but there are many associated factors:

Obstetrical
Immaturity
Hypoxia in labour
Chronic hypoxia in pregnancy
Birth trauma.

Paediatric
Immaturity
Hypoxia arising from RDS
Coagulation defects.

Treatment

There is no specific treatment, and protection of the fetus and neonate from periods of hypoxia offers the best means of prevention.

INTRACEREBRAL HAEMORRHAGE

Intracerebral haemorrhage is usually a consequence of hypoxial damage with subsequent haemorrhage from damaged blood vessels. This frequently causes significant long-term complications.

437

INTRACRANIAL HAEMORRHAGE

SUBDURAL HAEMORRHAGE

This is a rare condition in modern obstetric practice. It is liable to complicate any cranial injury, leading to haemorrhage over the cerebral convexity and to haematoma formation. Some localising signs may appear but the diagnosis is difficult, and the condition must always be borne in mind if cranial injury is suspected.

Bleeding arises from rupture of the cerebral veins in the subdural space. Blood extends over the frontal lobes and the first signs of cerebral irritation are usually irritability and convulsions. Retinal haemorrhages and abnormal eye movements will follow. Diagnosis is by the demonstration of blood stained CSF in the subdural space, and if a haematoma has formed decompression is required.

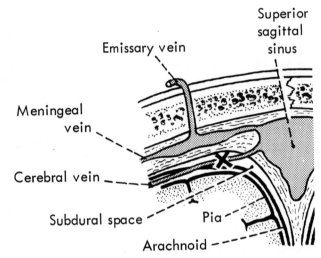

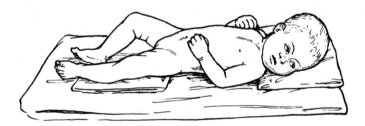

The picture shows the tonic deviation of the eyes which is a common sign.

INTRACRANIAL HAEMORRHAGE

TEARS OF THE DURA MATER

This injury is a consequence of excessive moulding and may occur in prolonged, unsupervised labours.

The fetal brain is protected against damage in labour by:–

1. Softness and moulding of membranous bones.

2. Ability of fontanelles to 'give' slightly on pressure.

3. Cushioning effect of cerebrospinal fluid.

4. Anatomical arrangement of dural septa with their free edges.

5. Plasticity of brain tissue.

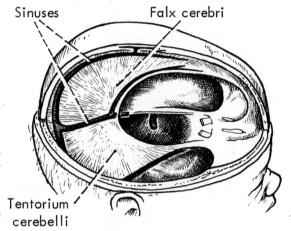

Sometimes however distortion is excessive and a tear of the free edge of the tentorium cerebelli occurs involving blood vessels. Death occurs from increased intracranial pressure, especially on the brain stem and medulla.

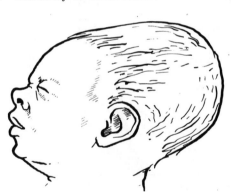

Moulding of the fetal head

This lesion is associated with difficult deliveries, such as high forceps, breech etc., but can occur after spontaneous vertex delivery. The signs and symptoms are those of apnoea neonatorum and definite diagnosis is made only at post mortem examination.

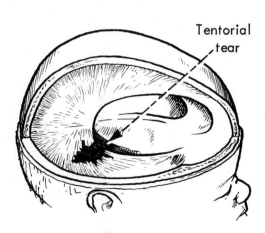

439

BIRTH INJURIES

FRACTURE OF LONG BONES

The bones most commonly broken are the clavicle, humerus and femur as a result of too forcible delivery. In the case of the clavicle there may be no signs at all and callus is felt 2 weeks later. In the case of the long bones the Moro reflex will be absent in that limb and X-ray will be required. In healthy infants callus formation is rapid and splinting is not needed.

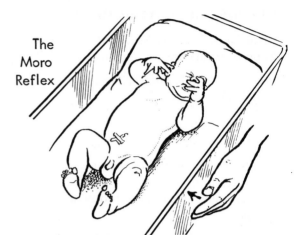

The Moro Reflex

The Moro Reflex — In response to a sudden noise or vibration, the arms and legs are extended and then approach each other with slight shaking movements.

DAMAGE TO THE BRACHIAL PLEXUS

This is caused by excessive lateral flexion of the neck during vertex or breech delivery.

1. **Erb's Palsy** C5,6   This is the commonest. Abductors and flexors of the upper arm are affected, and the arm hangs in the characteristic 'waiter's tip' position.

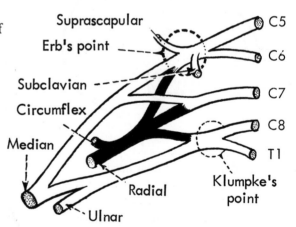

Suprascapular — C5
Erb's point — C6
Subclavian — C7
Circumflex — C8
Median — T1
Radial
Ulnar
Klumpke's point

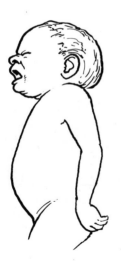

Erb's Palsy

2. **Klumpke's Paralysis** C8, T1 is rare. The hand is paralysed with wrist drop and absence of grasp reflex.

3. **Horner's Syndrome** — interruption of sympathetic supply in T1. Presents as ptosis, enophthalmos, meiosis of the pupil. This syndrome is liable to coexist with Klumpke's paralysis, but both injuries are rare.

Most degrees of injury may be left untreated. Severe injuries should be reviewed by an orthopaedic specialist.

BIRTH INJURIES

DEPRESSION FRACTURE OF THE SKULL

This may occasionally be caused by the tip of the forceps blade in difficult delivery. Usually no treatment is necessary but if cerebral irritation or paresis is observed, surgical intervention may be required.

Such injuries are best avoided by preferring section to difficult vaginal delivery.

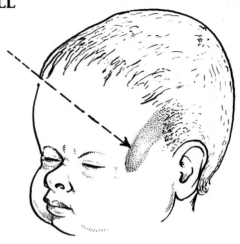

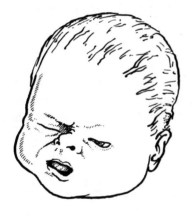

FACIAL PALSY

Paralysis of the facial nerve caused by pressure from the forceps made on the nerve as it emerges from the stylomastoid foramen. Recovery occurs in a matter of days, and any delay is an indication for further investigation.

STERNOMASTOID TUMOUR

A painless lump in the sternomastoid muscle, appearing in the first week of life. It has traditionally been attributed to trauma, but its aetiology is unknown. Torticollis is an occasional sequel; and the mother should be instructed to put the muscle on the stretch for 3 or 4 periods a day. This exercise may, at first, be painful to the baby.

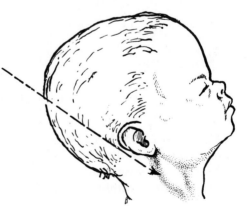

BIRTH INJURIES

SUPERFICIAL HEAD INJURIES

Minor abrasions may be sustained during forceps delivery or from the use of the vacuum extractor. They need only local treatment as a rule but dense connective tissue prevents vessel retraction and scalp wounds bleed freely.

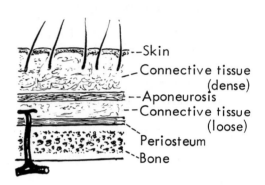

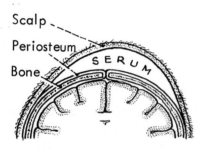

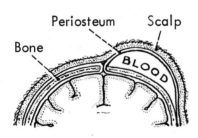

Caput succedaneum

CAPUT SUCCEDANEUM

('Substitute Head'). This is a normal occurrence caused by pressure of the cervix interrupting venous and lymphatic scalp drainage during labour. A serous effusion collects between aponeurosis and periosteum disappearing a few hours after birth.

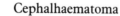

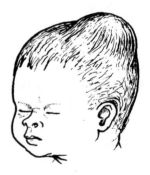

Cephalhaematoma

CEPHALHAEMATOMA is a collection of blood between periosteum and skull bone which is limited by the periosteal attachments at the suture lines. It is due to trauma and may not appear until several hours after birth. It should not be aspirated or drained and will normally be absorbed within a few weeks.

CONGENITAL DEFECTS

Many common defects are of unknown aetiology. Others can be explained by one of three mechanisms.

  A. Hereditary genetic defects.

  B. Chromosomal aberrations which may be familial.

  C. Incidental defect due to environment or of unknown aetiology.

Genetic counselling can be useful in regard to A and B. The need for such counselling sometimes arises during early pregnancy but usually it is sought after the birth of an affected child. Evaluation of the risks and possibilities is often a matter for the expert but the obstetrician and the general practitioner should be able to advise in straightforward cases.

A. HEREDITARY GENETIC DEFECTS.

Genes lie in specific location on paired chromosomes and a pair of such genes is known as a pair of alleles. If the alleles are identical the individual is homozygous.

1. **Dominant Genes**   These, as the name suggests, are 'strong' genes.

The presence of one such abnormal gene will over-ride the influence of a normal gene on the opposite chromosome and the disease will always be apparent. The individual is therefore usually heterozygous for the abnormal gene. 50% of offspring will be affected.

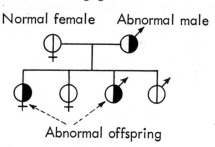

Examples: Achondroplasia, osteogenesis imperfecta, congenital spherocytosis, sickle cell anaemia and Huntingdon's chorea.

2. **Recessive Genes**   These are 'weak' genes. If only one allele of a pair of genes is abnormal and recessive its influence will be overcome by the normal gene on the opposite chromosome. Only if both genes are abnormal will the disease manifest itself. In a family both parents will require to be carriers and possess such a gene, i.e. both heterozygous, before the disease can be transmitted.

443

CONGENITAL DEFECTS

Recessive genes (continued)

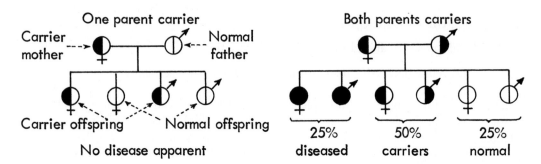

One parent carrier	Both parents carriers
Carrier mother — Normal father	
Carrier offspring — Normal offspring	25% diseased 50% carriers 25% normal
No disease apparent	

Examples: Most inborn errors of metabolism. These are numerous and affect various metabolic pathways. Their importance lies in the fact that if the defect is diagnosed early, the subsequent disease process may be prevented in some, but not all, by dietary means. This applies particularly to those genetic defects affecting carbohydrate and amino acid metabolism e.g. phenylketonuria. It does not however apply to the numerically most important member of this group — cystic fibrosis. The carrier rate for this condition in the United Kingdom approaches 1 in 20.

3. Sex-linked Recessive Disease This is a special situation where the abnormal recessive gene is linked to one sex chromosome, usually the X chromosome.

In the female the influence of the abnormal recessive gene on one X chromosome is counteracted by the normal more dominant gene on the second X chromosome. The female is therefore a carrier of the disease but not affected by it. The male possessing the abnormal recessive gene on his single X chromosome is affected since there is no opposition to its action. The family situation is

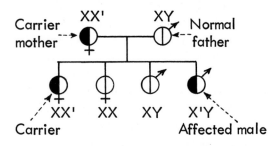

Carrier mother XX'   XY Normal father

XX'   XX   XY   X'Y
Carrier   Affected male

shown in diagram. 50% of female offspring will be carriers and 50% of males will show the disease.

Examples: Duchenne muscular dystrophy, haemophilia.

CONGENITAL DEFECTS

B. CHROMOSOMAL ABNORMALITIES

These are due to abnormalities arising during the maturation of the oocyte or sperm i.e. at meiosis. Errors at this time can cause unequal separation of the chromosomes resulting in germ cells which possess fewer or more chromosomes than normal. At fertilisation this abnormality is handed on to the offspring.

The commonest abnormality the obstetrician meets with is Down's syndrome (mongolism) due to an extra chromosome 21 (trisomy at 21). Diagnosis is made by karyotyping a culture of fetal cells obtained at amniocentesis or direct examination of tissue obtained by chorion villus sampling (see Chapter 6). The incidence of trisomy 21 increases with maternal age.

Maternal age	Risk of Trisomy-21
20-24	1 in 1,500
25-29	1 in 1,200
30-34	1 in 900
35	1 in 250
38	1 in 125
40	1 in 80
45	1 in 22

In a few cases the mongolism is due to an inherited chromosomal translocation and in all cases the parents should be examined for the defect.

Other examples of chromosomal abnormalities are Trisomies 18 and 13 and Turner's syndrome and Klinefelter's syndrome, both of which are defects of the sex chromosome.

Multifactorial Disorders (Familial diseases)

These result from a combination of multiple abnormal genes and the effect of embryonic and fetal environment. The risks or recurrence have been calculated on the basis of experience and are only approximate.

It is important when discussing the 'odds' with parents to give a balanced view, and to let the parents decide. A 1 in 20 chance of abnormality means a 19 in 20 chance of a normal child.

Condition	Chance of second affected child
Neural tube defect Anencephaly	1 in 20
Cleft palate	1 in 25
Congenital heart disease	1 in 30
Diabetes mellitus	1 in 12
Epilepsy	1 in 20

It will be obvious that in certain conditions, e.g. all dominant gene disorders, some sex-linked recessive gene conditions such a haemophilia and chromosomal disorders, the practitioner can give a general indication of possibilities. In many instances further investigation is necessary before venturing to give an opinion.

When in any doubt, the opinion of a medical geneticist should be sought.

CONGENITAL DEFECTS

Chromosomal Abnormalities   (continued)

At least three examinations can be made on the chromosomes of fetal cells obtained:

1. **Inspection of sex chromatin and determination of sex.** This is done directly on the sample obtained.

- - - - - Where the mother is a known carrier of a sex-linked recessive disorder such as a Duchenne's muscular dystrophy, male fetuses which have a 50% chance of being affected, can be aborted.

2. **Chromosomal Analysis** (Karyotyping). - - - - - This allows the detection of Down's syndrome (Mongolism) due to trisomy 21, and also some rare conditions such as 45XO (Turner's syndrome) or an additional X chromosome (Klinefelter's syndrome). Karyotyping may be offered in all cases where there is a history of an affected child or where the mother is 35 or over.

The nucleus is photographed after cell division has stopped, and the photographs of the chromosomes are arranged in order of size. The largest is called no. 1.

3. **Enzyme analysis.**

- - - - - This allows the diagnosis of many autosomal recessive diseases such as phenylketonuria. This investigation would only be done when there was already an affected child.

Such tests are complex and must be shared between many laboratories.

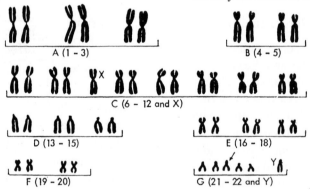

This is the karyotype of a male patient with Down's syndrome. Note the third chromosome at 21.

C. DEFECTS DUE TO ENVIRONMENT OR OF UNKNOWN AETIOLOGY

These are abnormalities which arise in individual pregnancies. Causes, such as infections during pregnancy or drugs given to the mother, can be recognised in some cases. In these instances parents can be assured that the defect is not familial. In others, although the aetiology is unknown, there does seem to be a familial factor operating as noted under multifactorial disorders, page 445.

CONGENITAL DEFECTS

The obstetrician and the midwife should have some knowledge of the prognosis for the commoner abnormalities seen at birth, so that they can answer the mother's questions and initiate treatment when necessary.

NEURAL TUBE DEFECTS

Most of these lesions are detected ante-natally by elevation of the maternal serum alpha-fetoprotein level or routine ultrasound (see Chapter 6).

The cause of neural tube defects is not known. There is a social gradient and geographical pattern — the North of England, Wales, Ireland and Scotland have a higher incidence than the South and East of England. Peri-conceptional vitamin deficiency has been postulated and is at present under active assessment.

Meningocele and Meningomyelocele

Herniations of meninges and spinal cord through a bony gap due to a mesodermal defect causing failure of fusion of vertebral arches (spina bifida) and failure of the development of posterior dura mater. It occurs usually in the lumbo-sacral region.

Meningocele

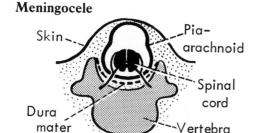

Herniation of pia-arachnoid is covered by skin (sometimes attenuated).
There is no paralysis and surgical closure can be delayed for 6 months.
Prognosis should be guarded until it is known for certain that nervous tissue is not involved. Otherwise the child will develop normally.

Myelocele

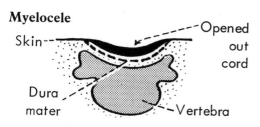

The internal surface of the cord is exposed.

Meningomyelocele

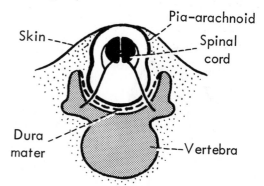

The cord is displaced as well as the membranes and neural epithelium forms the fundus of the sac. Skin cover is incomplete and infection likely unless closure is done within 24 hours. Paralysis of legs, bowel and bladder, and hydrocephaly, are normally present. An immediate surgical opinion should be sought to advise on the possibility of repair.

447

CONGENITAL DEFECTS

Neural Tube Defects   (continued)

Anencephaly

Anencephaly is the failure of proper development of the cranium and scalp. The face and base of the skull are present. It is usually diagnosed in early pregnancy and termination is offered as the condition is incompatible with life. Should the pregnancy proceed there is usually hydramnios, attributed to the inability of the fetus to swallow, the absence of fetal anti-diuretic hormone, and the secretions of the exposed choroid plexus and meninges. Anencephalic pregnancy without hydramnios may be very prolonged and this has been attributed to the absence of the fetal pituitary with its oxytocic hormone.

In labour the face is often the presenting part and shoulder dystocia is on occasion experienced.

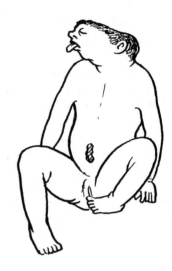

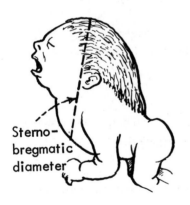

Sterno-bregmatic diameter

Iniencephaly

Iniencephaly is a condition giving a defect in the occipital bone in the region of the foramen magnum and fusing of the occiput to the ununited neural arches. The condition is incompatible with life.

Dystocia is rare due to associated hydramnios and premature labour. But if the pregnancy goes to term there may be gross disproportion as the sterno-bregmatic diameter tries to negotiate the pelvis. A destructive operation or Caesarean section will deliver the fetus.

448

CONGENITAL DEFECTS

Neural Tube Defects   (continued)

Hydrocephalus

Hydrocephalus is distension of the brain and skull due to increased pressure in the ventricles.

Physiopathology

CSF is secreted by specialised arterial plexuses called choroid plexuses mainly into the lateral ventricles. It passes thence to the IIIrd and IVth ventricles and through the median and lateral foramina of the IVth ventricle into the subarachnoid space. it is absorbed into the venous sinuses of the dura mater through protrusions of arachnoid called arachnoid granulations or villi (Pacchionian bodies).

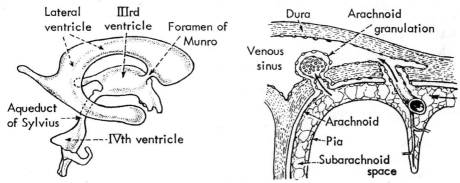

If the flow of CSF is obstructed, the pressure in the ventricles will gradually increase and the fetal head enlarges to such a size that delivery may be impossible without surgical interference.

Causes of obstruction

Blockage of the narrow connecting points between ventricles, or of the IVth ventricle foramina leading out to the subarachnoid space. Such blockage might be due to congenital abnormality, infection, or trauma, and as the CSF is confined to the ventricles it is known as an internal or non-communicating hydrocephalus.

Interference with the absorption of CSF due to an obstruction in the meninges or a venous sinus thrombosis in the dura mater. This can be congenital or infective, or traumatic in origin, and is known as an external or communicating hydrocephalus.

These distinctions principally concern the paediatrician who may be able to relieve the pressure in non-communicating hydrocephalus, but the obstetrician should be aware of the possibilities in mild cases. About 40% of cases of infant hydrocephalus are said to arrest spontaneously.

Well developed cases are easily diagnosed by palpation and X-ray or ultrasound, but mild degrees of hydrocephalus are very difficult to identify with certainty. If there is doubt, delivery should be by section even although there is a high chance of associated neural tube defect. When the diagnosis is definite the operation of craniotomy is employed (see Chapter 14).   449

CONGENITAL DEFECTS

CARDIAC LESIONS

Congenital heart lesions are second only to neural tube defects in frequency. Their recognition is increasingly important because of the great advances made in paediatric cardiac surgery in recent years. Diagnosis has also been improved by the development of neonatal echo cardiography.

Many lesions can be detected only by detailed paediatric assessment. The clinical presentation is often unclear but the following are indications for urgent paediatric opinion:

1. Respiratory difficulty — tachypnoea and tachycardia are present together with other evidence of cardiac failure.

2. Cyanosis.

3. Rapidly developing 'shock'.

4. Murmur detected.

CLEFT LIP AND PALATE

Lip or palate may be affected separately, but usually both are involved.
The mother should be told that a good cosmetic result will be obtained when the lip is repaired at about 4 months and that after the palate is repaired at about a year the child will be taught to speak normally. Spoon feeding may be necessary if sucking is weak, and the cleft should be kept clean.

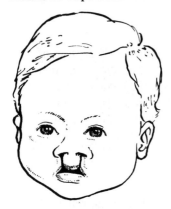

Bilateral cleft lip
('Hare lip')

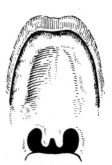

Cleft of soft
palate
(Bifid uvula)

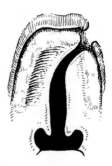

Unilateral cleft
palate

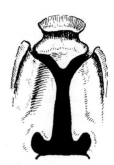

Bilateral cleft
palate

CONGENITAL DEFECTS

GASTRO-INTESTINAL TRACT

Oesophageal Atresia with Tracheo-Bronchial Fistula

The upper segment ends blindly at the level of T3-T4 and the distance of the blind end to the anterior alveolar margin is 10 cm.

It must be suspected antenatally in cases of unexplained hydramnios. In the neonate attempts at feeding lead to choking and cyanosis and there may be 'frothing' — excess of unswallowed mucus. If a sterile lubricated rubber catheter is arrested 10–12 cm from the alveolar margin, the diagnosis is almost certain. Suction should be continued and a paediatrician notified.

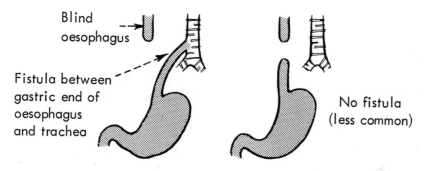

Blind oesophagus

Fistula between gastric end of oesophagus and trachea

No fistula (less common)

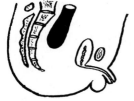

Failure of development of rectum

Imperforate Anus

There is a wide variety of congenital ano-rectal abnormalities and a relieving colostomy may be an emergency measure. The passage of faeces must be noted: but fistula is often present and the observer may be confused by small amounts of faeces passed per urethram or per vaginam.

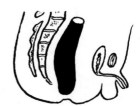

Cloacal membrane has failed to rupture

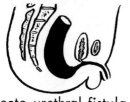

Recto-urethral fistula

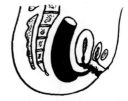

Recto-vaginal fistula

451

CONGENITAL DEFECTS

Gastro-Intestinal Tract (continued)

Exomphalos

Some of the abdominal viscera lie within the umbilical cord and there is incomplete development of the abdominal wall. (It is a persistence of the normal situation in the 10 week fetus.) The sac is a thin jelly-like membrane (the root of the cord) and the vessels of the cord run over the sac. The chances of repair depend on the size of the defect but prior to operation the sac must be kept moist with saline swabs to prevent drying and cracking.

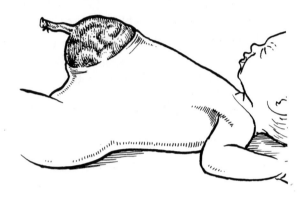

Gastroschisis

This term describes the presence of an abdominal wall defect with herniation of some or all of the abdominal organs.

TALIPES (CLUB FOOT) (L. talipes = walking on the talus or ankle).

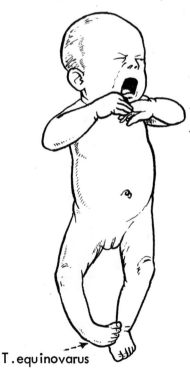

In true club foot there is always some resistance to complete passive correction. Treatment begins at birth in order to minimise the adaptive distortion of soft tissues and tarsal bones. The mother is taught to stretch and correct the deformity regularly and the baby must be referred at once to a paediatric surgeon. Operation is now seldom required.

ACCESSORY DIGITS

Small tags of flesh are common and can be removed by ligation. Fully developed extra digits must be surgically amputated at any time when the baby is big enough to withstand the operation.

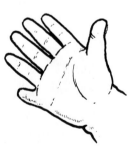

T.equinovarus

EFFECTS OF DRUGS ON THE FETUS

There are very few if any drugs which have been proved to have a completely predictable and unvarying effect on the human fetus when given to the mother. However certain drugs are recognised as being associated with a higher incidence of fetal injury or abnormality, and they must be used with the greatest care.

A drug should not be prescribed for a woman who is pregnant or may become pregnant during the course of treatment, unless the advantages it offers outweigh the possible risk to the fetus. In conditions such as epilepsy the risks associated with the medication have to be accepted as the effects of stopping the treatment would be unacceptable. Normal pregnant women require very little in the way of drug treatment.

Types of Injury to the Fetus

1. Mutations may arise in the ovum before or during fertilisation. These are usually lethal, resulting in abortion.

2. Embryonic cells may be damaged during differentiation by teratogens. The risk is greatest between three weeks and three months after the LMP.

3. Fetal growth may be retarded in the second and third trimesters, sometimes resulting in intra-uterine death.

4. Drugs given near term or in labour may have adverse effects after delivery.

The Thalidomide disaster

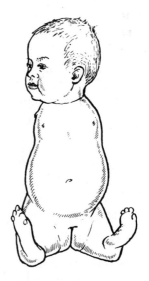

This drug was marketed in the late fifties as an effective and harmless hypotonic, but in 1961 after several hundred affected infants had been born, it was identified as the causal agent of phocomelia (failure of the long bones to develop: phoca, a seal). This disastrous episode did much to remind doctors and patients of the possible dangers of medication in pregnancy and create the present atmosphere of caution.

EFFECTS OF DRUGS ON THE FETUS

The adverse effects of some drugs have already been described on page 425 in relation to breast feeding.

The use of anticonvulsants, antithyroid drugs and anticoagulants during pregnancy has been described in Chapter 7.

The following drugs may also have adverse effects:

ANALGESICS

Aspirin should be avoided in high doses in late pregnancy as it interferes with platelet function and may increase the risk of haemorrhage. It may also cause premature closure of the ductus arteriosus. This also applies to other non-steroidal anti-inflammatory drugs.

ANTIPSYCHOTICS

Lithium has been associated with congenital malformations and neonatal goitre.

SEX HORMONES

The synthetic nor-progestogens used for oral contraception have been known to cause minor degrees of virilism in female infants, usually hypertropy of the clitoris which soon recedes.

Hormone pregnancy tests use short courses of synthetic oestrogen/progestogen to produce withdrawal bleeding if the patient is not pregnant. There is epidemiological evidence of an association with cleft palate and other abnormalities.

There is evidence from American experience of an association between carcinoma of the vagina in teenage girls and the administration of stilboestrol to the mother as a protection against abortion.

CYTOTOXIC DRUGS

These carry a high risk of teratogenesis.

ALCOHOL

Mothers who drink heavily are likely to produce babies showing some signs of the 'fetal alcohol syndrome' — small head, maxillary hypoplasia, eye deformities and abnormalities of the gastro-intestinal tract. The infants are undersized and hypotonic, and development is retarded. It should be noted that disulfiram (Antabuse) which may be given in treatment has been reported as having an association with limb deformities.

TOBACCO

Mothers who smoke have a higher incidence of abortion, pre-term delivery and perinatal death. Babies born to smokers are of a lower birthweight than those of non-smokers, and there may possibly be long term retardation of physical and intellectual growth. The damage to growth is probably the result of some constituent of tobacco smoke such a carbon monoxide, and the oxygen carrying capacity of the blood is known to be decreased.

CHAPTER 17

MATERNAL AND FETAL MORTALITY

MATERNAL MORTALITY

Maternal Mortality — death in childbirth — has for the last 200 years been a recurring tragedy that has caused public energies gradually to be directed towards the research, legislation, education and administration from which have evolved the high standard of maternity care which exists today. Childbirth is not yet completely safe, but maternal deaths are now so infrequent, that the incidence of fetal mortality has become the indicator of continuing improvement.

The Maternal Mortality Rate (MMR) is calculated as the number of deaths of pregnant women per thousand births live and still.

$$\frac{\text{Number of Maternal Deaths}}{\text{Number of Births (live and still)}} \times 1,000 = MMR$$

Deaths from abortion must also be included, and as they are added to the numerator only, the increase is not quite accurate. The true MMR would be:–

$$\frac{\text{Number of Deaths from Pregnancy}}{\text{Number of Pregnancies}} \times 1,000$$

This figure would be lower than the accepted MMR but is obviously unobtainable as neither abortion nor pregnancy itself is notifiable.

The numerator is also affected by definitions. Internationally, deaths occuring within 42 days of delivery are usually included, but in the United Kingdom the Confidential Enquiries into Maternal Deaths (see page 462) consider deaths occuring within 1 year of delivery.

MATERNAL MORTALITY

Mortality rates are published by the Registrar-General, and the first Report appeared in 1839. Not until 1874 was it compulsory to give the cause of death in a certificate; and in 1857 the Registrar for Birmingham stated that "No-one ever specifies deaths in childbed or from puerperal fever". Births have had to be notified only since 1907 (and stillbirths only since 1915); so 19th century mortality statistics must be accepted as an approximation.

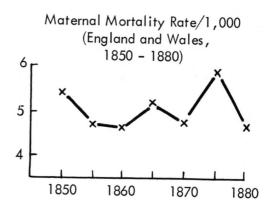

Maternal Mortality Rate/1,000
(England and Wales,
1850 – 1880)

These rates represented between 3 and 5 thousand deaths a year, about 60% from infection.

Some Causes of Death
in 1841

Puerperal Fever ⎫
Peritonitis   ⎬ "Metria"
Uterine Phlebitis ⎭
Flooding
Exhaustion
Debility
Convulsions
Mania
 - and simply -
Childbirth

From their inception, the reports of the Registrar-General deplored the deaths of so many women in childbirth — "the deep dark continuous stream of mortality" — and discussed the causes.

"The cases which cause the most distress to practitioners... are undoubtedly those deplorable and rare instances in which they communicate contagious diseases to their patients." (1841).

"A large proportion of the 500,000 English women who lie in every year and have any attendance at all, are attended by midwives who from one cause or another, probably delicacy in the national manners in points of this kind, receive no preliminary instruction in anatomy and other matters." (1841).

"A registered MRCS without any further qualifications has passed no examination in midwifery. Many are in large and successful midwifery practice; others it is to be feared must labour under disqualifications disadvantageous to themselves and to the patients". (1878).

457

MATERNAL MORTALITY

Maternal Deaths in England and Wales, 1875 (rate 6/1,000)	
Sepsis	2,662
Haemorrhage	1,038
Convulsions	538
Abortion	185
Mania	115
Ruptured uterus	36
Others	36
	4,610

Sepsis (puerperal fever etc.) was the most fatal complication. Spread by attendants from one patient to another had been described by Alexander Gordon of Aberdeen in 1795. ("It is disagreeable for me to mention that I myself was the means of carrying infection to great numbers of women.") In 1848 Semmelweiss published his results — a reduction in death rate in his clinic from 12% to 3% by making his students wash their hands in antiseptic before examining patients. Pasteur and Lister published their great discoveries; but the maternal mortality rate remained unaffected.

By the 1870's the mortality in the institutions was being attacked. Florence Nightingale had had to close the lying-in ward in King's College Hospital because of this, and she described in detail designs for an improved maternity unit which would be barred to medical students and the infections they might carry.

The superior results from Liverpool Workhouse shown in this table were correctly attributed to its isolation, absence of visitors, regular 'limestoning' of the wards by the paupers, and rigid segregation of pregnant women at all stages. In Florence Nightingale's recommendations there can be discerned the principles of organisation of present day maternity units at least until the era of antibiotics.

Institution	MMR/1000
King's College Hospital 1862 - 67	33.3
Queen Charlotte's 1828 - 68	25.3
Liverpool Workhouse 1867	9.0
England and Wales 1867	5.1
(from Florence Nightingale)	

MATERNAL MORTALITY

Maternal Mortality in 1910 (England and Wales). 3,191 deaths
(rate 3.6/1,000)

Sepsis	1,274	Inversion of uterus	8
Placenta praevia and flooding	612	Craniotomy	7
Convulsions	439	Hydrocephaly	4
Thrombo-embolism	334	Administration of	
Abortion	80	chloroform	4
Ectopic gestation	78	Instrumental delivery	3
Mania	48	Adherent placenta	3
Vomiting	38	Prolapsus uteri	2
Contracted pelvis	31	Rigidity of os	2
Ruptured uterus	28	Rupture of vagina	2
Malpresentation	16	Hydramnios	2
Caesarean section	15	Monstrosity	1

It will be seen that the main causes were:–

Sepsis: Haemorrhage: Toxaemia (Convulsions): Thrombo-embolism:
and Trauma.

At the turn of the century a slight improvement occurred, the result probably of several factors: a better understanding and application of 'Listerism'; an improvement in general hygiene and sanitation brought about by Public Health legislation; and the Midwives' Act of 1902, the first of many Acts which regulate the training and practice of midwives.

However a more dramatic and sustained fall was observed at the same time in Infant Mortality Rate; and by the 1920s, after the First World War, it became apparent that the risks of childbirth were not much less than they were 80 years before, while the scandal was proportionately greater.

England and Wales, 1880–1930

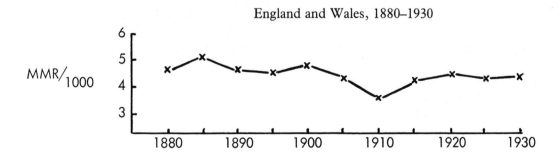

459

MATERNAL MORTALITY

With the founding of the Ministry of Health in 1919 a period of energetic official enquiry was entered into. Public Health antenatal clinics were instituted largely in the face of the medical profession's opposition, and repeated surveys were made and reported on. Eventually what had long been known was openly asserted; a large number of maternal deaths could be avoided if the standard of obstetric management were higher. A report in 1932 listed four 'Primary Avoidable Factors':–

1. Absence of antenatal care.
2. Errors of management.
3. Lack of reasonable facilities.
4. Negligence by the patient.

Committee on Maternal Mortality England and Wales, 1932		
3,059 Deaths Inquired Into		
Cause	Number	Percent
Sepsis	1,111	36.3
Toxaemia	506	16.4
Haemorrhage	450	14.8
Abortion	410	13.4
Shock and Trauma	319	10.4
Thrombo-embolism	206	6.8
Ectopic gestation	55	1.8

This table shows that the causes of death in 1932 were much the same as in 1910.

Deaths from Puerperal Infection (England and Wales) 1931–1940

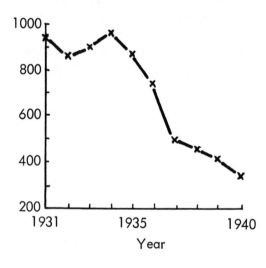

In the early thirties the mortality rate appeared static or even rising slightly; until in 1935 the antibacterial action of the sulphonamide Prontosil was demonstrated. It is the action of antibiotics, almost abolishing death from puerperal sepsis, and the development of blood transfusion services after the Second World War, that have made childbirth as safe as it is to-day.

MATERNAL MORTALITY

In 1937 a further Report made a series of recommendations — consultant training and supervision, provision of adequate maternity hospitals and antenatal clinics, flying squads, organisation of the Health Visitor service, and so on — which form the basis of modern practice.

Since then there has been continuous improvement, and maternal deaths are now referred to in actual numbers or the rate per 100,000, rather than percentages. There were 227 deaths in England and Wales in 1976–78 (11.9/100,000) and 44 in Scotland in the quinquennium 1976–80 (13.3/100,000).

The accompanying table shows the principal causes of maternal mortality in England and Wales 5 years before and after the Second World War.

In the years 1976–78, 227 maternal deaths occurred in England and Wales. The causes were as follows:

Pulmonary Embolism	45
Hypertensive Diseases	29
Haemorrhage	26
Anaesthesia	24
Ectopic	22
Abortion	19
Sepsis	17
Ruptured Uterus	14
Amniotic Embolism	11
Miscellaneous	20

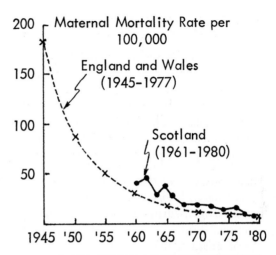

Year	1935	1950
Number	2,425	554
Abortion	27%	17%
Toxaemia	22	30
Haemorrhage	19	13·
Trauma etc.	23	16
Thrombosis	13	10
Sepsis	5	4

The Scottish figures for the quinquennium 1976–80 are very small (44) but in keeping with these:

Pulmonary Embolism	7
Haemorrhage	7
Anaesthesia	6
Amniotic Embolism	6
Abortion	5
Hypertensive Disease	4

The importance of pulmonary embolism as a cause of death is striking as is the relative advance (due to the decline of other causes) of general anaesthesia. Deaths from abortion have declined, a trend which began before the introduction of the Abortion Act.

461

MATERNAL MORTALITY

Confidential Enquiries into Maternal Deaths

Special Enquiries into maternal deaths have been carried out in the United Kingdom since the 1930s. The present system was introduced in England and Wales in 1952 and in Scotland in 1965. Since then a series of Reports, each covering several years, has been published. A consultant obstetrician in each region was appointed to act as assessor and subsequently assessors in anaesthesia were added. They were asked to consider the circumstances of each death and identify, if possible, avoidable factors. The identification of deficiencies by the Enquiries has, over the years, helped to improve the quality of the maternity services.

Deaths are classified as 'Direct' where death clearly resulted from complications of the pregnant state. 'Indirect' deaths are those arising from previously existing disease or disease which developed during the pregnancy, aggravated by the physiological changes of pregnancy. 'Fortuitous' deaths are those occurring incidentally during pregnancy but not in any way due to the pregnant state e.g. motor accident. The decline in numbers makes the maintenance of the confidentiality of these Reports increasingly difficult and the Scottish Report for 1976–1980 will be the last in its present form. It is intended to combine it with the recently instituted quinquennial review of Scottish Perinatal Mortality.

FETAL MORTALITY

Infant mortality has always been a matter of concern to society — in England and Wales in 1839 the mortality rate among children under three was 343 per 1,000 — but the obstetrician understandably feels a particular responsibility for stillbirths and neonatal deaths in the first week of life — the 'perinatal mortality'. As first week deaths are commonly attributable to factors arising during pregnancy or delivery, this combined death rate has been seen as an index of the standard of practice in institutional obstetrics.

STILLBIRTH

A stillbirth is a baby that does not breathe or show any other sign of life after being completely separated from its mother. In the United Kingdom the Stillbirth Rate refers to the number of stillbirths per 1,000 total births live and still. Stillbirth has been a notifiable condition since 1915, and registerable since 1927 (1939 in Scotland). The body may not be disposed of until the doctor has issued a Certificate of Stillbirth and the Registrar has issued a Certificate of Registration.

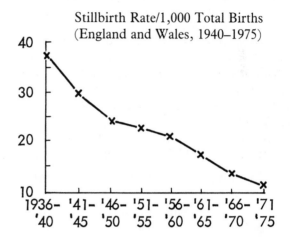

Stillbirth Rate/1,000 Total Births (England and Wales, 1940–1975)

The dramatic fall between 1940 and 1946 is attributed to the improvement in the nutrition of working class pregnant women affected by the wartime rationing system. Stillbirth rates have continued to fall steadily, and in Scotland in 1985 the rate was 5.5/1,000.

463

FETAL MORTALITY

INFANT MORTALITY RATE

Deaths of liveborn children are in the first instance included in the Infant Mortality Rate (IMR) which is the number of deaths of all children under a year per 1,000 live births.

The fall in IMR has resulted from the gradual improvement in domestic sanitation and hygiene which have accompanied the tremendous social changes of this century, the redistribution of wealth and increase in social expenditure.

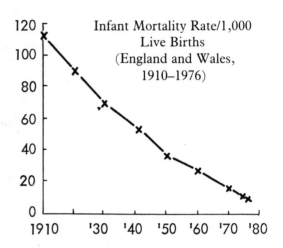

Infant Mortality Rate/1,000 Live Births (England and Wales, 1910–1976)

Included in the IMR are neo-natal deaths — all deaths under 4 weeks – and first week deaths. These groups now make up more than half the IMR.

PERINATAL MORTALITY RATE (PMR)

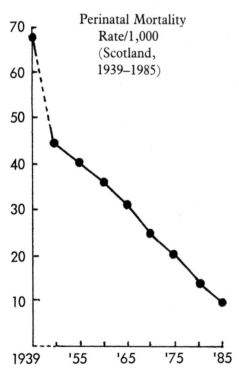

Perinatal Mortality Rate/1,000 (Scotland, 1939–1985)

PMR is the number of stillbirths plus first week deaths per 1,000 births live and still. This statistic is of the closest interest to the obstetrician and paediatrician since it records deaths of their patients, and the PMR for a maternity unit is to some extent a measure of the standard of care provided. Many factors have combined to produce the dramatic improvement in the perinatal mortality rate — improved general health, fewer patients of high parity and improved antenatal and intrapartum care. To some extent, the fall may be seen to be artificial as the excellence of neonatal paediatric care will prolong the life of some babies beyond the first week and thus beyond the defin-ition of perinatal mortality. Similarly the use of prenatal diagnosis and termination of pregnancy in potentially lethal conditions has reduced deaths from fetal deformity. For these reasons some authorities advocate the introduction of a new measure of perinatal wastage which would include mid-trimester abortions and neonatal and infant deaths which appear to be perinatally related.

FETAL MORTALITY

Perinatal Mortality (Continued)

The principal causes of perinatal death in Scotland were analysed in a nationwide survey for 1977-81 and this perinatal review has now been established on a permanent basis.

Classification of the deaths was that described by Baird in 1954 and used in the British Births Survey. The distribution of causes of death in 1981 was as follows:

	%
Low birth weight (less than 2500 g — no complication in the mother)	31
Fetal deformity	23
Normal birth weight (greater than 2500 g — no complication in the mother)	12
Antepartum haemorrhage	12
Toxaemia	9
Maternal disease	5
Trauma	3
Rhesus Incompatibility	2
Other	3

The classification may usefully be extended to separate growth-retarded babies from pre-term and differentiate types of antepartum haemorrhage and maternal disease.

Perinatal mortality rate by maternal age and parity (Scotland 1977–81)

	0	1	2	3+	Total
Under 20 years	17.1	12.6			16.9
20–24 years	13.9	10.6	11.4	18.2	12.6
25–29 years	13.1	9.3	10.4	17.9	11.3
30 and over	17.2	10.7	12.3	23.0	14.8
Total	14.7	10.2	11.5	21.5	13.1

It will be seen that the highest perinatal mortality rates are found in women of all ages having their 4th or subsequent child and in women having their 1st baby before the age of 20. Social class is a measurement of education, physical development and diet and women in social classes I and II have lower perinatal mortality rates than those in social classes IV and V. The poorer reproductive performance of women below the age of 20 is due in part to a preponderance of mothers from social classes IV and V. Older age groups will contain more women of high parity, and the risk of intercurrent disease complicating pregnancy increases with age.

CHAPTER 18

CONTRACEPTION

HORMONAL CONTRACEPTION

Hormonal contraception takes 3 forms:

1. Combined (oestrogen/progestogen) pill.
2. Progestogen-only pill.
3. Progestogen injections.

COMBINED PILL

This is by far the commonest form of oral contraception (OC). About 3 million women in the United Kingdom are said to be 'taking the pill'. It is the most effective form of contraception apart from sterilisation, and, for many women, the most acceptable aesthetically. A pill is taken daily for 21, 22 or 28 days depending on the formulation and a withdrawal bleed will normally occur in the pill-free days or during the 7 placebo days of the everyday preparations.

Mode of action

(a) The pill prevents ovulation. FSH secretion is depressed so that normal follicular development does not occur and the LH peak is abolished. This is mainly due to oestrogen but progestogens can also suppress ovulation, at least in large doses.

(b) The endometrium does not develop normally and the absence of a corpus luteum prevents the preparation of an endometrium suitable for implantation. There is a 'pseudo-atrophy' so that even if ovulation occurs implantation is unlikely. This is a combined effect of oestrogen and progestogen.

(c) Changes in cervical mucus make sperm penetration less likely. This is a progestogen effect.

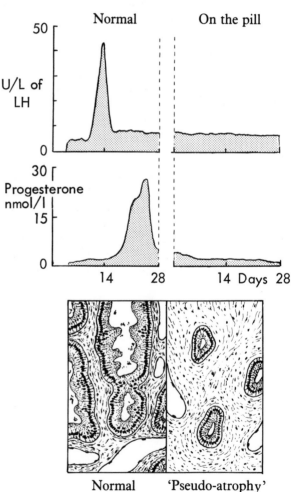

Normal endometrium   'Pseudo-atrophy'

HORMONAL CONTRACEPTION

Combined pill (continued)

Constituents

The combined pill is made up of one of two oestrogens, either ethinyloestradiol or its 3-methyl-ether, mestranol, which is less potent. All contain between 20 and 50 micrograms of oestrogen. Six progestogens are in common use. Their potency, as measured by their effect on the endometrium, varies considerably. They are (with the amount contained in different preparations):

1.	Desogestrel	0.15 mg
2.	Ethynodiol Diacetate	1.0–2.0 mg
3.	Levonorgestrel	0.15–0.25 mg
4.	Lynestrenol	2.5 mg
5.	Norethisterone	1.0 mg
6.	Norethisterone Acetate	1.0–4.0 mg

Most pills are monophasic i.e. contain the same amount of oestrogen and progestogen throughout the cycle. There is, however, one biphasic preparation and several triphasic pills which aim to mimic the normal cyclical variation in hormone levels. Unopposed oestrogen is not given at any time however.

Choice of pill

There are currently about 30 different combined preparations. Usually a preparation containing 30 or 35 micrograms of oestrogen will be prescribed but the aim is to find, for the individual patient, the preparation which gives good cycle control without side-effects. In general, increasing the dose of progestogen (or using a more potent one such as Norgestrel or Desogestrel) will reduce menstrual loss. Poor cycle control may require alteration to 50 micrograms of oestrogen. The phasic pills have the lowest total dose of steroid and may be preferred for older women. They also, however, have a reduced margin for error if pills are omitted.

HORMONAL CONTRACEPTION

Combined pill (continued)

Major side-effects

A great deal of clinical and laboratory research and epidemiological analysis all go to support an association between the combined contraceptive pill and venous thrombo-embolism, myocardial infarction and stroke. Widespread metabolic effects can be demonstrated in pill users and among the effects of these appears to be an increase in venous thrombosis and arterial disease. Nevertheless it must be remembered that the risks are very small and most of the information we have derives from higher dose pills than presently used. It is to be hoped therefore that the present generation of pills will reduce the incidence of serious complications.

Thromboembolism

This appears to be due to the oestrogen component and is dose related, hence the introduction of low-dose oestrogen or progestogen-only. Even the low-oestrogen pills are associated with a significantly higher risk in women over 25, and hypertension and obesity are predisposing factors.

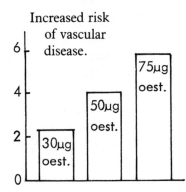

The risks are directly dose-related to the amount of oestrogen taken, and also to the amount of progestogen.

Myocardial infarction and stroke

It has been claimed that OC users run a fourfold risk of these diseases, especially women over 35 who smoke. Arterial disease is attributed mainly to the effects of the progestogens. It has been known for some time that OCs alter the characteristics of lipoproteins in the direction of vascular disease. Low levels of high density lipoprotein-cholesterol (HDL-C) are produced by many of the progestogens used (oestrogens appear to increase HDL-C), and new progestogens have been introduced in which this effect has been reduced.

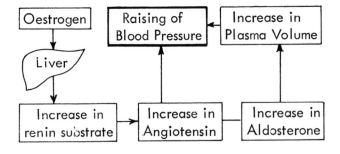

Hypertension

OCs gradually raise the blood pressure, sometimes to the hypertensive range. The blood volume is increased by fluid retention, and the secretion of angiotensin is increased.

470

HORMONAL CONTRACEPTION

Combined Pill   (continued)

Minor side-effects

Oestrogen	*Oestrogen and Progestogen*	*Progestogen*
Breakthrough bleeding	Weight gain	Acne Depression
Nausea	Post-pill	Dry vagina
Painful breasts	amenorrhoea	Loss of libido
Headache		Insulin resistance
		(This is not a minor complication in diabetes)

Cancer and the Pill

Progesterone stimulates mitotic activity in breast endothelium, and evidence has been published which suggests that long-term oral contraceptive users before age 25, especially with the more potent progestogens, may incur an increased risk of subsequent breast cancer.

Evidence has been offered to suggest that long-term oral contraceptive users run a greater risk of cervical cancer and dysplasia, perhaps because the steroid hormones reduce immunity to antigenic causal factors. Long-term users should certainly have regular cervical cytology examinations.

Prolonged oral contraceptive use depresses mitotic activity in the endometrium and follicular maturation in the ovary, and these effects are considered to offer some protection against cancer of these tissues.

Contraindications

Below are listed the commonly accepted contraindications to the pill and the circumstances in which special precaution should be taken. It must be remembered however that few of these contraindications are absolute and the risks of the patient using the pill have to be set against the possibly increased risk of pregnancy if an alternative method is employed. Absolute contraindications are cardiovascular disease, liver disease and breast cancer.

Contraindications	**Special precautions**
History of cardiovascular disease	Collagen diseases
Hypertension	Otosclerosis
Heavy smoking	Diabetes mellitus
Obesity	Sickle cell disease
Migraine	Surgical operations
Chronic hepatitis	Severe varicose veins
Breast cancer	History of depression
Endogenous depression	Age over 35

471

HORMONAL CONTRACEPTION

Combined Pill   (continued)

Failure of the pill

The failure rate of the combined pill is very small, between 0 and 1 per cent, and there is often an avoidable factor.

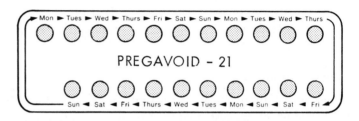

1. The patient may forget to take the pill. Packing by the pharmaceutical firms is ingenious but not foolproof. If one pill is missed, two are taken the next day.

2. Gastroenteritis, perhaps following dietary indiscretion, may impair absorption.

3. Certain groups of drugs such as anticonvulsants, usually phenytoin and phenobarbitone, and the antibiotic rifampicin are known to increase the metabolic activity of hepatic enzymes, and increase the rate of excretion of contraceptive steroids. (Cf. the treatment of neonatal jaundice with phenobarbitone).

4. Several antibiotics including ampicillin are associated with an increase in breakthrough bleeding, and pregnancy has been reported. Oral contraceptives are conjugated in the liver, excreted in the bile, and partly reabsorbed. If gut bacteria are inhibited by antibiotics, reabsorption may not occur, leading to increased bowel excretion but lower circulating levels of steroids.

Clinical supervision

1. A detailed medical and family history should be taken to identify risk factors.
2. General physical examination to include weight, blood pressure, breast and pelvic examination and a cervical smear if due.
3. Assessment at 3 months to determine side-effects and check the blood pressure.
4. Six-monthly breast and blood pressure check.
5. Pelvic examination and cervical smear 3-yearly.

HORMONAL CONTRACEPTION

PROGESTOGEN-ONLY PILL

This pill contains no oestrogen and is sometimes known as the 'mini-pill'. A small dose of progestogen is taken daily without any break.

It produces its contraceptive effect by its combined action on the endometrium and the cervical mucus (see page 468).

Its contraceptive effectiveness is less than the combined pill, failure rates of 2–3/100 woman years being commonly quoted. Better results have however been reported (see page 481).

Indications

1. Oestrogens contraindicated or otherwise unsuitable.
2. Age over 35 years.
3. During lactation.
4. Diabetic patients.

The main advantage of the progestogen-only pill is the absence of major metabolic disturbance and its main disadvantage (apart from an increased pregnancy rate) is disturbance of the menstrual cycle. If pregnancy does occur there is an increased risk that it may be ectopic. Clinical supervision should be as for the combined pill.

PROGESTOGEN INJECTIONS

Two long-acting compounds are now available for long-term users in this and many other countries. They are Medroxyprogesterone Acetate 150 mg every 3 months and Norethisterone Oenanthate 200 mg 2-monthly. They inhibit ovulation and have the usual progestogen effect on the endometrium and cervical mucus. Pregnancy rates are generally less than 1%. The only significant metabolic effect appears to be a reduction in HDL-cholesterol which also occurs in oral progestogens. They are suitable for use in patients who might take the progestogen-only pill with the extra benefit of reliability and the avoidance of pill-taking. Their main side-effects are menstrual irregularity and amenorrhoea. In addition there may be some delay in the return of fertility following discontinuation of the treatment. Pregnancy is unlikely for 8–9 months after the last injection.

THE INTRA-UTERINE DEVICE (IUD)

An IUD is made of polythene and copper (gold, silver and stainless steel have also been used) and is sufficiently flexible to be drawn into an introducer for insertion into the uterine cavity.

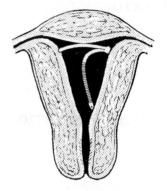

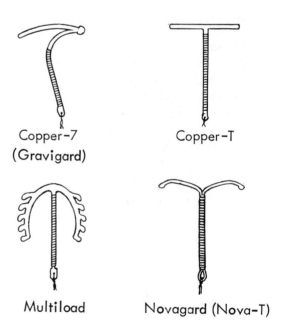

Lippes Loop

The Lippes Loop which is available in different sizes is the only 'inert' intra-uterine device obtainable in this country. It is made of polythene and is a little bulkier than the copper-containing coils and therefore perhaps more likely to cause heavy periods. In theory the loop should give prolonged use but recently there have been reports that these inert devices predispose to colonisation with actinomyces-like organisms, especially actinomyces-Israelii, in long-term users. It may be advisable therefore that even inert IUDs should be changed at intervals of no more than 5 years.

Copper-containing IUDs incorporate a winding copper wire which is said to increase contraceptive efficiency. Their thinner diameter makes them easier to insert, and it is claimed that the menstrual loss is smaller.

Because of the gradual absorption of copper, these IUDs are renewed every 2–5 years. Copper IUDs produce local concentrations of copper salts which apparently give some protection against bacterial contamination.

Copper–7
(Gravigard)

Copper–T

Multiload

Novagard (Nova–T)

THE INTRA-UTERINE DEVICE

MODE OF ACTION

This appears to be by preventing implantation. An inflammatory reaction is certainly induced in the endometrium, and there is an increase in serum immunoglobulins, suggesting an immune reaction. Endocrine patterns are unchanged, but the luteal phase is often shortened by about two days, perhaps because of an increased secretion of prostaglandin.

PRINCIPLE OF INSERTION OF IUDs

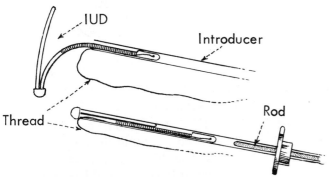

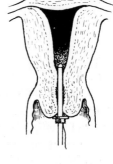

1. The IUD is first of all folded and pulled into a plastic tube called the introducer.

2. The introducer is then inserted into the uterus.

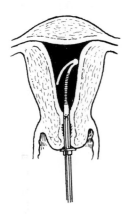

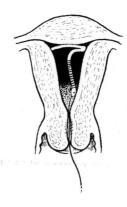

3. The IUD is forced out of the inserter by a rod ...

4. ... and takes up its position in the uterus.

INTRA-UTERINE DEVICES

TECHNIQUE OF INSERTION

1. The cervix is exposed, swabbed and grasped with a tenaculum forceps.

2. The introducer is inserted and the IUD expelled into the cavity. The thread is then cut, leaving about 2 inches in the vagina.

   With very nervous women some sedation or even an anaesthetic may be required.

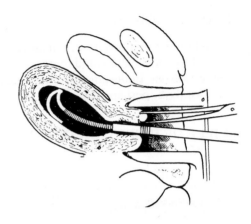

COMPLICATIONS OF IUDs

1. Increased menstrual loss

The cause may be the increased fibrinolytic activity which occurs round the IUD. It can be minimised by the use of antifibrinolytic agents such as aminocaproic acid or tranexamic acid. Antiprostaglandin agents such as mefanemic acid or diclofenac are also effective.

2. Infection

There is an increased risk of pelvic inflammatory disease, especially during the first year, and inert IUDs are associated with actinomycosis infection if retained for long periods. There is disagreement about how long an IUD should be left if symptomless, but extraction is often more difficult after several years in situ, and changing the IUD at 3–5 yearly intervals seems sensible.

3. Pregnancy

This is about 1 to 1.5 per 100 woman years, and is most likely in the first two years. The risk of ectopic pregnancy is greater in IUD users and has been calculated as 1.2 per 1000 woman years.

4. Expulsion

There is a 5 to 10 percent incidence, usually in the first 6 months.

5. Translocation

The IUD passes through the uterine wall into the peritoneal cavity or broad ligament. It is thought that this begins at the time of faulty insertion, and once diagnosed by X-ray should be removed at laparoscopy.

CONTRAINDICATIONS TO IUD CONTRACEPTION

1. Existing pelvic inflammatory disease.   2. Menorrhagia.
3. History of previous ectopic pregnancy. 4. Severe dysmenorrhoea.

POST-COITAL CONTRACEPTION

POST-COITAL CONTRACEPTION ('Morning After' Contraception; 'Interception')

Effective post-coital contraception has been sought for many years, usually in the form of douching with various liquids which have been unsuccessful because of the rapidity with which the sperms leave the vagina for the cervical canal and uterus. Modern methods are extremely effective if started early enough.

High dosage oestrogens

Ethinyloestradiol 5 mg, or diethylstilboestrol 50 mg taken daily for five days in divided doses starting within 72 hours of coitus. These dosages cause nausea and vomiting which may be so severe that the patient cannot continue with treatment, and it is possible that levels of antithrombin III may be reduced, contributing to an increased risk of thromboembolism.

Method of action

Corpus luteum function is depressed and the preparation of the endometrium for implantation is prevented.

Double Dose of OC Pill

Two tablets of $50\mu g$ ethinyloestradiol and $500\ \mu g$ levonorgestrel (Eugynon-50 or Ovran) are taken within 72 hours and repeated in 12 hours. This treatment is much better tolerated.

Complications of Hormone Treatment

1. Pregnancy may not be prevented and there is a theoretical risk that the embryo may be affected.
2. If pregnancy occurs, there is an increased risk of ectopic pregnancy.

Insertion of IUD

This method can be used for up to 5 days after coitus. It offers the advantage of being free from patient failure and should be offered when hormonal treatment is contraindicated, but like steroid hormones it should not be used if there is a history of previous ectopic pregnancy.

ETHICAL CONSIDERATIONS

The distinction between contraception and abortion depends on the age at which the individual is considered to have come into existence — at fertilisation or nidation — and whatever method of post-coital contraception is used, there can be no certainty as to the point at which interference with the natural process took place.

BARRIER METHODS

VAGINAL DIAPHRAGM (Dutch Cap)

This is a rubber diaphragm which when smeared with spermicidal cream will prevent sperms from reaching the cervical canal. It is less efficient than oral contraceptives or IUDs unless used strictly according to instructions; but it has no side-effects.

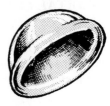

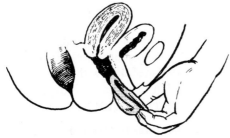

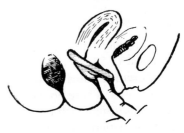

1. The diaphragm is smeared with spermicidal cream round the edges and on both sides, and guided into the posterior fornix.

2. The front end is tucked up behind the symphysis.

The diaphragm must not be removed until six hours after intercourse, and if intercourse is repeated in that period more cream must first be injected with an applicator. An alternative to the diaphragm is the more closely fitting cervical or vault cap.

VAGINAL SPERMICIDES

Spermicidal agents are inserted in the vagina in the form of creams, pessaries, gels or aerosols. One dose of spermicide must be injected before each act of coitus. The method is simpler in practice than the diaphragm, but probably less reliable.

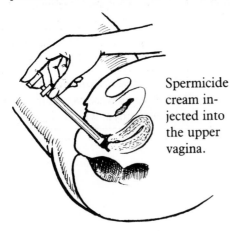

Spermicide cream injected into the upper vagina.

THE SPONGE

A disposable plastic sponge is inserted into the vagina and can be left in situ for at least 24 hours. Sponges need no fitting, are comfortable and, when impregnated with spermicidal cream, offer an effective barrier.

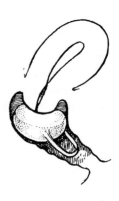

NATURAL METHODS

THE RHYTHM METHOD ('Safe Period')

The woman must take her temperature every morning and watch for the sustained rise which indicates ovulation. Such graphs are not now accepted as being very precise indicators, but women with regular periods can usually identify the peri-ovulatory time with a fair degree of accuracy.

If the evidence suggest ovulation, say between the 12th and 14th days, 24 hours are allowed for ovum survival and 3 days should be allowed for the survival time of sperms in the genital tract, these times being all suppositions. This means that coitus must be avoided from the 9th to the 15th day and a 24 hour safety margin at either end increases the avoidance period from the 8th to the 17th day inclusive.

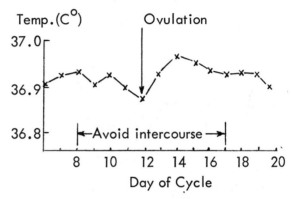

THE OVULATION METHOD (The Billings' Method)

The woman is taught to identify the peri-ovulatory phase by noting the vaginal sensations associated with changes in cervical mucus.

This method provides the same opportunities for coitus as the Rhythm method, but should be more accurate.

In practice, more protection would be afforded by a combination of arbitrary distinction between safe and unsafe days, and a close observation of physical signs and symptoms.

Say 5 days	Menstruation	
2–3 days	'Early Safe Days'	Sensation of vaginal dryness
4–5 days	Moist Days – **Not Safe**	Increasing amounts of sticky mucus
2 days	Ovulation Peak – **Not Safe**	Copious, clear 'slippery' mucus
3 days	Post-ovulation Peak – **Not Safe**	Gradual decrease in secretion
11 days	'Late Safe Days'	Minimal secretion

MALE METHODS

COITUS INTERRUPTUS

This means withdrawal of the penis just before ejaculation. It is widely practised and probably adequate for couples of low fertility, but some sperms must enter the vagina, and withdrawal at the point of orgasm is unnatural.

SHEATH (Condom, 'French Letter')

A thin rubber sheath fits over the penis. It interferes with sensation and is liable to come off as the penis is withdrawn after the act, but it is a very efficient method if used correctly.

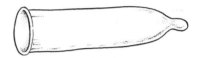

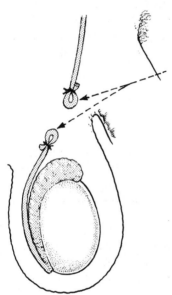

VASECTOMY

The vasa deferentes can be divided by a simple operation done under local anaesthesia.

1. It takes several months for the storage system to become clear of sperms and a few non-motile ones may persist whose significance is uncertain. It may take a year before the ejaculate is completely sperm free.

2. About 5% of patients demonstrate minor complications, including vasovagal reactions, haematoma and mild infection. There are occasional reports of severe infection.

3. Possible long term complications include the development of sperm autoantibodies, and there is often great difficulty in reversing the operation if this should be required.

Extensive scrotal and penile haematoma following vasectomy.

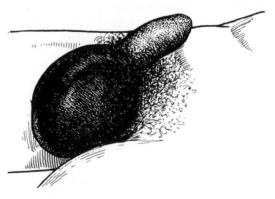

Female sterilisation is described in Chapter 14.

FAILURE RATES IN CONTRACEPTION

There are four factors affecting the failure rate for any method of contraception.

1. Inherent Weakness of the Method.

    For example the rhythm method which depends on the accurate determination of the time of ovulation can never be as reliable as OC.

2. Age

    With all methods, the failure rate declines as age increases.

3. Motivation

    Every method depends on the determination of the woman to use it correctly. Thus pills may be forgotten, diaphragm users 'take a chance', even with IUDs a suspicion that the device is out of place may be ignored. Social class affects motivation.

4. Duration of Use

    The failure rate, especially with occlusive methods, declines as duration of use, and therefore habit, increases. This observation is also true of IUDs, perhaps because the IUD becomes more effective the longer it is in place. Prolonged use is itself an indication of good motivation.

Table of failure rates

The following table is taken from Vessey et al (1982) and their figures are based on the prolonged observation of over 17000 women, all 25 and over, and about 40% of whom were in social class I or II.

Method	Number of accidental pregnancies	Number of woman-years of observation	Failure rate per 100 woman-years
OC			
$50\mu g$ oestrogen	61	37412	0.16
$30\mu g$ oestrogen	21	7749	0.27
Progestogen only	21	1756	1.2
IUDs			
Saf-T-Coil	85	6791	1.3
Copper-7	34	2200	1.5
Diaphragm	485	25146	1.9
Condom	449	12492	3.6
Coitus Interruptus	45	674	6.7
Chemicals alone	36	303	11.9
Rhythm Method	25	161	15.5

INDEX

INDEX

INDEX

INDEX

INDEX